THE AMERICAN HEALTH FOUNDATION
GUIDE TO LIFESPAN HEALTH

THE AMERICAN HEALTH FOUNDATION GUIDE TO LIFESPAN HEALTH

A Family Program
For Physical and Emotional Well-Being

Contributing Editors:
Ernst L. Wynder, M.D.
Mario A. Orlandi, Ph.D.

Co-ordinating Editor:
Mary Boyle

**This book was based in part upon
contributions to Multimedia by the following:**

Michael Argyle, D.Sc., Christiaan Barnard, M.S., Ph.D.,
John Conger, Ph.D., Frank Falkner, M.D., F.R.C.P.,
Marjorie Fiske, D.Sc., Ray Hodgson, Ph.D.,
John Illman, Jerome Jaffe, M.D., Robert Kastenbaum, Ph.D.,
Leonard Kristal, Ph.D Christopher Macy, B.Sc.,
Robert Petersen, Ph.D., Rhona Rapoport, Ph.D.,
Robert Rapoport, Ph.D., Martin Richards, Ph.D.,
Charles Spielberger, Ph.D., Leonore Tiefer, Ph.D.,
Peter Trower, M.A., Barbara Notkin, M.A., Sheldon White, Ph.D.

DODD, MEAD & COMPANY
New York

This book was devised and produced by
Multimedia Publications (UK) Ltd

Editors: Jo Cheesewright, Ela Ginalska
Production Director: Arnon Orbach
Designer: Julian Holland
Picture Researchers: Anne Marie Ehrlich, Sarah Waters
Artists: Roger Twinn, Steve Wilson

First published by Dodd, Mead & Company Inc.
79 Madison Ave, New York, NY 10016
First Edition

Library of Congress Cataloging in Publication Data
Main entry under title:

The American health foundation guide to lifespan health.

   Bibliography: p. 275
   Includes index.
   1. Developmental psychology.   2. Health.   I. Wynder,
Ernest L.   II. Orlandi, Mario.   III. Boyle, Mary.
BF713.A465   1984   155   84–4026
ISBN 0–396–08373–0

Black and white and colour origination: D.S. Colour International,
Ltd, London
Typesetting: Tradespools Limited, Frome
Printed in Spain by Graficromo SA

Contents

Introduction	**6**
Before birth and birth	**12**
The biology of pregnancy	14
A child is born	21
Infancy	**24**
Feeding	26
Sleeping and crying	30
What newborns can do	35
Girl or boy?	39
Learning to move and think	43
Learning to speak—the end of infancy	50
Childhood	**56**
How a child's thinking develops	58
Relating to other people	63
Going to school	72
Coping with children's problems	88
Adolescence	**96**
A time for becoming	98
Sexual behaviour	108
Adolescents and their parents	114
Taking drugs	118
The importance of the peer group	124
Psychological problems	127
Ready for adulthood	132
Young adulthood	**136**
Employment, study or neither	138
Partners for life?	146
Sexual reactions and problems	154
Pregnancy and motherhood	165
Birth—a family event	174
Life with infants and children	182
Middle age	**188**
The changing family	190
Love and intimacy	193
A mid-life crisis?	198
When depression strikes	204
Losing a partner	209
Work—the later years	214
Old age	**224**
Changing bodies and minds	226
Reacting to problems	240
Love and intimacy in later life	248
A home full of strangers	251
Taking our leave	256
Glossary	**264**
Useful addresses	**270**
Further reading	**275**
Index	**278**
Picture credits	**287**
Acknowledgements	**287**

Introduction

Despite recent scientific advances, human development remains an awe-inspiring mystery. Throughout history writers and students from practically every culture on earth have been fascinated by the phenomena related to biological and psychological growth processes—from conception and birth through adulthood to death. Beliefs in many societies regarding human growth and development have been greatly influenced by culturally defined myths and folklore. In other societies, such as our own, this topic has become the focus of intensive interdisciplinary scientific research. The past decade has witnessed enormous strides in our understanding of the human body, its growth processes and its relationship to the mind. A new consensus is emerging regarding the role of individual behaviour patterns in guiding the course of growth and development—a consensus which offers exciting opportunities to young and old alike. *American Health Foundation Guide to Lifespan Health* is a comprehensive introduction to these opportunities. It is the underlying premise of this book that *any* individual, regardless of age, inherited deficiencies, or present health status, can benefit immensely from the adoption of a healthy lifestyle. It's never too late to start down the road to better health—or too early!

Growth, development and predetermination

The general observation that various developmental events (such as puberty) take place at a predictable age in most individuals has led scientists to suggest that the course of human development is largely governed by biological processes, and that these processes are genetically programmed. This orientation in terms of growth and maturation suggests that, given certain minimal prerequisites such as appropriate nourishment, early development will proceed according to a highly specific series of predetermined events. These processes, referred to collectively as "growth", were thought in the past to continue through adolescence until a developmental plateau was reached sometime during early adulthood. Subsequent change later in life was viewed from this perspective as a decline in function or simply as "ageing" rather than a continuation of development or growth. This deterministic view of growth and development would seem to be borne out by the observation that the *stages of life*, that everyone experiences from early childhood through

adulthood to old age, are an inevitable aspect of human existence. However, this view does not account for the fact that individuals who are the same age chronologically, can vary widely in their overall health status and general well-being. Recent research has shown that factors other than chronological age, genetic disposition, or infectious disease must be taken into consideration when trying to account for a person's health status. An overwhelming amount of data indicates that these additional factors are *behavioural* and that the *lifestyle* we lead plays a particularly important role in determining the course of our development. This is encouraging, because if all developmental events were genetically predetermined we would have little justification or rationale for trying to influence or improve the course of our biological and psychological growth, or to improve our general well-being. Life, in that case, could be regarded as a treadmill that we walk along from birth to death, passively accepting our condition as something over which we have no control. Thousands of individuals, however, have already decided that such a view is overly pessimistic. They have joined the health and physical fitness revolution, a social movement that is based specifically upon the premise, and the personal experience, that the course of human development can be significantly influenced by lifestyle decisions. In what sense then, and to what extent, can one continue to grow through life?

The lifespan developmental approach

Developmental events are largely, though certainly not entirely, determined through genetic inheritance; and many, though certainly not all, aspects of growth and ageing can be influenced by the lifestyle one selects. A scientific and philosophical perspective has emerged that reconciles these apparently disparate facts of life. This perspective is called the *lifespan developmental approach*. Though the first major work on human development from this perspective was published in 1777 by Tetens, a German philosopher, it is only within the past decade that this approach has received widespread attention. The lifespan approach is more of an orientation to the study of human growth than a specific theory, and as such, it is based upon a number of important assumptions. The first assumption is that human development is an interactive, dynamic process that continuously integrates environmental and behavioural factors with genetically determined factors. This means that while the general patterns and sequences of developmental events, including ageing, are highly predetermined, there is a great deal of flexibility within the system. The second assumption is that this dynamic, interactive process is in operation from the moment of conception until death. This implies that many significant aspects of development continue to be altered throughout life and that "growth" is a lifelong interactive process that continues during adulthood and even into old age. With this perspective in mind, both the motivation and the rationale are apparent for attempting to influence the course of human development through lifestyle change. The lifespan developmental approach, therefore, embodies a scientific rationale for growing throughout life via appropriate behavioural changes. This approach does not, obviously, suggest that the ageing process can be literally halted or reversed, but rather that the natural ageing process can be postponed to a great extent, and a great amount of youthful vigour retained through lifestyle reorientation.

A great deal of scientific evidence has accumulated in support of the lifespan approach and it is now widely accepted that a variety of environmental and behavioural factors significantly influence the course of human growth and development.

At first glance, the division of the lifespan into a number of stages is deceptively simple. It is, however, a hazardous exercise. How many stages should there be? Ultimately, the decision is arbitrary. More important, by what criteria are we to define a "stage"? Our society places great emphasis on age, but a person's age *per se* is of little value in helping us to understand his or her behaviour. A more popular way of using the term "stage" is to refer to sets of events—both within the individual and in the environment—which tend to occur at certain points in the life cycle. But this, too, can be problematic. Which events should we choose as being significant? Events which, with rare exceptions, naturally occur at certain times (for example, puberty) should not be confused with events such as retirement or children leaving home, which tend to occur at certain points in the life cycle only because of the way our society is structured and which, of course, never actually happen to a good many people. There is a danger here that we will come to see such social events as naturally associated with certain ages and that we will fail to appreciate that reactions to naturally occurring events such as puberty are profoundly influenced by social norms.

We may also come to view the groups contained within different life stages as much more homogeneous than they really are and fail to see important similarities between people at different life stages.

Why then is this book divided into seven stages? Firstly, because it does represent the lifespan as it is experienced by the majority of people in industrialized societies. Secondly, because it provides a useful, if imperfect, framework for presenting what is known about people of different ages. Each "stage" is presented from the point of view of the main character; when other groups are discussed, it is usually in terms of their relationship to the person at the stage being discussed. Inevitably, readers will disagree about the placing of certain events, which only demonstrates the difficulty of defining a "stage."

Optimum health and lifestyle factors

Health, when viewed from the perspective of lifespan growth, represents a potential level of functioning and a state of physical and mental well-being that can go far beyond the mere absence of disease. In the past, most people viewed health as simply the condition which resulted automatically from successfully avoiding disease. Physicians were relegated to the role of technicians who assumed responsibility for curing diseases through surgical or pharmacological intervention. Little or no responsibility was placed upon the patient for his or her health status, and very little mention was ever made of "preventive medicine". This was understandable at one time, when most diseases were caused by infectious agents and the need was greatest for practitioners of "curative medicine". Since the turn of the century, however, there has been a dramatic shift in the leading causes of death in the United States. During the 1800s and early 1900s, infectious diseases such as influenza, pneumonia and tuberculosis were the most common causes of death. Today, however, the most common causes of death are heart disease, cancer, strokes and accidents—all of which have been correlated with personal behaviour patterns and lifestyle and which are, therefore, to a greater extent preventable. In fact, it has been estimated that 90 per cent of all deaths today are caused by factors over which the medical care system has little control, and over which individual patients have a great deal of control through lifestyle reorientation. The changing trends in patterns of disease have brought about concomitant changes in social values. No longer do most individuals believe in the

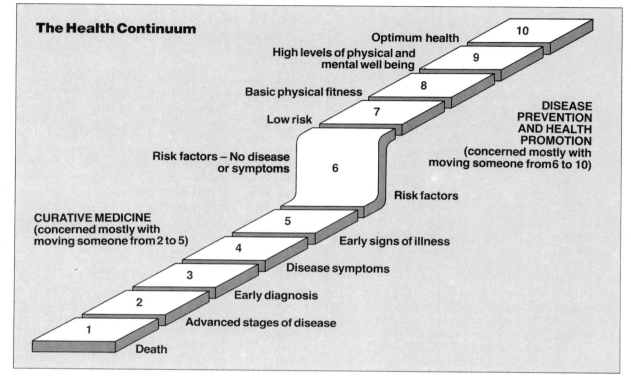

The Health Continuum

- Optimum health — 10
- High levels of physical and mental well being — 9
- Basic physical fitness — 8
- Low risk — 7
- Risk factors – No disease or symptoms — 6
- Risk factors
- 5
- Early signs of illness
- 4 — Disease symptoms
- 3 — Early diagnosis
- 2 — Advanced stages of disease
- 1 — Death

DISEASE PREVENTION AND HEALTH PROMOTION (concerned mostly with moving someone from 6 to 10)

CURATIVE MEDICINE (concerned mostly with moving someone from 2 to 5)

unlimited capability of medical science to repair any damage to their bodies that careless living might produce. A sense of responsibility has been accepted by some individuals, who now view their health and well-being as a gift that can either be conserved or wasted according to the lifestyle that one selects. Others, however, only worry about their health when they lose it, and this, unfortunately, is often too late to do anything about it. This realization has created a shift in emphasis for many health professionals from disease treatment to prevention and health maintenance. In the process, it has presented all concerned with a formidable challenge: to attain the optimum health levels possible throughout the lifespan, utilizing healthy behavioural principles. In other words, preventive medicine challenges us to be as healthy as we possibly can be within the limitations over which we have no control, such as age and genetic inheritance.

Many types of behaviour have been implicated as risk factors for specific major mental and physical disorders, and these are, therefore, the areas where lifestyle changes can be most effective in preventing disease and promoting health. One of the major goals of this book is to provide the reader with pertinent information about these health-related behaviours and their impact on health throughout

the lifespan. While some of these factors are briefly described below, they are considerably expanded in the chapters which follow.

The triangle of health

Our health, from birth until death, is primarily determined by a combination of three types of factors: those that we inherit (genetic factors), those that we come into contact with in our daily living (environmental factors), and those that we bring about ourselves through our personal behaviour (lifestyle factors).

It is important throughout our lives to frequently take stock of our health status and to determine which of the various factors influencing our health are under our control and which are not. For example, though many genetic deficiencies, such as certain enzyme or hormonal imbalances, can be corrected through medical treatment, many others cannot. The greatest potential for influencing the course of human growth and development lies in the control of environmental and behavioural influences on health. Since, essentially, both of these types of factors involve aspects of lifestyle, the key to gaining control of your personal health and well-being can be said to lie in *behaviour change*. What are some of these lifestyle factors that are closely related

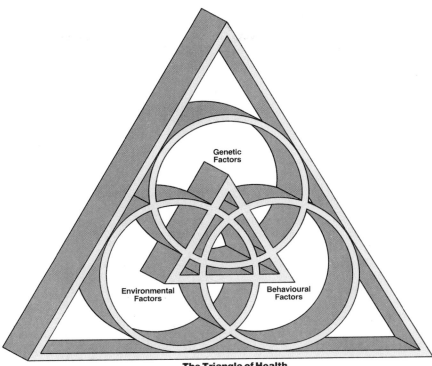

The Triangle of Health

to health; areas where changes in behaviour are most likely to be effective in influencing growth and development?

*Cigarette smoking

Cigarette smoking is the largest single preventable cause of ill health and premature death in the United States. It is the major single cause of cancer death and is an etiological factor for coronary heart disease and peripheral vascular disease. It is the single most important cause of chronic obstructive pulmonary disease and is associated with increased risk of atherosclerosis as well. Cancers of the bladder, liver and pancreas are more common in cigarette smokers, and smoking is also a risk for peptic ulcer. Overall, smokers have a 70 per cent higher death rate than non-smokers, and each year more than 300 000 premature deaths in the United States alone are linked to tobacco. For example, those who smoke and also take oral contraceptives increase their risk for coronary heart disease and some forms of cerebrovascular disease. Mixing alcohol consumption with the smoking habit leads to increased risk for oesophageal cancer and cancers of the larynx and oral cavity. In conjunction with various occupationally related substances, such as asbestos, smoking increases the likelihood of lung

and laryngeal cancer. In addition, smoking is estimated to contribute to as many as 225 000 deaths from coronary heart disease each year in the United States. Furthermore, smoking is the major identifiable cause of accidental death and injury resulting from residential fires. The evidence is clear: if you or someone you love smokes cigarettes, then quit as soon as possible; if you do not smoke, then don't ever start.

*Alcohol consumption

While the consumption of alcoholic beverages in moderation is often thought to be relatively harmless, "problem drinking" and overt alcoholism can lead to serious health problems. Approximately 10 million adults in the United States or 7 per cent of those 18 or older, are considered to be problem drinkers. In the 14 to 17 age group, problem drinkers are estimated to comprise 19 per cent of the total population and to number over 3 million. Ten per cent of all deaths in the United States involve alcohol. Cirrhosis, which is one of the ten leading causes of death today, is largely attributable to excessive alcohol consumption. Various cancers, including those of the liver, mouth, oesophagus and pancreas, are all linked to alcohol consumption, and a wide range of birth defects have been attributed to maternal drinking during pregnancy. In addition, the economic costs to society, both direct and indirect, which result from alcohol misuse and related accidents are staggering—a figure which was estimated at nearly $50 billion in the United States in 1977. Obviously, controlling your alcohol consumption is another way in which you can gain control of your health and well-being.

*Nutrition

Proper nutrition is a prerequisite for health maintenance and optimal health throughout the life cycle. *Undernutrition* results from diets which are deficient in essential nutrients. *Overnutrition* results from the consumption of more calories than the body requires for growth and maintenance. Either eating pattern can lead to serious health problems, and yet both can be corrected by changing one's behaviour. Current data in the United States indicate that, among individuals aged 20 to 74, approximately 24 per cent of women and 14 per cent of men are obese, or clinically diagnosed as overweight, a condition which has been correlated with a variety of illnesses and a large number of premature deaths each year. Average intake of total fat, saturated fat and cholesterol is considered excessive among 35 per cent of adults in the United States, and is considered a behavioural risk factor for coronary heart disease and some forms of cancer. A significant percentage of pregnant or lactating women have iron deficiency anaemia or folic acid deficiency. Average daily sodium intake among adults in the United States is 4–10 g per day which is considered to be approximately twice the optimum level for good health. Refined sugar consumption is believed to be causally linked to dental caries, particularly among children and adolescents. Diets which are deficient in dietary fibre have been shown to be linked to a number of cancers of the gastrointestinal tract. Learning to avoid certain foods, for example, those that are high in fat content, high in sodium content, high in sugars, and high in total calories should be an integral aspect of everyone's health maintenance programme. In addition, understanding the specific dietary requirements of certain population groups (such as iron requirements for pregnant or lactating women, and calcium requirements that increase as we get older) can lead to added health benefits throughout the lifespan.

*Exercise

Although the health benefits from exercise are not completely understood, scientific research con-

tinues to support the value of regular physical activity for both the treatment and the prevention of a variety of health problems, including: coronary heart disease, obesity, hypertension, osteoporosis and stress. A comprehensive exercise programme can include a variety of lifestyle changes that are easily achieved, such as increasing the amount that one walks each day. Recent research has shown that a variety of problems normally associated with ageing, such as osteoporosis and a variety of joint inflammation disorder, can be minimized through regular exercise. A number of suggestions are offered in the chapters that follow that will help to make exercise a regular part of your lifestyle throughout the lifespan.

*High blood pressure management

High blood pressure, or hypertension, can lead to serious illness and premature death. It is estimated that 60 million Americans have high blood pressure. Of these, approximately half require treatment and half are considered borderline and in need of periodic medical examinations that include blood pressure monitoring. Treatment normally consists of a combined regimen of anti-hypertensive medication and dietary change to reduce sodium intake. Untreated hypertension is a major cause of stroke and can also lead to heart disease and kidney failure. Having your blood pressure checked regularly is another action that you can take to prevent serious illness and premature death.

*Accident prevention

Accidental injury is the leading cause of death among individuals who are between one and 44 years of age; and for the 15- to 24-year-olds, injuries account for 55 per cent of all deaths. Nearly half of all accidental deaths result from automobile accidents and the rest are related to burns, poisoning, falls and a variety of other causes. In addition to these fatalities, an even larger number of people suffer from non-fatal accidents that require medical treatment. While this represents an enormous burden upon individuals and society in general, it should also be noted that the vast majority of these injuries are preventable. Accident prevention, if it is to be effective, should begin in the home and should recognize known high risk groups, such as burns among children aged 10 and younger, automobile accidents among teenagers and young adults, and fatal falls among those 75 and over.

*Stress management

Because stress is such an accepted part of twentieth

century lifestyles, a number of illnesses that are believed to be related to stress have come to be known as the "diseases of civilization". These include, among others, coronary heart disease, hypertension, stroke, a number of gastrointestinal disorders and possibly cancer. Available data support the contention that individuals who consistently deal with the sundry obstacles of life in a confrontational, compulsive and impatient manner tend to have a higher incidence of these illnesses. However, since the manner in which we cope with life stress is largely under our control, these stress-related illnesses are preventable. Successful stress management involves (a) learning to identify the symptoms and causes of unhealthy stress, (b) learning to cope with stressful situations in a healthy, productive way and (c) adopting a general lifestyle that is conducive to good health, and that minimizes the potential for stress to have deleterious effects. The recommendations for lifestyle reorientation that are made throughout this book will help young and old alike to manage the harmful effects of stress.

The behaviour changes outlined above are only a few of the many opportunities that are available to those who have decided to take control of their health and well-being. This book has been written in the hope that readers will gain an appreciation for the profound influence that they can have on their growth and development, from early childhood throughout adult life.

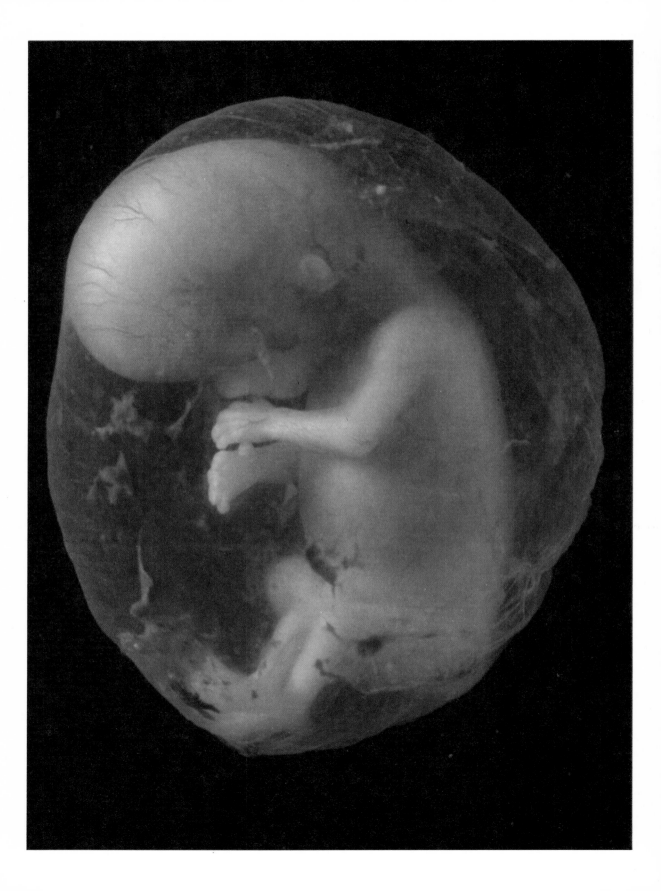

Birth

Our birth is but a sleep and a forgetting:
The Soul that rises with us, our life's Star,
Hath had elsewhere its setting,
And cometh from afar;

William Wordsworth

The events of conception, gestation and childbirth have always fascinated us and it is easy to understand why. Until recently, conception and gestation were mysterious processes, and remain so in many societies; childbirth, too, was surrounded with secrecy but at least a large number of people knew something of what went on, even if they preferred not to share their limited knowledge. The outcome of gestation was, and still is, uncertain; babies differ in sex, in constitution and in health. But the outcome is clearly important. All parents-to-be want their child to be physically perfect. In societies less developed than ours, the sex and the health of the child may be of enormous economic importance; at some points in history, it has been a matter of life or death for the mother or child.

These three factors—lack of knowledge, uncertainty of outcome and importance of outcome—are exactly those conditions which foster the development of myths and folklore, which are attempts to predict and control them. Beliefs about childbearing therefore differ from culture to culture and change only very slowly in the face of scientific knowledge. We now have greater control over these processes than was believed possible even forty years ago. Recent scientific advances have raised important ethical issues at every stage of childbearing from pre-conception (should couples be encouraged to choose the sex of their child?) to conception (what is the legal status of an AID child?), gestation (under what circumstances should foetuses be aborted?), birth (how much control should the mother have over the place and manner of birth?), and post-birth (what efforts should be made to keep handicapped children alive?). Perhaps because of the speed of scientific progress, these issues have only recently become topics of public debate; we are as yet nowhere near resolving them.

Left: The miracle of life—a human foetus within its amniotic sac

The biology of pregnancy

None of us can predict how our lives will end, but at least we can be certain how they began—as a single cell formed by a female ovum (egg) fusing with a male sperm. This process of fertilization is the culmination of a complex series of biological events. For the mother these begin with the release of a ripened ovum or egg (ovulation) somewhere around the fourteenth day of the menstrual cycle. The egg is transported from the ovaries through one or other of the Fallopian tubes, each of which is about 4 in (10 cm) long. It is carried downwards by contractions within the tube and by a current formed by the beating of tiny, hair-like structures called cilia. The egg will be available for fertilization for only about 12–24 hours immediately after ovulation.

In the father's body, production of sperm cells is a continuous process—as many as 500 million sperm mature daily. From the testes, sperm pass into the epididymes (storage tanks consisting of some 20 ft (6 m) of coiled tubes) and it is here that the sperm mature. From each epididymis, the mature sperm cells move into one or other of the two 16 in (40 cm) tubes known as the vasa deferentia. From here, the sperm cells move into the seminal vesicles which not only store sperm, but also produce fluids, sugars for nourishing the sperm, and prostaglandin. The prostate gland contributes acids, trace elements and enzymes to the sperm to form a thick milky fluid—the semen.

At the climax of sexual intercourse, the seminal vesicles pour semen into the urethra for ejaculation. The urethra expands to two or three times its normal width, producing an explosive feeling, while powerful muscular contractions propel the semen out of the penis in a series of about half a dozen surges.

In a single ejaculation, there may be as many as 350 million sperm deposited around the cervix or neck of the womb. These sperm face a formidable journey, thousands of times greater than their own length.

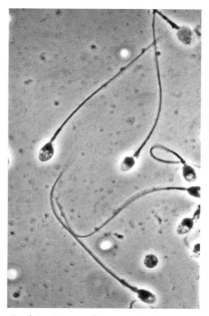

In this picture of sperm (greatly magnified—each one is only 1/500 in or 0.05 mm long) the heads and necks are clearly visible.

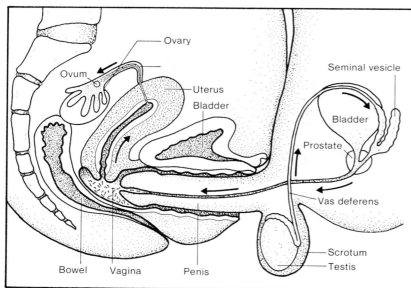

Ovary
Ovum
Uterus
Bladder
Seminal vesicle
Bladder
Prostate
Vas deferens
Scrotum
Testis
Bowel Vagina Penis

The journey of the sperm to the ovum
The sperm have to travel 12 cm (almost 5 in) through the uterus to penetrate the ovum in the Fallopian tube. Of the millions ejaculated, only a few thousand survive in the uterus and even fewer reach the Fallopian tube. They live for 24 to 48 hours. But a successful journey can be made only during two days on either side of ovulation, as only then can they penetrate the mucus present in the vagina.

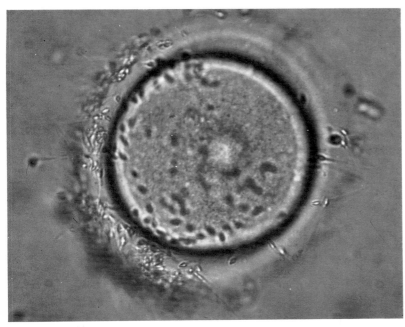

Many sperm attempt to penetrate and fertilize the ovum (egg) in one of the Fallopian tubes, but normally only one manages to break through the protective outer cover.

Not surprisingly, the task they face is reflected in their structure. Each sperm is about 1/500 in (0.05 mm) long and is divided into five parts: head, neck, mid-piece, tail and end-piece. The head is packed with chromosomes, which potentially make up half the genetic component of the new life formed; the rest of the structure is designed to propel the sperm cell towards the egg. The cylindrical neck is believed to account for the long whip-like movements of the tail that keep the sperm mobile. The mid-piece contains the mitochondria, tiny power houses which release the energy necessary for movement.

The first task for the sperm cells is to penetrate the cervix, and there will be many casualties at this stage. The "successful" cells swim forwards at a speed of about 1/10 in (3 mm) a minute, by contracting in length, first along one side of the tail, then along the other. Sperm differ in their speed and strength of movement, so that perhaps only 200 000 or so will eventually reach the Fallopian tubes. Of these, about 100 000 will enter the wrong tube, and of those which enter the tube containing the egg, only about 100 may reach it.

A sperm may spend several hours in the female before it is able to penetrate and fertilize the egg. During this time it undergoes changes which make penetration possible. These include the shedding of the acrosome, the thin cap encasing the head of the sperm cell. The acrosomal cap is believed to contain an enzyme which dissolves the protective outer cover of the ovum, making sperm penetration easier. This cap-shedding is not only restricted to the sperm which eventually penetrates the egg, but also affects the doomed sperm around the egg. This act of self-sacrifice is not without purpose—the enzyme from just one cap would be insufficient to break down the ovum membrane, but the enzyme from many thousands produces a strong concentrated enzyme mass. Contrary to popular opinion, it does take more than one sperm to produce a baby!

It could be said that the process of fertilization leaves a great deal to chance. There is no mechanism to guarantee contact between sperm and egg; new life hangs quite literally in the balance of random movement of sperm and egg in the Fallopian tube. In lower plants, by contrast, sperm are directly attracted to eggs. In bracken, for example, the eggs secrete malic acid to draw sperm to them. In humans, however, once the egg has been penetrated by a sperm, it usually resists overtures from any other sperm except in occasional cases of twins and in rare cases which result in the death of the embryo.

The first cell
The solitary cell formed by fertilization contains all the material necessary for the creation of a new human being. The control centre of this process is the cell nucleus, where the blueprints for life are stored in the form of 46 chromosomes—a large collection of genes—arranged in 23 pairs of different shapes and sizes. There are many thousands of genes within a cell—exactly how many is in dispute—and every body cell which eventually arises from this single cell contains the same set of genes.

The developing foetus
Fertilization takes place in one of the Fallopian tubes and the fertilized egg spends several days there before implanting itself in the wall of the uterus. During this time, the cells divide steadily. About 30 hours after fertilization the ovum divides into two cells; a second division occurs some 20 hours later, giving four cells and by the time of implantation there are about 150 cells. At this stage, the embryo is called a blastocyst and a series of changes affecting its outer layer brings about the formation of the placenta, the organ which provides the embryo with nourishment from the mother's bloodstream.

This is a hazardous time for the embryo. Many embryos do not develop normally—in fact fewer don't than do. About 10 per cent fail to implant, and of those that do about half are aborted spontaneously, usually without the mother knowing. Most of these losses are attributable to abnormalities in the embryo or in its nutritive and protecting environment.

The role of genes
We have seen that every body cell carries exactly the same information in its nucleus as 23 pairs of chromosomes. Within a muscle cell, for

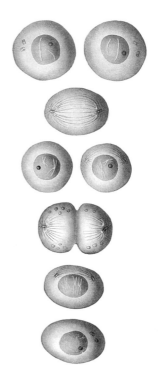

Division of cells by meiosis
Cells in the ovaries and testes divide by this special process to produce daughter cells with half the number of parent chromosomes. The cell first splits into two, each cell receiving one chromosome from each pair (23 chromosomes). These two cells then divide again—this time the strands (chromatids) in each chromosome pull apart (23 chromatids). The process is completed when each chromatid duplicates itself—the four daughter cells now have 23 chromosomes.

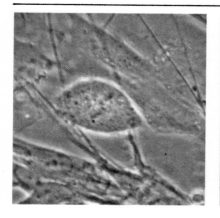

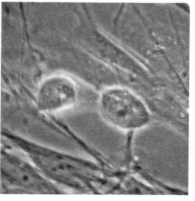

Nerve cells dividing by mitosis
As the embryo develops, the cells become specialized to form the different tissues and organs of the body, e.g. blood, skin, muscles, etc. This process is called differentiation, and involves the activation of some of the information encoded on the chromosomes while some remains dormant. Once the cells specialize, like the nerve cells shown here, they will divide by mitosis to produce other nerve cells.

example, there are instructions for the construction of a blood cell or a nerve cell—in fact for every cell. But the muscle cell ignores every instruction but its own.

Because genes control the behaviour of cells, they also control physical appearance which is, after all, the result of cells behaving in certain ways. The whole process of cell division and differentiation, of determining the structure and function of cells, is masterminded by the genes on these chromosomes, which are made of deoxyribonucleic acid (DNA).

Each parent may have contributed half of the genes within the cell nucleus, but the new baby will almost certainly look more like one parent than the other, or like neither! The reason is that genes, like people, can be described in comparative terms as "good", "bad",

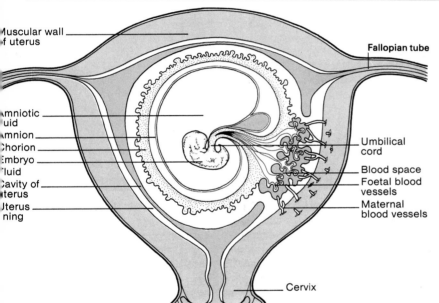

Muscular wall of uterus

Fallopian tube

Amniotic fluid
Amnion
Chorion
Embryo
Fluid
Cavity of uterus
Uterus lining

Umbilical cord

Blood space
Foetal blood vessels
Maternal blood vessels

Cervix

The developing foetus

As the foetus develops, the uterus stretches and becomes more muscular in preparation for birth. The embryo is surrounded by a sac containing amniotic fluid and enclosed by two membranes, the amnion and the chorion. It is joined to the placenta on the uterus wall by the umbilical cord. Here the mother's and the foetus's bloodstreams are in close proximity, but separate, and the foetus makes use of the mother's organs of respiration, digestion and excretion. The cervix is sealed by a mucous plug.

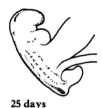 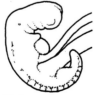 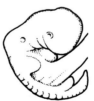 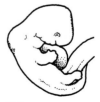 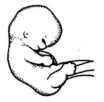

25 days
The first 60 days are the most crucial period of development. After 25 days the embryo is a soft piece of tissue. A swelling contains the brain, and other bulges become the jaws and mouth. The mid-section contains a developing heart.

28 days
The largest organ is now the heart, which pumps blood round the body and into the placenta through the umbilical cord. The brain and nervous system grow; the stomach begins to form; and the tail, already forming at 25 days, is growing.

32 days
Limb development begins. The bones and muscles eventually grow from 25 pairs of tissue segments (somites) on the trunk. At this stage the embryo is very sensitive to any drugs or germs in the mother's bloodstream.

34 days
Buds which will be arms and legs continue to develop, as does the tail. Rudimentary eyes appear and the nose takes shape. The brain becomes more elaborate and the cranial nerves (which control the head) start to form.

41 days
The head and arms grow rapidly and the hands show the outline of fingers. The eyes develop and the external ear begins to form. The heart and the liver—which begins to produce blood—bulge above the umbilical cord.

47 days
The head grows rapidly and the neck, ear and ear canal can be seen. The eyes, already with retina and lens, are open and eyelids grow. The mouth has lips, tongue and 20 teeth buds. The heart is not seen; the tail disappears.

"recessive" or "dominant". Everyone carries some genes which have not found expression in themselves, but which may have been expressed in their parents or grandparents and may subsequently be expressed in their children.

Brown-eye genes, for example, are dominant over blue-eye genes: a brown-eyed parent may carry the genes for blue eyes as well as brown, but a blue-eyed parent cannot carry brown-eye genes. Two blue-eyed parents, therefore, can expect to have only blue-eyed children, but if one parent has two genes for brown eyes and the other two genes for blue eyes, their children will have brown eyes. Two brown-eyed parents, however, might both possess the recessive blue gene and are likely to have one blue-eyed child in every four.

Inheritance of characteristics determined by a large number of genes is much more complicated. Children tend to be more average than their parents. For example, most children of very tall parents tend to be tall, but less so than their parents. On the other hand, a child of two short parents may be quite tall—provided both parents are carrying some of the many genes for tallness.

The genes contributed by the mother and father at conception form the new baby's *genotype*. However, the environment—including the uterine environment—has a profound effect on how this genotype will eventually be expressed, so the term *phenotype* is used to refer to the physical and psychological characteristics that the person actually displays. Your phenotype is the expression of only a small part of your genotype.

Detecting abnormalities

Many abnormalities in the growing foetus can be detected by examining the cells taken from it. Body cells are constantly dying and being replaced. Some cells in the intestinal lining, for example, live for only one and a half days, white blood cells survive only a few days, while oxygen-carrying red blood cells survive for about four months. Dead cells from the growing foetus are discarded into the fluid (the amniotic fluid) which surrounds it in the womb.

The process known as amniocentesis consists of inserting a very fine needle into the mother's abdomen, drawing off some of this fluid and examining the foetal cells it contains. Over 100 abnormalities, including spina bifida and many chromosomal abnormalities (see pages 54 and 55), can be detected or ruled out by this process. It does not guarantee that the baby will be 100 per cent healthy, as not all abnormalities can be detected from cell examination. The process does, of course, reveal the baby's sex by detecting the XX or XY chromosomes, but most parents prefer to be kept guessing till the birth!

Smoking and alcohol

Because everything consumed by the mother during pregnancy will eventually reach the foetus via the placenta, there is special concern about the effects of drugs on the developing baby. Nicotine and alcohol are two examples of substances which can affect the baby's development. Smoking in pregnancy, for example, can reduce full-term foetal weight by, on average, 5 oz (142 g) and causes a 30 per cent rise in perinatal deaths (deaths within 24 hours of birth). Why smoking in pregnancy should reduce birthweight is not fully understood, but it may affect placental bloodflow and foetal nutrition.

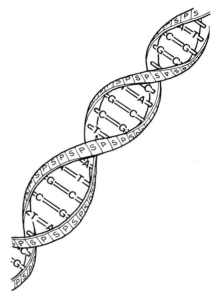

The structure of DNA
Above: The "spiral staircase" of the DNA molecule. Its sides consist of sugar and phosphate and the steps are combinations of four nitrogen-containing compounds—adenine, thymine, cytosine and guanine (A, T, C, G). Below: The molecule reproduces itself by separating down the middle and picking up new A, T, C and G units to form identical new spirals.

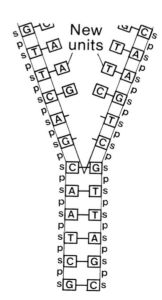

Concern about the effects of alcohol on foetal development can be traced to the time of Aristotle, who noted that drunken women often bore feeble-minded children. The effects of excessive alcohol consumption during pregnancy are now recognized by the label *foetal alcohol syndrome*, a collection of features which includes poor development of parts of the upper lip, nose and eyes, and mental retardation. One problem in determining the effects of alcohol *per se* on the foetus is that heavy drinking is often associated with other factors such as poor nutrition, smoking, maternal ill-health and stress, which themselves may have deleterious effects on the growing baby both before and after birth. It is now thought that even small amounts of alcohol can harm the foetus, especially if taken on a regular basis, and that there is no safe level of alcohol consumption during pregnancy.

Premature babies

Traditionally, for want of a better method, foetal age is usually counted from the first day of the menstrual period before conception—on average two weeks before fertilization. The most frequent "age" at birth is 280 days or 40 weeks (38 weeks of true foetal age), but there is considerable variation, with babies born between 259 days (37 weeks) and 293 days (42 weeks) being regarded as normal.

Babies born earlier than 37 weeks are known as pre-term babies and, until recently, all babies weighing less than 5½ lb (2500 g) at birth were termed premature regardless of their physical health or length of gestation. Now babies who are less than 5½ lb (2500 g) are known as low birthweight babies! Take the cases of baby Leonard and baby Peter. Baby Leonard, born at 36 weeks, weighed 5½ lb (2500 g), a perfectly normal weight for his gestation age. Baby Peter also weighed 5½ lb (2500 g) but he was born at 40 weeks and his weight was below the normal range for his gestational age.

Babies such as Leonard will catch up perfectly well without showing any adverse effects from their earlier exposure to the outside world. However, so-called "small for dates" babies may not fully catch up with babies in the normal range, though they will close the gap a little. Some fail to grow as tall as full-term babies and may also be mentally impaired to varying degrees.

Ultrasound

The worst time for small-for-dates babies is the tail end of pregnancy when growth should be rapid. Many doctors are now recommending induction of such foetuses at 36 or even 34 weeks. But how can such babies be identified?

The most effective method is to use ultrasound. This technique can be used to determine growth trends at any stage of pregnancy. Very high frequency sound waves—so high that they cannot be heard—are beamed at the foetus and echoed back. The time taken for the echo to return is measured. The size of the foetal head can be measured by scanning with a number of beams and feeding the findings into a computer. Similarly, though with less accuracy, ultrasound is used to measure foetal abdominal circumference and length from head to buttocks. More than 90 per cent of small-for-dates babies could be detected if all babies were measured from head to buttocks between the ages of 6 and 12 weeks, for head width between 13 and 20 weeks, and abdominal circumference at 32 weeks.

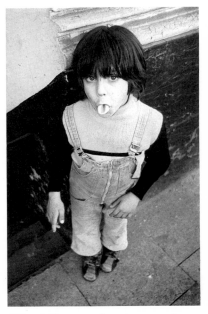

The ability to curl one's tongue is determined by a dominant gene— only if both genes in the appropriate pair are recessive will the trait be absent.

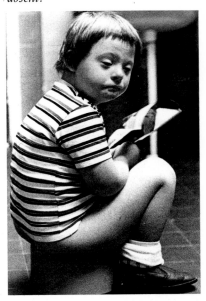

Down's syndrome (mongolism) is the result of a chromosomal abnormality, originating at conception. People with this condition have 24 pairs of chromosomes rather than the normal 23.

Multiple births

About one in every 80 pregnancies results in twins. They are either identical or, more frequently, fraternal. Identical twins develop from the segmentation of one zygote (fertilized ovum) and are genetically identical, while fraternal twins develop from two separate zygotes and are no more alike than brothers and sisters generally. The likelihood of giving birth to twins is partly determined by heredity; and fathers and mothers in their thirties are more likely to produce twins. Twins are more likely to be miscarried than are single babies, and difficult births are more common.

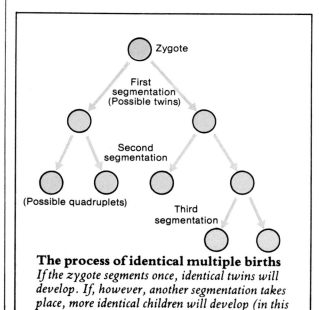

Two of a kind—identical twins.

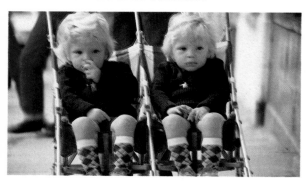

The process of identical multiple births
If the zygote segments once, identical twins will develop. If, however, another segmentation takes place, more identical children will develop (in this case, identical quintuplets are possible). Such babies are at risk during pregnancy and birth.

IDENTICAL TWINS

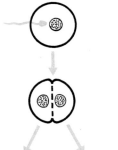

A single fertilized egg segments to form identical twins. Identical twins therefore carry the same chromosomes and genes.

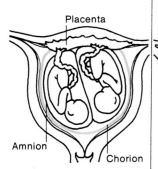

Heads down, they share the placenta and lie in separate amniotic sacs inside the chorion membrane.

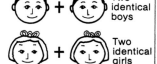
Two identical boys
Two identical girls

Having an identical heredity, identical twins are always of the same sex.

FRATERNAL TWINS

The fertilization of two different eggs results in fraternal twins. These twins therefore carry different mixtures of chromosomes and genes.

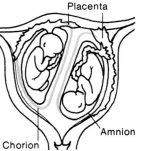

One with head down and one breeched, they have separate placentas, amniotic sacs and chorion membranes.

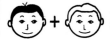
Two boys
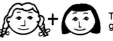
Two girls
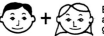
Boy and girl

They can be a boy and a girl.

A child is born

How does a baby react to the process of birth? There is no single simple answer to this question. We can look, first, at the physical and psychological effects of the birth process itself and, second, at the influence of events of the immediate post-birth period on the baby's later development.

The birth process

Strange as it may seem to us in the outside world, birth, as far as some of the newborn's physiological functions are concerned, is an incident without special significance. It is merely part of a steadily changing sequence of events regulated by biological clocks. For example, the maturation of the nervous system seems to be unaffected by birth, judging by brain-wave activity as measured by an electroencephalograph. The electroencephalogram, or EEG, of a baby born at 30 weeks will be much the same five weeks later as that of a baby born at 35 weeks.

Similarly, the experience of pre-term birth does not precipitate any switch over from foetal haemoglobin to adult haemoglobin (haemoglobin is the pigment which gives blood its red colour and is the means by which oxygen is carried from the lungs to the cells; foetal and adult haemoglobin have different molecular structures). This switch usually occurs in about the 36th week in preparation for birth, but it is not triggered by birth.

Cardiovascular and respiratory systems are the ones most altered by birth. Failure to breathe normally in the crucial period just after birth is a common cause of neonatal death or brain damage. However,

The newborn baby—the umbilical cord has been severed, but the amount of contact enjoyed by mother and baby immediately after the birth may have some influence on their future relationship.

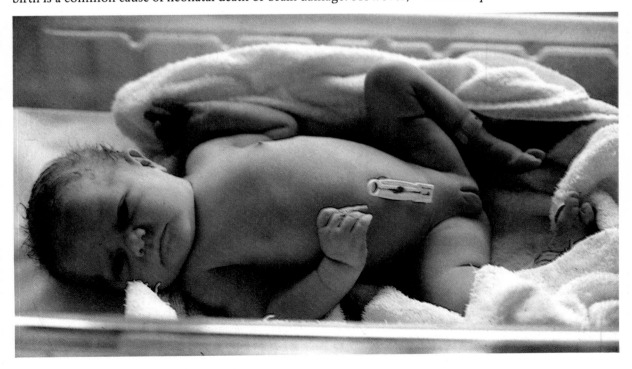

contrary to popular opinion, newborn infants are better able to withstand oxygen deprivation than are children or adults. Many neonatologists now think that failure to start breathing may arise from pre-existing brain damage.

Certain obstetric interventions may carry some risk to the baby. Painkillers or anaesthetics taken by the mother during birth all pass through the placenta to the baby. This may result in a baby who is irritable, or less alert or responsive to particular stimuli. Forceps delivery, which occurs five times as often in induced as in natural births, carries a slight risk of brain damage, but it has to be weighed against the damage that might result if the birth were not helped along.

It is always difficult, however, to separate out the effects of events at birth from other factors known to affect a baby's development. Mothers who do not prepare well for the birth by, for example, attending antenatal classes, may require more painkillers, be less able to co-operate or more likely to be delivered by forceps. These same mothers may also have looked after themselves less well.

The psychological effects of birth

Some psychologists and psychiatrists have suggested that the birth experience—with its connotations of crushing and suffocating, and sudden exposure to external stimuli—is one of life's most traumatic events and that it profoundly affects a person's future psychological wellbeing. There is very little evidence, however, to support this point of view; indeed it is difficult to know what kind of evidence would support it. Perhaps we should expect babies born by Caesarian section, who are taken directly from the womb by surgery, to be better adjusted! Adults who claim to relive their birth under hypnosis seem to be responding more to the demands of the situation or to their idea of what birth might be like than to any true memory of their birth.

This is not to say that the birth experience should not be as calm and relaxed as possible, for both mother and baby. The advantages of a relaxed birth, however, may lie in the fact that less obstetric intervention may be needed and that the mother and baby may be more responsive to each other.

The mother–infant bond

Is there a natural or instinctive bond between a baby and its mother? And does early disruption of the bonding process affect a baby's development? There is certainly evidence from animal experiments and natural observation that, in some species, if the young are removed from their mother for a short period soon after birth, she rejects them completely when they are returned to her. Obviously, this does not happen with humans, but it does seem that early separation of mother and infant influences the quality of care the baby receives.

In a classic study, a group of mothers were given a period of unlimited contact with their babies immediately after birth. The mothers laid their babies on the bed beside them so that they could look into their eyes. Then, talking to their babies softly, the mothers began to explore them gently with their hands. When these babies were older, their mothers were still taking more time and trouble caring for them. They were doing this more lovingly than mothers

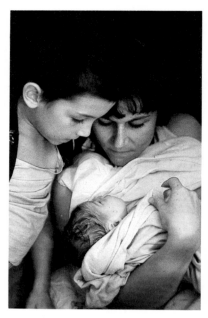

A mother and newborn baby need to have the opportunity to develop responsiveness to each other as the baby meets an increasing amount of environmental stimuli and, later, a more complex network of relationships.

whose babies had been removed from them in standard American fashion. It still remains to be shown that the babies derive some lasting benefit from this early extra care, particularly as a replication of this study in England showed that early differences in the quality of care disappeared after six months.

An important way in which the infant can quickly gain resistance to infection is by being put to the mother's breast immediately after birth. A study by Klaus and Kennel showed that, given complete freedom, many mothers do this naturally. Unless the baby is depressed by painkilling drugs given to the mother during labour, he or she will often suck vigorously for a time. Milk will not be present in the breasts yet, but the baby will receive colostrum, a clear and slightly sticky fluid containing proteins, which transfer some immunity to infection from mother to baby. This early sucking stimulates the production of milk in the breast and may well be important for the baby in "fine tuning" of the sucking actions.

There are, moreover, sound physical reasons why early contact between mother and infant should be encouraged. Our skins are covered by a rich flora of bacteria and yeasts. Technically these are infections, but they are harmless—indeed, they are probably beneficial. A baby is born without flora, but rapidly acquires it by contact with adults. If the baby's first contacts are with the mother and father, it will be from them that the skin flora comes. If, however, this early contact is prevented or curtailed, the flora will come from whoever handles the baby; doctors or nurses, for example, may be carrying disease-causing bacteria. Early contact with parents protects against such infections, because once the skin is colonized it is more difficult for new, and possibly damaging, kinds of bacteria to be admitted.

Newborn babies, then, have already been exposed to a considerable amount of environmental stimuli before, during and immediately after birth. How these will affect what the babies achieve and the kind of people they become remains to be seen; human powers of adaptation, however, are impressive and there is a great deal of evidence to suggest that what happens later—even much later—in life will profoundly influence future wellbeing.

Myths and old wives' tales

The myths and customs surrounding childbirth seem to derive mainly from three fears: fear of the "contamination" of blood (particularly menstrual blood); fear of the unknown spirit sources of life; and fears for the welfare of the child.

The blood taboo is echoed in Christian countries today in those denominations where women have to be "churched" to "purify" them after childbirth. In many cultures men were, and still are, specifically excluded to protect them from the dangerous powers of the "life force" present at the birth. And fears for the child led pregnant women to avoid certain things; for instance, to see a rabbit feeding would ensure that the child was born with a hare-lip. The new-born had to be protected from evil spirits and it is thought that long christening robes, once so popular in England, derive from the wish to disguise the baby as an adult.

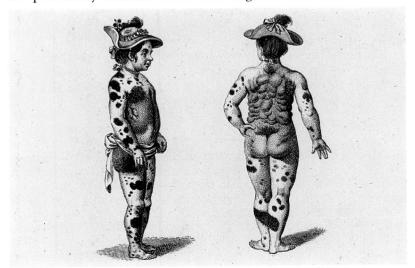

This engraving was made in 1793 and depicts a child covered in deer-like hair. The deformities were attributed to the fact that, during pregnancy, the mother had been involved in a quarrel concerning a stag.

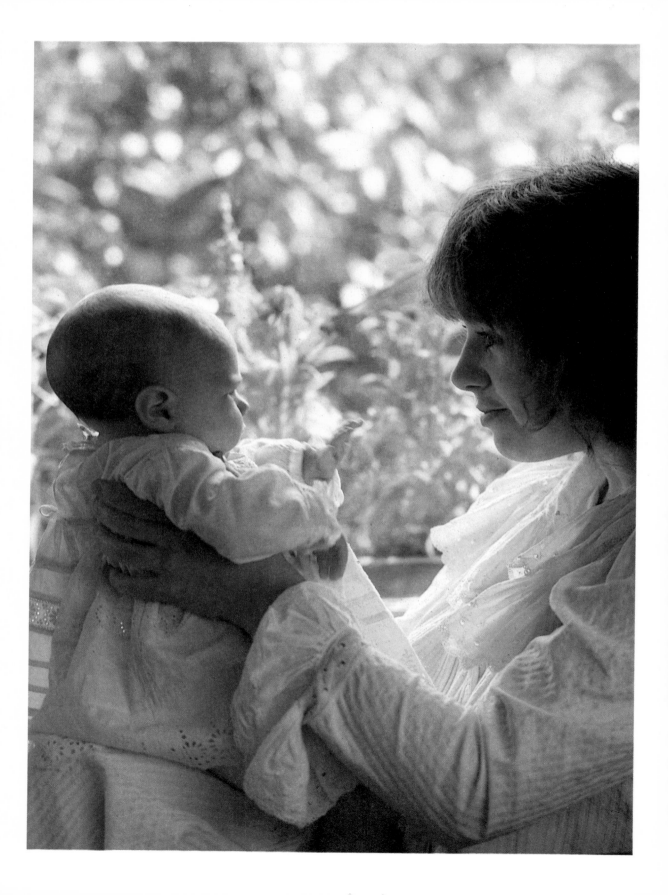

Infancy

How to fold a diaper depends on the size of the baby and the diaper.

Dr Benjamin Spock *Baby and Child Care*

Is he developing normally? Shouldn't she be walking by now? Questions like these are common and often reflect distressing parental concern. Parents may worry about a less-than-average rate of physical development or be proud about rapid development in one area. But different rates of progress do not necessarily signify much—every normal child gets there in the end. Growth is a target-seeking process. The passage of an infant along his or her "growth curve" is comparable to that of a missile directed at a distant target. Just as two missiles may follow slightly different paths and both hit the target, two children may have slightly different courses of growth but both end up with almost the same physique.

Differences in the rate of maturation are apparent even before birth. Some children play out their growth allegro, others moderato, a few lentissimo. It seems that heredity is to a large extent responsible for setting the metronome but environmental influences, especially nutrition, also play a part.

Does growth occur in spurts or is it a smooth, continuous process? Except during adolescence, development is more continuous than sporadic. This applies as much to motor development as to mental ability. This is why it is unwise to set hard and fast standards of growth and development.

The wise parent, while paying attention to any signs that may spell danger for the child, accepts that his or her relationship with the infant is not subject to hard and fast rules, but will vary from the so-called "norm". Parenting is not so much a matter for doing things by the book, but rather playing it by ear—improvising our lines as we go along. After all, this is a new relationship in which both players are inexperienced.

Left: A life begins, and the world is a source of many new and often strange experiences

Feeding

Feeding is a central activity with a new baby, so it is hardly surprising that a great deal of attention has been devoted to how it "should" be done. Most of the controversy about infant feeding can be reduced to two basic questions: should the baby be breast- or bottle-fed, and what pattern of feeding should the new mother adopt?

Unfortunately the answers that are often given to these questions are determined more by fads and fashions than by good supporting evidence. All too often the answers are also dogmatic, and hint at the possibility of dire consequences for the baby's future if one or other method and pattern of feeding is not adopted. Conversely, many books on child care hedge their bets on the subject of feeding, often giving highly equivocal advice such as "breast is best but the bottle is just as good". Given that no two mothers will face the same set of problems, the best approach is, perhaps, to give information rather than advice, so that every mother can make up her own mind and choose what she thinks will be best for herself and her child.

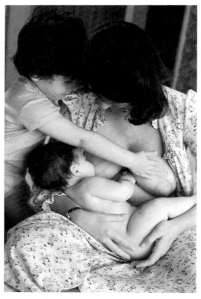

Breast-feeding can help strengthen the bond between mother and baby. It can also be a source of great interest to other children in the family.

Breast versus bottle

There is little doubt that breast milk is ideally suited to the needs of the human infant. For the first few days after birth, babies live off their own fat stores. Around the fourth or fifth day, they often go through a period of restlessness and crying, which marks the time they first become hungry. As one might expect, natural selection has arranged things so that those demands for food are met by the production of breast milk.

Human milk is a very complicated mixture of fats, proteins, sugars, minerals and water that can satisfy all the baby's food requirements for the first year or so of life. However, breast milk does more than this: both milk and the colostrum produced by the breasts in the first few days after the baby's birth are rich in antibodies that help protect the baby against infection. Breast milk also makes the alimentary canal a very hostile environment for bacteria. The iron contained in breast milk is bound in special protein, which ensures that almost all of it is absorbed into the baby's bloodstream, leaving too little in the alimentary canal to sustain harmful bacteria. Bottle milk, by contrast, contains larger amounts of iron, but in a form that is poorly absorbed, so that most of it passes straight through and is eliminated in the faeces. As a result, breast-fed babies tend to be more resistant to illnesses.

Babies who are not breast-fed may become sensitive to cow's milk. Their immune systems react to some of the proteins in the milk passing through the wall of the gut into the bloodstream. This permeability to "foreign" proteins disappears after the first few weeks, but before that even a single formula feed can cause problems in the small minority of babies that are affected. Research has also linked asthma and eczema to bottle-feeding. For asthma, it has been shown that symptoms can be relieved by putting the child on a diet free of cow's milk.

Over the 50 or so years that cow's-milk formulae have been available, their composition has changed, so that they now resemble human milk more closely. Long experience has shown that they do provide adequate food for a baby, but their composition is not identical to that of human milk. Fierce arguments still continue about the importance or otherwise of these differences. The most important probably concerns the risk of infection which, with modern sterilizing techniques, is minimal in industrialized countries. On the other hand, for the poor and malnourished of the Third World, bottle-feeding amounts to a death sentence for many babies. However, although bottle-feeding may not usually *introduce* infection, it provides no extra protection against it. As we have seen, the addition of an iron supplement to cow's-milk formulae may even encourage bacterial growth in the gut.

The behaviour of mothers of both bottle- and breast-fed babies plays an important part in determining the composition of their baby's food. The composition of breast milk varies with what the mother eats. Because many drugs—including nicotine and alcohol—and environmental contaminants that the mother takes in will reach the baby, breast milk is not always as natural and wholesome as it seems. A breast-feeding mother should always get her doctor to check that any drug prescribed for her is safe for the baby.

When powdered milk is used to make up a bottle feed, it is vital that instructions about diluting the powder with water are followed carefully. Samples of bottle milk made up by nurses and mothers in English maternity hospitals have shown that there is a strong tendency to put in too much powder on the assumption that, if two scoopfuls are good for a baby, three must be even better. However, just the opposite is true. The problem is that milk contains salts, and to get rid of these through the kidneys the baby must have water. An over-concentrated feed does not provide enough water, and so the excess salts accumulate in the body.

This process, if it continues too long, can have serious consequences. The first sign of *hypernatremia*, the technical name for this condition, is that the baby becomes fretful and cries a lot. If this is misinterpreted as hunger, and the baby is given more over-concentrated food, the problem gets worse. It is always worth remembering that babies, especially if bottle-fed, may be thirsty as well as hungry, particularly if the weather is hot, or the house warm.

Psychological factors

Much has been said and written about the importance of the close physical relationship of breast-feeding for the emotional development of children. However, research evidence has repeatedly failed to support this assumption. Although a great deal may be gained by a close physical relationship between infants and their parents, this is neither ensured by breast-feeding nor precluded by bottle-feeding. Both breast- and bottle-feeding mothers can make feeding a time of physical closeness with their babies.

It has been suggested that breast-feeding mothers show more affectionate behaviour towards their babies, but to suggest that these differences have to do with breast-feeding *per se* is to ignore the fact that mothers differ enormously in their overall attitude and behaviour towards their children; the decision to breast-feed may be a consequence rather than a cause of a more affectionate attitude towards the baby. A mother who for good practical reasons decides to bottle-feed need not fear that she is depriving her child of affection.

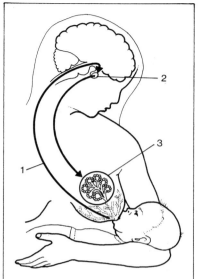

How milk gets to the baby
Nerve impulses from the nipple (1) stimulate the pituitary gland (2) to release prolactin into the bloodstream. This causes the cells of the alveoli (3) to swell with milk.

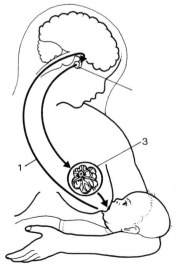

How milk is "let down"
Nerve impulses (1) stimulate the posterior of the pituitary gland (2) to release oxytocin. This causes muscles (3) to squeeze milk to the nipple.

Feeding patterns

The composition of milks from various mammals varies quite widely, depending not only on the diet of the mother but also on the feeding patterns and growth rate of the infant. Tree shrews, for example, feed their young every 48 hours, and rabbits every 24 hours; and the milk of these species has a high protein and fat content. Young tree shrews and rabbits also suck very fast, ensuring nourishment in minimum time.

Human milk contains a much lower amount of protein and fat— identical amounts, in fact, are found in the milks of anthropoid apes. Human infants also suck relatively slowly, suggesting that both the mother's milk and the baby's sucking are adapted to a pattern of very frequent feeding.

This pattern is found in pre-agricultural or hunter-gatherer societies such as the Bushmen of the Kalahari and the Australian Aborigines, and even amongst many agricultural and pastoral societies. Observations of mothers in the Kalahari, for example, have shown that their babies suck at the breast about every 20 minutes. This pattern of continuous feeding is, of course, only possible if mother and baby are in almost constant contact.

In our society, by contrast, parents are more distant from their babies and our idea of meals eaten at set times is applied to babies from the moment they are born. Being very adaptable, babies can accustom themselves to restricted feeding, but there are limits to this. For most babies and mothers, feeding less frequently than every three hours, with one feed missed at night, makes the establishment of breast-feeding very difficult.

Frequent feeding is especially important in the first week or two of lactation, firstly because it can avoid the period of restlessness and crying when the baby first becomes hungry, secondly because it avoids the sometimes painful engorgement of the breasts which occurs when the milk comes in, and thirdly because the level of production of milk is set to some extent by the demands of the baby. With too infrequent feeds, the production of milk may never rise to the level required to sustain the very high growth rate of a young baby.

Forming a habit

Sometimes mothers are reluctant to provide very frequent feeds at this time for fear that they will set a pattern which may be difficult to cope with later. They may also feel that unrestricted feeding may not be in the infant's best interest; the unfortunate phrase "demand feeding" tends to reinforce this idea, with its implication that the infant is trying to exert its authority and make unreasonable demands. Given the speed with which adults try to satisfy their own food demands, this seems rather unfair! In any case, even with total demand feeding, the frequency of feeds soon begins to decline.

Artificial feeds are more concentrated than breast milk. This makes it possible to bottle-feed satisfactorily—at least from a nutritional point of view—every four hours, which would be too widely spaced for breast-feeding.

Like most things to do with babies' lives, the "right" pattern of feeding is the one that the mother and baby work out between themselves to suit their own style of living. Parents should distrust anyone, however eminent, who is dogmatic on this subject.

BREAST V. BOTTLE

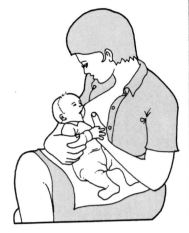

Breast-feeding

Human milk is ideally suited to the needs of babies. It contains all that is required by the baby for the first year or so of its life. And it gives him or her a natural immunity to almost all common childhood diseases.

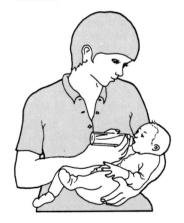

Bottle-feeding

Bottle-feeding, on the other hand, may leave the baby more vulnerable to infections and some babies may be allergic to cow's milk. However, by using a bottle the feeding can be shared between two or more people.

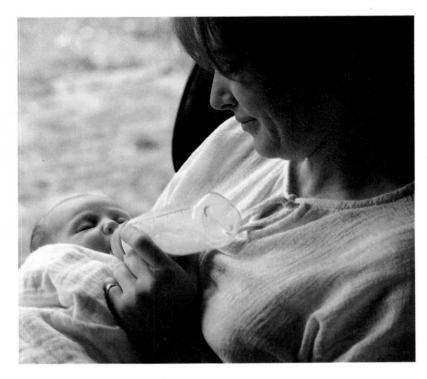

Bottle-feeding allows greater flexibility for the mother both in sharing the feeding with others and in adjusting the time between feeds, as artificial feeds are more concentrated than breast milk.

Weaning

Sometime in the first year, parents will begin to give solid foods to their baby. As with everything else to do with infant feeding, this topic has been beset with controversy and rapidly changing fashions. A few years ago in Britain, some professional advice suggested that babies should begin eating solid foods in the first couple of weeks after birth. Today, the recommendation is for solid foods to be started at three or four months. Breast milk, in fact, provides a perfectly adequate diet for a baby for the whole of the first year, and the same is probably true for the artificial milks.

When solids are introduced, these need not be the bland and sometimes rather tasteless commercially available baby foods. Parents may find these much more troublesome and expensive than giving a baby some of the food from their own meals. Babies' chewing powers are rather limited, so it is wise to ensure that any food given is either put through a blender or sieved. There is no good reason for assuming that the taste perception of infants is any different from that of adults. Parents should experiment with the wide variety of the foods that they themselves enjoy. Babies will quickly spit out anything that does not give them pleasure!

The idea that the experience of weaning is a psychologically traumatic one for the infant originated with Freud. Like assumptions about the importance of breast-feeding, research has failed to substantiate these claims. Abrupt weaning might come as something of a surprise to the infant and be distressing if it is accompanied by a reduction in close physical contact. However, weaning is usually a gradual process, and parents can easily ensure that they continue to maintain a high level of physical contact with their baby.

Sleeping and crying

Throughout the first year, the commonest complaint of parents is that their baby wakes frequently and cries a lot. It is hard for parents not to feel that they are somehow causing the crying. And as their own sleep gets disturbed, worry can be compounded by exhaustion.

Perhaps the first point to establish is: how much do babies sleep? Probably less than is commonly thought. On average a newborn baby sleeps for about 12 to 14 hours in each 24 and this drops to 10 hours or less by the end of the first year. These are average figures; there is a good deal of variation and many babies sleep more than this or less.

Sleep is not evenly distributed through the day and night. Within a week or so of birth a circadian (more or less 24-hourly) pattern begins to develop, so that sleep is most likely between midnight and 6 am—a trend that most parents encourage!

Many babies are particularly fretful between 6 pm and midnight. No satisfactory explanation has been given for this evening colic. Even though it is important that adults find time for themselves, it may be better, given a wakeful baby, to aim for, say a 9 o'clock bedtime rather than one at 6 or 7 o'clock. If babies are placed in infant seats, where they can see what is going on, they will often be quite content to sit and watch people move around them. Daily routines are very much an individual matter and everybody needs to work out their own system, making the best balance they can between the needs of all the household members.

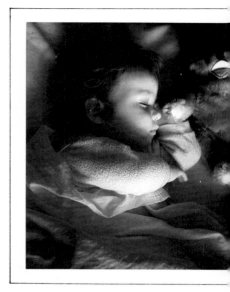

Types of sleep

In both babies and adults, sleep is a very complicated mixture of activities which occur in rhythmical cycles punctuated by "awake" periods. These may occur every two hours or so through the night.

The different types of sleep are accompanied by changes in the electrical activity of the brain, which can be distinguished on an electroencephalogram (EEG). There are basically two types of sleep: quiet or deep sleep, and rapid eye movement (REM) sleep. By watching a sleeping baby, it is quite easy to see which of the two states is reigning. On falling asleep, a baby (like an adult) first goes into quiet sleep, in which breathing is regular and the body still. As a baby moves into REM sleep, breathing becomes irregular and shallower, at times stopping completely for a few seconds. This can be very frightening for parents who see it, but it is quite normal. During REM sleep, babies may twitch and move. Smiles, facial grimaces and sucking movements are common, as too are startles. If you watch a baby's eyes during REM sleep, you can often see bursts of flickering movements of the eyeball. These are clearly visible through the eyelids.

Waking states

We can categorize a newborn's waking activity into three states, but the boundaries are not quite as clear-cut as those between the two sleeping states. These are "quiet alert" (eyes open, no large body movements), "active" (eyes open, body movements) and "crying".

Research has shown that in Western societies infants cry an average of 1–2¾ hours a day. This crying is often thought of as an

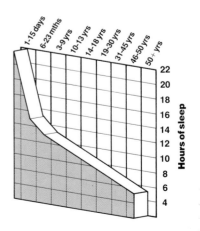

The amount of sleep taken in 24 hours varies not only from individual to individual, but also with age, as this graph (showing common sleep times) illustrates.

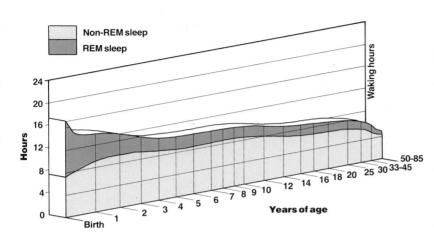

Average daily REM and non-REM sleep
Just as the overall length of sleep decreases with age, so also does the proportion of REM (rapid eye movement) sleep. For a baby, over half (indeed up to 70 per cent) of all sleep may be REM sleep. As far as is known REM sleep has the same recuperative function for babies as for adults; the large amount taken by very young babies may be accounted for by the wealth of new experiences filling their waking hours.

inevitable part of infancy, but cross-cultural studies suggest that the amount of crying is culturally determined. Infant crying, in fact, is rare in societies which practise demand feeding and where the infant is in almost continuous contact with the mother. This is not to say that these infants never become fretful, but that the mother is able to respond to subtle distress cues such as facial expression and body movements before these escalate to crying. When crying does occur, it is treated as an emergency signal and responded to swiftly—within about six seconds. In Western cultures, by contrast, response to infant crying is delayed from 5 to 30 minutes or ignored altogether. This may lead to prolonged crying when the child is older.

There are probably other reasons, apart from the mother's early interpretation of distress cries, why crying frequency differs across cultures. These may be related to factors which foster the "quiet alert" state in infants.

The habituation process
It is noticeable that babies become quiet when their attention is caught by an interesting sound or object. Unless especially interesting, new objects lose their novelty after a few minutes and babies are likely to become more restless and to scan with their head and eyes for new things to look at. This gradual loss of apparent interest in things as they become familiar is known as *habituation*. It is a very important process, because it allows us to respond selectively to the world around us, rather than being overwhelmed by the multitude of stimuli we face.

Most babies are capable of habituation right from birth—and probably before birth. You can see this for yourself with a simple experiment. If a baby is awake, a sharp noise usually produces a startle response—a jerk of all or some of the limbs. But if you continue to make a noise—say, snapping the fingers—about every 10 or 15 seconds, the response will gradually decline and disappear. When it has disappeared, it will return in response to another sound, showing

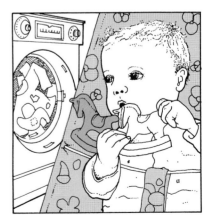

Wakeful or fretful babies may be happier placed in the midst of the activity of others, rather than being put to bed or in a room on their own.

EMOTIONAL OUTBURSTS

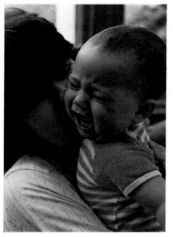

Changes to routine or environment may be a solution to infant crying, as may traditional calming techniques such as swaying and cuddling.

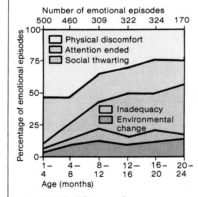

In 1935, Blatz and Millichamp observed the emotional outbursts of five infants and charted the changes in frequency and in the nature of their causes (1 = physical discomfort; 2 = attention ended; 3 = social thwarting; 4 = inadequacy; 5 = environmental change). The graph shows that their number falls with age, as does the proportion caused by physical discomfort.

that the effect is not simply due to tiredness. Similar experiments can be done with other senses—sight, feel and taste.

A baby who spends large amounts of time on his or her back, with only the ceiling or the sides of the cot to look at, will quickly habituate to these stimuli and become restless. In those cultures where infants are in almost continuous contact with the mother, they are faced with an ever-changing array of visual, auditory and tactile stimuli. Parents can easily increase the amount of visual stimuli to which their infant is exposed not only by moving the baby around, but also by introducing pictures (even on the ceiling), mobiles, or other patterns which are visible from sitting and lying positions. Changing patterns of auditory stimulation can be provided from the radio, adult speech or just everyday household noises.

The capacity to amuse oneself

Babies very quickly become aware of the effect of their own actions on the physical and social world. This will be considered in more detail later, but the simplest form of the process is worth mentioning now: in everyday terms, it is the capacity to amuse oneself. A number of experiments demonstrate this capacity in infants. In one series, babies were provided with foot panels which operated a switch when they were kicked. This was linked to a mobile which moved when the foot panel was kicked. This set-up provided hours of amusement for babies who repeatedly kicked the panel to set the mobile moving.

Another experiment showed that it was the fact that the baby caused the mobile to move that was important. Two babies were linked in tandem. Baby A had a foot panel which not only moved his own mobile but also another one over the cot of baby B. Baby B had a foot panel which was not connected to either mobile. Baby A continued looking at his mobile for much longer than baby B. When the babies were reversed so that baby B was controlling both mobiles, it was baby A who lost interest first.

Babies live in a world that is full of things that can be acted on in just the same way and, indeed, provide much more exciting possibilities than the simple feedback loop of the kicking panel and mobile. Hands can be moved to hit rattles hanging in the cot, or to make shadows on its side. Kicking can move blankets or shake the cot, producing interesting sounds.

Sucking is soothing

Babies will often quieten and soothe themselves by sucking. Feeding often has this effect. But sucking a thumb, a fist, the teat of an empty bottle or a dummy can be equally effective.

Often babies choose a particular blanket or toy which they hold or stroke while comfort-sucking. A favourite blanket may be reduced to a small shred of frayed material before it is finally abandoned by a toddler. Mothers may try to withhold these objects for fear that the baby's attachment to them is abnormal, but this is rarely the case.

Rocking the cradle

Perhaps the most widely used means of calming a baby in our culture is through movement—not surprising, as it is an extremely effective means of soothing, and of inducing a "quiet alert" state. Until the present century, most cradles in Britain were made with crescent-shaped rockers so they could be moved from side to side. For some reason, despite their effectiveness, these are seldom seen today except in museums or antique shops. A small fortune probably awaits the manufacturer who copies one of these old designs! Rhythmical sounds are also soothing for infants. Most lullabies have a slow rhythm which is similar to the frequency with which cradles are rocked.

Rhythmical sounds are also effective. Light or classical music—or even the purring of a vacuum cleaner—can have a marked calming effect.

Wrapped in swaddling clothes

Another calming technique that has more or less completely disappeared from industrialized societies is swaddling. Until the eighteenth century this was used in almost all societies in temperate, but not tropical, regions and even today it persists in a good many cultures—in the Middle East and among some American Indians, for instance. Many paintings of the Virgin and Child illustrate how it was done. The basic principle is to wrap up the baby tightly, with the legs together and the arms held by the baby's side.

Used with care, swaddling can be employed advantageously with babies in industrialized societies. By being tightly wrapped in a sheet or blanket, a fretful child can be helped into a peaceful sleep. For the technique to be effective, it seems important to start using it in the first few weeks of life. An older child, unused to such restriction, may fight against it. Swaddling with a thin sheet is very effective if a baby is restless in very hot weather, probably because it cuts down body movement.

Fleecy lining

One effective means of calming an unswaddled baby is to vary the texture of bed covers. Recently the effects of laying pre-term babies on lambswool fleeces, rather than on cotton sheets, have been studied. Lambswool is soft, and a baby can sink into it, so getting more skin contact than hospital sheets offer. The change of bedding had quite marked effects. Crying and movement were reduced and growth rates increased.

Parents can use lambskins at home for their babies. The fleeces are washable and can be obtained in most countries.

Baby and parents in the same bed

As living standards have risen, babies have increasingly been placed in rooms of their own. Some parents have reduced this segregation by having their babies sleep with them. This arrangement does not suit every parent, but the advantages are obvious, especially if the baby is being breast-fed. Fears about the baby witnessing sexual intimacies between the parents are often rationalized by statements about the dangers of lying on or smothering the baby. In fact, these dangers are minimal and a baby may be safer in the parents' bed than say, on the living-room floor or shut up in a room alone.

Sleep problems

Several surveys have indicated that more than 20 per cent of one-year-olds regularly wake at night. Exhausted and short-tempered parents can suffer an ever-widening circle of problems that can have very

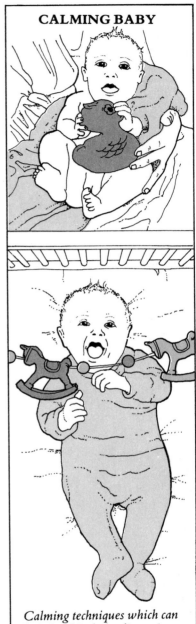

CALMING BABY

Calming techniques which can be helpful include: distractions in the baby's environment, which can be a mobile or toy; comfort sucking such as thumb-sucking; singing or other rhythmical sounds or movement; the old-fashioned practice of swaddling; and soft bed coverings.

serious consequences. What can be done? Perhaps the first step is to find out just how much the baby is sleeping. It may be that the total amount of sleep is average, but the timing out of step with the parents' routine. Both the baby's and the parents' routine may have to be changed so that a compromise between their sleep patterns is reached. However, the most crucial factor is what sleep-problem babies do when they wake. Babies and adults wake at intervals during the night, stir a bit, and go back to sleep. Sleep-problem babies cry when they wake.

Most babies cry during the night on some occasions—during teething, for example, this may happen much more often. However, it seems that babies who regularly wake at night have been fretful as newborns and active and responsive throughout their first year. The problem therefore is unlikely to have arisen through parental mishandling—a common professional assumption. It is worth noting, however, that in older infants prolonged crying may be a result of the parents having delayed their response to the infant's crying in the first six months.

A bored baby is a fretful baby

The usual advice given to parents whose babies continue to wake and cry at night is to give either more or less feed at night on the often unfounded assumption that the babies wake from hunger or "colic".

If we are right in thinking that the real problem is not a failure to sleep enough, but more a question of what babies do when they wake up, it may be more useful to think of some of the techniques already mentioned for calming a baby. He or she may be given some means of self-quieting—a suitable object to suck, for instance, or a more interesting visual and tactile world in his or her cot.

The root of night waking may lie with the kind of society we have constructed. Babies vary, and some infants have probably always shown the behavioural features that characterize night wakers.

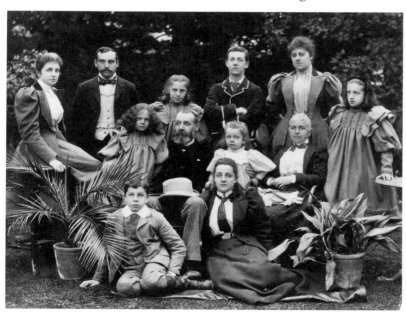

We expect babies to conform to daily timetables and their mothers to look after them in isolated circumstances. In earlier times, when work was largely centred in and around the home, living arrangements were more flexible, and there were often relatives or servants around to share child care. Attitudes towards child care were probably not as ambivalent or coloured by anxiety as they are today, so that night crying could be ignored more easily and was not such a cause of worry.

What newborns can do

The years of dependence

The most obvious feature of an infant's world is his or her total and direct dependence on older members of society. From an evolutionary viewpoint, a long period of childhood dependence is a fairly recent characteristic of the human species and sets us apart from even our closest primate relatives, the great apes. Evolutionary biologists and anthropologists have suggested that this long dependence is the key to human evolution: it is seen as providing a period in which to learn the social skills necessary for the maintenance and development of our complex social life and culture.

The giant step

The great importance of culture and learning in human evolution is made plain by the ability of a baby to move from the Stone Age to industrialized society in a lifetime. The first human societies that made use of stone tools appeared about 500 000 years ago. However, this evolution did not occur uniformly in all parts of the world. Even today cultures which represent an essentially Stone-Age society still persist. People who have made the transition from these hunting and gathering societies to our own industrialized world show that the transition can be made in a lifetime, especially if the move begins in childhood. Evolving from simpler human social groups to those of the industrialized world does not, therefore, involve biological change, but is the result of cultural developments passed on from generation to generation.

Adaptation is the key

Infant behaviour can be roughly divided into those patterns which are an adaptation to the special dependent world of infancy and those which are precursors of adult behaviour. It is through adaptation to the world of infancy that adult patterns emerge.

Perhaps what is most astonishing about human babies is that they are able to adapt so well to such varied cultures and child-rearing techniques. Physical and intellectual development across cultures is surprisingly similar, with milestones such as age at walking and talking being almost the same. It seems that, despite the culture they are born into, babies are able to construct their own environments for development.

This, together with babies' flexibility, allows similar development from dissimilar environments. It used to be thought that such similarity could only be the result of innately programmed development. What we now understand is a kind of paradox: similarities and regularities in development arise not from pre-programmed inflexibility but from pre-programmed flexibility, a flexibility that allows infants to use different environments in very variable ways to achieve the same ends. It is this plasticity that is innate in human infants.

Communication and games

The basis of human communication, both verbal and non-verbal, is a series of social rules by which we interact and understand a multitude of cues and signals. During infancy, by definition, we cannot speak,

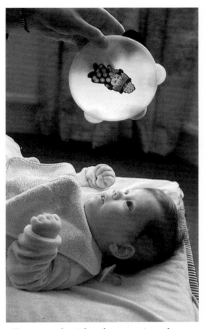

Compared with other species, the human baby's period of dependence is a long one, possibly because of the complexity of social skills which need to be acquired. Infants respond to those around them from the very beginning and soon have a well-developed social life and communication system—this is the start of the process by which human skills are transmitted from generation to generation.

but we can communicate many of our needs and intentions quite clearly and can play our part in games and other fairly complicated social interchanges.

Getting the right response

Infants discover their social world by observing the responses they receive to their actions. Responses tell babies what their actions mean to those people around them and allow them to modify their actions to produce more desirable responses. Even an apparently simple link between action and effect is quite complex and rich in learning opportunities.

A baby cries. What happens? Nothing, perhaps, because the "caretaker" decides that the cry is not one of hunger or serious distress. The most likely response is for the parent to pick up the baby and feed it. But the chances of being picked up depend on the length of time since the last feed. Soon after a feed, a baby is likely to be picked up because the parent thinks it is still hungry or has wind. Three-and-a-half to four hours later, it will be picked up because the parent thinks the crying represents hunger. The chances of parental response are also much higher in the daytime than at night. So even this simple example shows how much babies can potentially learn about their social world from the way in which their cries are or are not responded to. Other research shows that infants will reliably increase or decrease responses such as crying, smiling, sucking, moving and vocalizing, depending on how and in what pattern their parents react.

Crucial timing

Timing is a vital characteristic of all social communication. Right from birth an infant's behaviour has a rhythmical structure, and the caretakers' actions are built round this, so providing the beginnings of the mutual timing structure seen in all social encounters. For example, a baby does not suck continuously, but in a series of bursts separated by pauses. The behaviour of a breast-feeding mother seems to fit around this rhythm: she is much more likely to talk to the baby in the pauses between bursts of sucking. This kind of interaction provides the infant with an opportunity of learning the first rules of communication.

Playing games

From these first coordinated activities, social interaction quickly develops and becomes more complicated. Around six or eight weeks, infants begin to smile more frequently, and then go on to build their smiling into more complicated social exchanges. A typical game is for an adult to sit face to face with an infant and get him or her to smile and laugh by moving the head towards and away from the baby. The baby looks intently at each approach and eventually smiles. Then the baby often turns away from the adult for a little time before turning back to signal readiness to begin a new sequence. It is easy to show that the infant has an expectation of what is going to happen next by changing the sequence in some way. At a few months of age, in situations like this, babies show a clear sense of surprise. Indeed, this is a common component of games such as peek-a-boo. In these social games, an infant needs both familiarity with the games partner to provide predictability and an element of novelty and surprise which

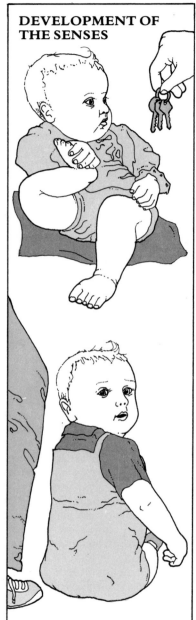

DEVELOPMENT OF THE SENSES

A very young baby has some sophisticated skills, including the ability to follow a moving object with the head and eyes or—if the movement is small—with the eyes alone. Also, a baby can usually locate a voice speaking softly and out of sight.

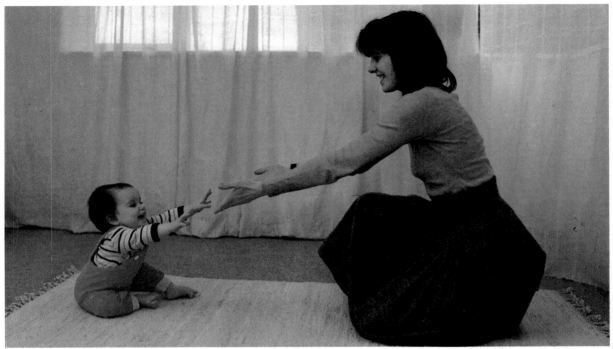

eventually leads to more complex sequences. Parents provide this variability by changing their games as the infant gets older.

Learning the rules

We can divide the things that infants learn in their social encounters into two categories. Firstly, there are rules and conventions known to all members of the culture, such as the expression of emotion, and the meaning of words and gestures—in fact, all the social knowledge we need to behave appropriately in varied social situations. Secondly, there are all the private and particular shared means and rituals of behaviour that go on between two people who know each other well.

At first, the infant is restricted to familiar relationships and to learning individual idiosyncrasies. But by moving between several familiar relationships and by encountering strangers, the common features begin to merge and so knowledge of the culture begins to be built up. Over-exclusive mother–infant relations impede this development and it is notable that shyness is often marked and prolonged in infants who have social experience of few adults.

Imitation

Much adult behaviour—probably more than most people suspect—is a product of imitation. This is a far from simple reaction. You must perceive what another person is doing and translate this into a parallel action of your own. There have been long disputes among psychologists about the age at which babies begin to imitate. In the first few months, quite a lot of imitation occurs in adult–infant interactions, but most of this is the adult imitating the baby. The early imitations produced by infants are restricted to the limited range of actions that are in a baby's social repertoire. Thus, it is fairly easy to train a baby of

Babies will anticipate the fact that they are about to be lifted or supported, responding with pleasure.

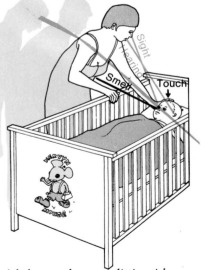

A baby soon learns to distinguish people, particularly its mother or whoever else looks after it. Babies will develop different styles of interaction with different people, and seem able to adapt to several regular minders.

a few months to stick out its tongue when you do, but it is impossible at this age for a baby to imitate your blinking, or other complex motor movements. These early imitative actions, however, are the prologue to a process which will eventually result in children whose gestures, speech, movements and manners are remarkably like those of people around them!

The limited value of games

The social games of infancy emphasize the ways in which infants are able to use widely differing experiences to reach the same developmental goals. In spite of their varied social experience, most children develop the major social skills at roughly the same time. One reason for this is that the routine caretaking to which every infant is exposed involves social interaction and games. It may be less fun, but a situation in which a baby is being persuaded to take food is as valuable for social learning as any of the games described earlier!

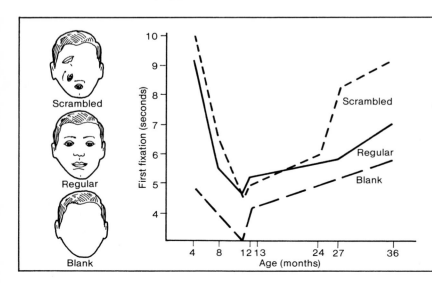

From birth, babies' social interaction becomes more and more complicated, until they are able to participate in games with adults. Early games involve the baby's ability to anticipate what is going to happen next, though at a few months of age surprise becomes a common feature, in games such as peek-a-boo.

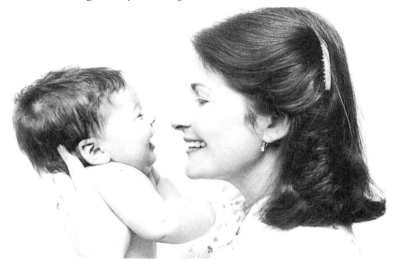

In an experiment by Jerome Kagan, babies of different ages were shown realistic, scrambled and blank masks of the human face, to see how much attention they gave them, measured by the length of time they fixated (stared at) them. The youngest (four months) paid great attention, probably because the masks did not look exactly like anyone they knew. Then there was a decline, but at twelve months the attention picked up again, probably because the babies now saw something odd in the faces.

Girl or boy?

We have seen that an important function of social interaction between infants and adults is to convey information to the infant about the rules and consistencies obvious or implicit in people's behaviour. One very important part of this information concerns the range of beliefs and expectations about how members of each sex behave and the social roles they adopt. Sexual identity can be defined as a person's image of himself or herself as male or female and its beginnings can be seen in infancy.

Sexual identity is a social construct, but it is obviously closely related to biological phenomena. With rare exceptions, girls develop a female identity and boys a male one. Sexual identity is a fundamental aspect of our lives. Test this out for yourself by trying to describe an imaginary person without making them male or female. It is virtually impossible. In industrialized societies, women tend to be stereotyped as passive, weak, submissive, intuitive and decorative, while men are seen as aggressive, powerful, rational and independent. These descriptions actually refer to positions on an imaginary scale rather than to absolutes, so that women are seen as more passive than men, men as more aggressive than women, and so on.

Of course, like any stereotypes, these are not accurate descriptions or aspirations for many people, though in very broad terms they reflect the places the two sexes occupy in our current social system.

An area of controversy

In looking at the emergence of gender identity, we must hold both the general and the particular in mind: the ways in which child-rearing is formed and shaped by institutions and prevailing social assumptions, and also the ways in which children are affected by the particular relationships they form with people immediately around them. The issues involved in such discussions are deeply controversial.

Roughly speaking, there are two sides: the nativists, who believe that gender is fixed by biology and inevitable, and the environmentalists, who see gender as a product of social learning. The first would argue that it is a fact of biology that women are best fitted for the rearing of children and that this is the principal aim and function of their lives. Those on the other side would say that this is neither natural nor inevitable, but the result of growing up in a society where these particular assumptions about women's roles are heavily reinforced. To support this view they may well cite cultures in which expectations and roles are different. A nativist might counter this kind of evidence by suggesting that genetic differences between populations may account for variations in behaviour.

However, as we saw on page 18, it is impossible to know exactly what a person's genetic make-up is—all we can see is the phenotype: the outcome of genes and environment. To debate whether this outcome is a result of genes *or* environment (or to try to determine which is responsible for which characteristic) is pointless: genes and the environment do not add together, but are intertwined and intermingled from the moment of conception in the most complex way imaginable, and continue to intertwine and intermingle at every step in the development process.

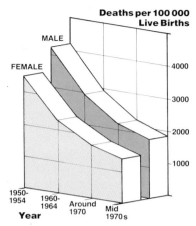

Distinctions between the sexes exist from the moment of conception. More boys than girls are conceived, but male foetuses miscarry more often than female ones. In addition, more boys than girls die within a year of birth, as is illustrated in the graph, which shows the death rate for infants aged under one year. (Figures taken from combined data for more developed countries.)

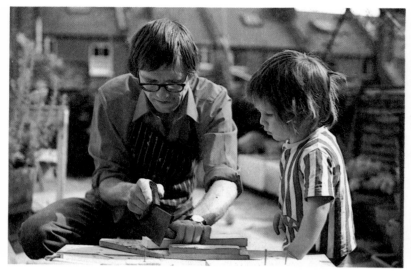

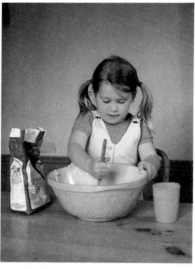

Children appear to develop gender identity—the acting out of their particular sex—by the age of two or three. Their behaviour increasingly *conforms to the roles that society dubs "masculine" or "feminine"—for example, in the choice of toys and games. But it is very difficult to* *establish how much this is conditioned by the male and female roles they see played out around them.*

Sex differences in infancy

In terms of growth, and indeed of survival, there are sex differences throughout foetal life and infancy. More boys than girls are conceived, but male foetuses more often miscarry. Both perinatal deaths and those in the first year of infancy show an excess of males. The reasons for this mortality difference between the sexes are not yet well understood.

When we turn to behavioural differences, we move into less certain territory. What we can conclude is that sex differences in the behaviour of newborns are very small. Certainly, nobody is going to be very successful if they try to tell the sex of babies from their behaviour. Likewise, there are few differences in facial appearance and body build.

Some studies, but by no means all, have shown differences in the way parents handle babies of each sex. What parents do with infants not only reflects their own beliefs about what is appropriate, but also differences in infant behaviour. As development proceeds, these effects will intermingle and reinforce each other in such a way that it is impossible to say which came first.

The gap widens

By the end of infancy, sex differences are consistent and striking. For example, if you take any phase of language development—say, the production of the first word—this will occur, on average, three to four weeks earlier in girls. It is not understood why this should be. Some parents seem to talk more to their daughters; possibly this accelerates the development of speech. On the other hand, there is some evidence that, in girls, some parts of the brain mature earlier. However, this cannot be seen as a simple "cause" of girls talking earlier, as brain development could well be influenced by differing parental treatment of boys and girls. Similarly, parents may talk more to girls because girl babies babble more. As with all developmental processes, everything seems to depend on everything else, and it is difficult or even impossible to say that there is any simple cause of any observable difference between the sexes.

The anatomy of sex

A baby's sex is noted at birth from the appearance of the external genital organs. In a few very rare cases hormonal and other abnormalities can mean that the anatomy of the external genitals is a misleading indication of the child's true sex, as expressed in the chromosomes of every cell in the body. In such cases the child may be brought up as a member of the opposite sex. Studies of such children show that the sex of assignment, the sex they are thought to be at birth and treated as during development, is of overriding importance in determining behaviour. So gender identity seems to be largely a product of treating a child as a boy or a girl.

Children vary a good deal in the age at which they begin consistently to refer to themselves as a boy or a girl, but the evidence points to the fixing of gender identity at a surprisingly early age. Part of this evidence comes from the study of children who, because of abnormalities, have been reared as members of the opposite sex. When such mistakes are discovered, the abnormality is usually corrected surgically, changing the child's anatomical sex to that of his or her chromosomes. If this is done before the age of two or three, the transition is usually fairly easy, but at later ages there can be considerable psychological turmoil, suggesting that gender identity is already well formed by this time.

Sex stereotyping

This process is often treated rather superficially, leading many parents to assume that the worst aspects of stereotyping can be avoided by not providing the typical "sex-appropriate" toys or books and by making special efforts to treat sons and daughters in the same way. There are two problems here. However much parents modify their own behaviour, children still grow up in a world where sex stereotyping and sex-role differentiation are the rule rather than the exception. For example, nursery and primary school teachers are almost always women, doctors are usually men, and male nurses are rare. Outside the home, punishment for deviation from prescribed roles may outweigh any rewards offered by the parents.

Secondly, we still know very little about the actual processes by which sex roles are learned or, indeed, what actually is learned. It is usually assumed that boys learn to be more aggressive, girls less ambitious and so on.

Paula Caplan, of the University of Toronto, has suggested that one of the crucial differences between boys and girls is that girls are much more concerned than boys with gaining approval from others. She has shown that girls' aggressiveness and the amount of effort they put into a task tends to fluctuate according to whether there are adults present. If her theory is correct, then its implications are very far-reaching. It would be extremely difficult for parents to become aware of what exactly they are doing to encourage this difference, far less to eradicate it. But this is not to say that attempts to change things within the home are futile: the blurring of sex roles opens up more possibilities to the children and shows that sex roles are socially determined and not fixed for all time.

Learning a sex role

By a child's second birthday, sex differences in behaviour are quite marked. In nurseries where many toys are available, boys will probably be pushing cars around, playing chase or building brick towers, while the girls may be sitting painting or playing with dolls in a doll's house. Girls are also more likely to stay close to the (female) teacher and to talk to her more. Furthermore, these differences will almost certainly be reinforced by the teacher's reaction to the children's activities.

Children, above all, are intensely interested in social conduct. They watch others and then try things out for themselves. This kind of identification is particularly strong between children of similar ages; as play with other children increases, so too do opportunities for adopting stereotyped behaviour.

As an antidote to this, an infancy and childhood in which both parents deliberately take on most aspects of the traditional maternal and paternal roles is likely to leave a child, whether a boy or a girl, with a much richer sense of what is possible and desirable in later life. This is one of the reasons why most psychologists welcome the movement towards more equal parental roles.

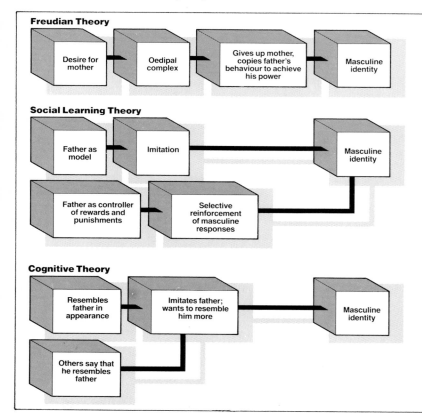

Freudian Theory

Desire for mother → Oedipal complex → Gives up mother, copies father's behaviour to achieve his power → Masculine identity

Social Learning Theory

Father as model → Imitation → Masculine identity

Father as controller of rewards and punishments → Selective reinforcement of masculine responses

Cognitive Theory

Resembles father in appearance → Imitates father; wants to resemble him more → Masculine identity

Others say that he resembles father

MASCULINE IDENTITY

There are three major theories of how gender identification (boys behaving in "masculine" ways and girls in "feminine") develops. In the case of the male, according to Freud, a small boy has a childish sexual desire for his mother. In order to avoid retaliation from his father, he temporarily renounces his mother, and starts to imitate his father, with the ultimate aim of overthrowing him. Social learning theory also sees the boy as imitating his father, but because he is powerful, to be admired, and a source of rewards and punishments, which reinforce the boy's masculine behaviour. Cognitive theory suggests that a boy imitates his father because he has a realization or "cognition" that he shares maleness with him.

Learning to move and think

Newborn babies are largely observers, albeit active ones, of the world around them, dependent on other people to move them around. By the close of infancy, however, most youngsters can walk, hold and manipulate objects and are becoming increasingly independent. The development of physical and mental capabilities is closely related, but, as we shall see, both of these take place within a social context.

Can newborns walk?

The basic pattern of movement required for walking is present in a newborn baby and can easily be demonstrated. If a newborn is supported under the arms, leaning slightly forward with the soles of the feet touching a firm surface, he or she will usually perform walking movements. Sometimes it is necessary to stroke the top of one foot to get the first step. Some psychologists have argued that the walking of newborns is not a reflex pattern, because the stepping pattern seems to be adjusted to the surface the baby is walking on, and that it is even possible to get babies to step over objects. Others are less convinced. Either way, it is clear that the newborn "knows" the basic pattern of movement required for walking.

Newborn babies can crawl too. If you put some support behind babies' feet as they make crawling movements, they are able to push themselves forward. The interesting thing about these early move-

The basic patterns of movement required for crawling and walking are obviously present in the newborn baby. They then disappear before re-emerging when the infant starts to crawl and walk independently.

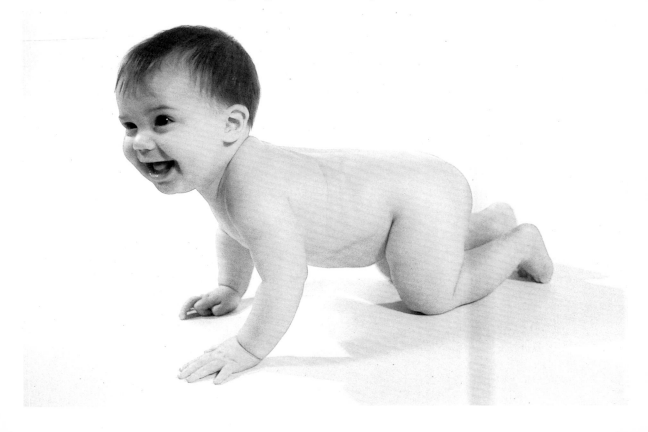

ment patterns is that they become difficult to elicit after a few months and are not seen again until the baby walks independently. This period of quiescence presumably results from evolutionary pressure to increase the infant's dependence on its caretakers.

Average age for motor milestones

Pre-war American developmental psychologists spent much of their time examining large numbers of children to establish the average age at which various points in development, the so-called motor milestones, were reached. The results of these studies gave the impression that the milestones represent a constant progression: sitting unsupported at six months; standing supported by furniture at eight-and-a-half months; walking alone at eleven-and-a-half months, and so on.

However, there is great variability in the ages at which each stage is reached and even in the sequence of the stages. Walking, for instance, is quite normal at any time between 9 months and 18 months.

The effect of stimulation

That specific encouragement and opportunity for movement can accelerate motor development was demonstrated in the United States by Dr Myrtle McGraw. She worked with a series of twins, providing stimulation for only one of each pair. As the films she made testify, not only did the stimulated twin always reach the motor milestones earlier, but she was able to produce quite remarkable physical skills and competence at very early ages. One of her more dramatic film sequences shows a two-year-old roller skating with an assurance and skill that many adults never achieve.

Similarly, some cultures, in East Africa for example, have been found to have accelerated motor development compared to the norms in Europe and America. These cultures tend to place a good deal of emphasis on physical development. At the other extreme, we have the example of Navajo children, who spend much of their first year strapped to a cradleboard, yet walk independently at a slightly earlier age than white American children. These experiments are yet another illustration of the adaptability of the human infant. Infants are provided with varying opportunities for physical exercise, yet all of

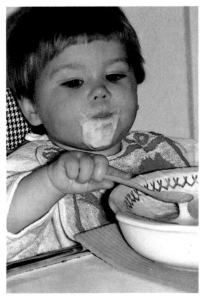

A small child's attempts to feed him or herself, usually after fourteen months, aid the development of coordination and locomotor movements through a process of trial and error.

Motor development

Infants usually go through a progressive sequence of motor development, which results in their being able to stand and walk. The pattern of behaviour—rolling over, sitting up, crawling, pulling up, walking—seems the same regardless of the individual training or encouragement given. The rate of progress, however, varies widely. There may be four or five months difference in the age at which one child learns to walk as compared to another.

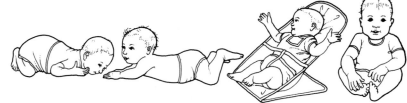

0.4 months
A baby's actions are mostly reflexive. When laid down the baby cannot change position but will extend his limbs.

1.6 months
Lying face down, the baby can lift his head for a few seconds at a time. Face up, he will watch his own hands.

2.3 months
The baby can raise his head and chest when lying flat, and turns his head to sound. Kicking is vigorous.

5.3 months
The head is now self-supporting and the baby can sit up unaided. There is control of simple, grasping movements.

them, except those with rare abnormalities, successfully walk.

With specific instruction and practice, however, physical skills which are not universally developed can be taught at surprisingly early ages. Swimming is a good example. Newborns will make "dog paddle" movements if suspended in water and will raise their heads to keep their noses clear of the water. If given frequent practice, it is possible to get children swimming quite effectively by the second half of the first year. If swimming is encouraged at this time, the pleasure derived from water usually persists throughout childhood. However, if swimming practice is not given during the first year, a fear of water seems to set in and it is then often difficult to teach children to swim until they are six or seven years old.

Reaching and grasping

The finer-grade hand and finger movements involved in grasping and reaching follow the same kind of pattern of development as locomotor movements. Under suitable conditions, newborns can orientate their arms towards an interesting object. Hands and fingers often point quite accurately towards an object, and crude hitting movements may be made. But at this age a baby can only grasp an object if it is placed in the palm of his or her hand.

Controlled reaching and grasping of objects does not usually occur until towards the middle of the first year, but frequent practice seems to accelerate development of control. However, by the second half of the first year, reaching does become important, not least in social games. Offering and exchanging objects with social partners become a very significant part of an infant's social encounters. Such games help to focus the attention of the infant and adult on the same object, and this may be important in the first stages of speech, because it ensures that both are "talking" about the same thing.

Piaget's theories

In infants, the development of physical skills is linked very closely with that of mental abilities. The person who did most to show the links was the late Jean Piaget, who devoted a lifetime's work to the subject. His theory was that development took place in two main stages. At birth, he suggested, infants are totally *egocentric*: they can't

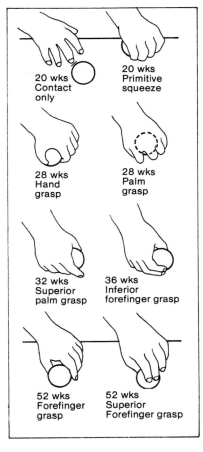

Development of grasping

The reflexive fingergrip of the newborn is lost after 16 weeks, and the infant masters a variety of different grasps during the first year.

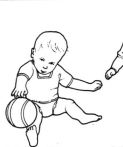

6.6 months
The baby sits with a straight back and begins to reach for objects. If held up, he can put some weight on his feet.

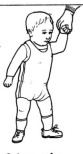

8.1 months
The baby can crawl and will stand supported. He can grasp with thumb and fingers to hold on to the support.

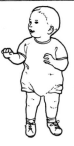

9.6 months
The baby is able to pull himself up to a standing position and with firm support can take his first few steps.

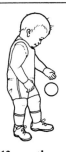

11 months
Standing is independent. The baby cannot yet walk alone, but will creep sideways, holding on to furniture.

12 months
The baby can stand or sit down without help, and may begin to walk without support or when held only lightly.

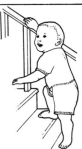

16.1 months
The child will climb or descend stairs with a combination of creeping and walking, holding on to the stair rail.

tell the difference between themselves and the rest of the world. Gradually, however, the growing infant learns, through trial and error, that there is a separateness between his or her feelings and actions and those of other people. Piaget called this the *sensori-motor* stage (*sensori-* = feelings, *motor* = actions). For him, the end of this stage marks the end of infancy.

In his original experiment, Piaget used the game of hide-and-seek. He took some object that a child was playing with and hid it under a cushion. He was able to show that, up to the age of seven ·months, the infant would not look for the hidden object, seemingly losing all interest in it. But, after this age, the infant would continue to search for the object and remove the cushion to find it. In other experiments, Piaget showed that there was a stage in the sensori-motor period when infants first begin to work out different ways of getting what they want: a typical example might be that of a favourite toy just out of reach. There comes a moment at which the infant learns that he or she can use some other object to bring the desired toy within reach.

The strength of Piaget's theory is that it underlines the positive role that infants play in their own development. They learn about the world by acting on the world. Its weakness is that it underplays the effect of social surroundings on the development process. There is evidence to show, for example, that infants can recognize the existence of individuals—and know whether a particular individual is there or not—before reaching the stage of understanding that a "lost" object may be hidden elsewhere. Games such as "peek-a-boo", may, in short, be a vital first step on the way to hide-and-seek.

Assessing ability

Intelligence tests for both adults and children now use a method of computing IQ which expresses, in statistical terms, a person's deviation from the average performance of others of similar age, rather than a "quotient". The term "intelligence quotient" was retained because people were familiar with it and because average performance for each age was arbitrarily called 100. So when we say that a child has a high IQ, we simply mean that he or she is able to answer questions that, on average, only older children tend to answer correctly.

The general principles of infant testing follow those of early intelligence tests, described on page 87. Infant tests are usually called developmental tests and the quotient a DQ or developmental quotient. Instead of asking questions, the tester assesses such things as physical co-ordination, manipulation of objects and social responses. Each item in the test is given an age level and the DQ is calculated in the same way as an IQ:

$$DQ = \frac{\text{mental age}}{\text{chronological age}} \times 100$$

The results of developmental tests can be highly variable, even across a short timespan. This is probably because performance is influenced by the baby's state.

Because of this variability, it is unwise to use the tests in isolation to predict infants' future development. In fact we can make more accurate predictions for things such as school performance, IQ and

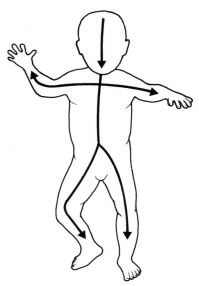

Developmental directions
As an infant learns to move and gain control of his body and limbs, there are two main directions of development: cephalocaudal and proximodistal. **Cephalocaudal development** *occurs from the head downwards (literally—head to tail);* **proximodistal development** *occurs from the midline of the body outwards, towards the hands and feet (literally—near to far). The progressive developments in each direction are more or less simultaneous and follow typical patterns. For example, control of head and eye movements precedes the ability to roll over or sit up. Reaching and stretching of the arms is in voluntary control before the hand and fingers can be used to grasp effectively. These developmental directions can be traced in many aspects of the baby's progress throughout the first year.*

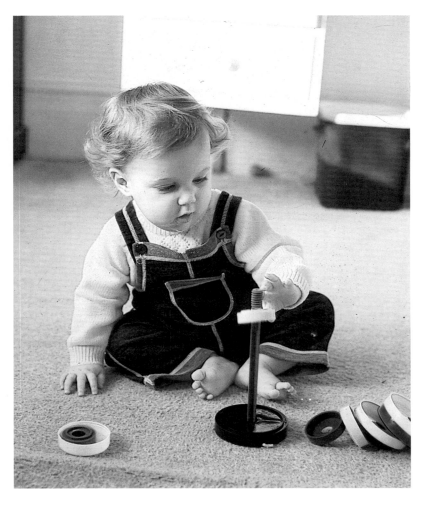

The ability to reach and grasp objects does not usually occur before the age of six months. Children's toys are often designed to stimulate and develop control of such skills.

eventual employment from the average IQ of the infant's parents. Once again, this points to the importance of the social world in determining a child's development. Of course, predictions of this kind assume that the infants are healthy and will develop normally, and that their environment will not undergo any major upheavals during this period.

Handicapped infants

Where a baby is born with a known handicap, informed guesses about possible futures can be made on the basis of the knowledge of development in similar children. However, it should not be thought that just because a diagnostic label can be given to a child, a very accurate prediction about outcome can be made. The huge variety of factors which influence normal children also affect the development of those with abnormalities. In fact, outcome is more variable for handicapped children partly because, for them, specific teaching may be necessary to learn what normal children achieve by their own efforts in any reasonable environment. Sidney Bijou, an American developmental psychologist, has shown clearly how the natural consequences of a handicap—say, being unable to walk—interact with the reactions of those around the child in a circular way, with the result that the child acquires far fewer social and intellectual skills than he or she might, in theory, have done. There is an unfortunate tendency among both parents and professionals to attribute all such deficits to the handicap. Indeed, it is only relatively recently that the term "ineducable" was dropped as a description of some mentally handicapped children.

Children who are born blind or who become blind as young infants provide a good example of the circular process which Bijou talks about. These children often show delayed and abnormal speech patterns which, research has suggested, stem from the limited social interaction these children often have in infancy. Blind babies tend to be rather unresponsive and do not provide as much pleasure for parents and others as normal children: in popular jargon, they don't turn their parents on. However, if parents understand these processes and have plenty of emotional support in their very difficult situation, many of these effects can be avoided and the child's speech will be relatively normal.

Handicapped children vividly demonstrate, by default, just how active a part infants play in their own development, in the creation of their own psychological world. If a child is damaged, these active development processes are interrupted; special steps have to be taken to provide what infants cannot create for themselves.

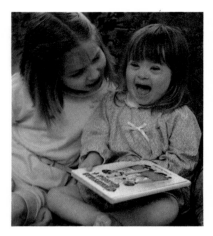

A handicapped child cannot make the same contribution to his or her own development and requires more and different help from others to compensate for this.

Early intervention

In recent years, systems of developmental assessment have been set up in many communities. These are designed to identify those children who might benefit from some kind of intervention or special education. In some cases, early assessment may prevent the development of abnormalities which, once entrenched, are very difficult or impossible to correct. Deafness is a good example. As deaf children cannot hear speech, they cannot learn to speak themselves. However, the ease of language acquisition after the provision of a hearing aid depends greatly on age. If an aid is given before a year or 18 months, speech may well develop relatively normally. But if the aid is given later, speech may show many peculiarities which can persist for a lifetime. It appears that there is a sensitive period for the acquisition of language, after which learning becomes much more difficult.

This idea is supported by studies of children who have suffered brain injuries. The long-term effects of even quite severe injuries suffered in the first two years of life may be fairly mild, whereas the same injury at a later age can cause more serious impairment. At the earlier age, the brain is still plastic: intact areas can to some extent take over the functions of injured areas. However, as development proceeds, the brain becomes set in its patterns, and compensatory processes become less and less efficient.

This early ability to recover from injury emphasizes once again that infants, despite their apparent vulnerability, are very resilient, and that developmental processes can reach common goals in alternative ways. As adults, we may be better at using our wits to minimize the effects of damage or hostile environments, but our capacities for biological compensation are more limited than those of babies; gradually, one facility takes over from the other as we age.

The development of movement and language

	MOTOR DEVELOPMENT	VOCALIZATION AND LANGUAGE
12 weeks	Lifts head and chest when lying face down; weight supported on wrists and elbows; reflex actions gradually disappearing but not immediately replaced by voluntary control.	Responds to being spoken to or touched by smiling and making sounds known as cooing, vowel-like sounds given out in 15–20 second phases; crying is less than in earlier weeks; listens intently to sounds other than speech such as bells, rattles, musical toys.
16 weeks	Head self-supporting when lying or held in a sitting position; rolls over and kicks; grasping without control of thumb.	Follows sounds with head and eyes; increased response to speech; sounds emitted include laughing and chuckling noises as well as continued cooing.
20 weeks	Sits up with support at first.	Vowel sounds of cooing interrupted by sounds with the character of consonants (m, ng, s, f) but vocalization as yet bears no direct relationship to adult speech.
6 months	Sits up without support, will reach forward and take weight on hands; direction of reaching is confined; gaining control of hands in grasping and letting go; when held up will put some weight on feet but cannot stand.	Cooing develops into babbling, vowels and consonants mixed in single syllables (ma, mu, di); no apparent pattern in the recurrence of sounds within the flow of babbling.
8 months	Crawls and will stand holding on to a person or stable object; grasping becoming more refined, using fingertips and thumb.	Syllables repeated (ma-ma, ba-ba-ba) frequently in babbling; utterances acquire some intonation and are used as signals of feelings or requirements; tone and general meaning of words such as yes, no, 'bye are understood.
10 months	Pulls up to standing position and can step sideways when holding on to a support; hand and eye co-ordination rapidly developing.	Sound play, such as clicking or bubbling, interspersed with previous forms of vocalization; some attempts to imitate sounds and differentiate words and syllables; attempts to imitate words are rarely successful.
12 months	Walks independently or held only by one hand; sits down on floor from standing position.	Repeated syllables used in forming words (mama, dada, baba) and some words are more or less successfully imitated; one or more recognizable words uttered; simple sentences, requests and commands understood.
18 months	Walks confidently but with a stiff and impulsive gait; climbs stairs holding support; grasping ability fully developed, able to handle spoon, cup and so on in feeding.	Vocabulary increasing but still combined with babbling, now gaining complexity in intonation and variety of sound—also called jargon, apparently used as conversation but meaningless; words used singly; pictures of familiar objects named; sound games enjoyed, with attempts to join in; understanding still well in advance of speech.
24 months	Moves easily between sitting and standing; can run, with a tendency to fall suddenly; walks up and down stairs putting same foot forward at each step.	Vocabulary of 50 or more words, now sometimes combined in simple two or three word sentences spontaneously created; interest in language and communication increases—words heard are repeated and stories are listened to with attention.
30 months	Good command of balance, able to jump, stand on one foot, walk on tiptoe; in control of independent finger movements and can use hands efficiently in playing.	New words learned every day and vocalization used to convey definite communications; adult speech well understood; sentences put together using a basic grasp of grammatical rules, not by imitating adult phrases.

Learning to speak—the end of infancy

Though the beginnings of speech mark the end of infancy, it is during that period that the foundations of this remarkable achievement are laid.

It would be an exaggeration to say that we understand how children learn to speak, but the recent flurry of activity of developmental psychologists and linguists seems to have established the broad line of what is involved.

Our first assumption has to be that babies have a predisposition to learn to speak, just as they are predisposed to walk or to become members of a social species within a culture. We do not know all that is involved in this predisposition, but the ability to relate to other people is likely to be at the heart of it. At first, the structure of social interactions is provided by the parents. They respond in predictable ways to infant behaviour, but gradually the infants begin to play a more active part and some of the initiative passes to them. This is possible because they begin to try to make sense of their social world by searching out the rules and regularities. Even in apparently simple day-to-day interactions such as feeding and dressing, the foundations of language are already being laid. Not only do they involve rule-learning, but paying attention to speech and responding to speech sounds that adults make. This selective attention to speech sounds is another part of the human potential for language learning. Of course, infants do not understand what is being said, but they learn, by association, the meaning of particular tones of voice and inflections. For example, quite young babies become upset and cry if people around them become angry and raise their voices.

Baby talk

When people, including even young children, talk to infants, their speech changes in characteristic ways. They use short, simple sentences, and often repeat words and phrases. The pitch of the voice is higher, and intonation is more varied. There are several probable reasons for this. An obvious one is that we do not have a lot to say to babies. Often we are simply affirming our presence as a social partner, communicating for the sake of it, rather than transmitting a vital message.

This is the cradle of communication in which infants begin to learn about their social world. The modified—simplified and exaggerated—speech to infants is an ideal teaching device and shows several parallels with body-language, which also shows simplifications and exaggerated features when directed at infants. Notification seems to make rule-learning easier, while the exaggerations and emphasis hold the infant's attention.

First words

As the end of their first year approaches, infants produce their first recognizable word. Very often this is the name of one of the more significant figures in their social world and is usually uttered in their presence. At first, words are produced as if they were an optional extra to the social understanding that is created by gesture and non-language sounds. But words are important to the adult, who usually

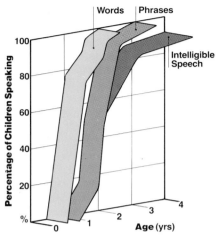

Speech development

Most infants begin to say whole words by about 44 weeks, rapidly followed by two-word phrases. With the onset of more complex constructions individual differences become more marked; only 65 per cent of children use intelligible speech by the age of two. Speech acquisition is influenced by aptitude, presence or absence of siblings and parents, parental behaviour and other environmental factors.

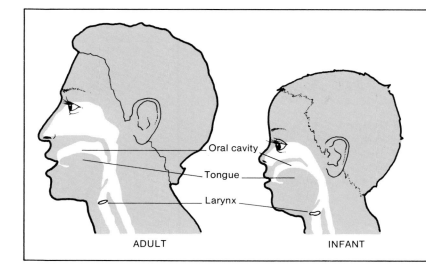

Oral cavity

Tongue

Larynx

ADULT   INFANT

Development of the vocal tract
The sounds a baby can make at birth are limited by the structure of the vocal tract. Variations of sound in adult speech depend upon movement of the tongue within a relatively large oral cavity (far left). In the infant (left) the tongue is restricted because it occupies more space in the oral cavity. The larynx is high in the throat. During the first four months of life the vocal tract matures. After that, the baby can begin to produce sounds closer to recognizable speech.

sees them as a landmark, and they serve as a great stimulus for further social exchange. Gradually, infants begin to refer to things that are not present. Though their command of language is still extremely limited, they have taken the first faltering steps as members of their culture. They have used language to extend their communication beyond the here and now.

Interpreting words
At the single-word stage, the meaning a child attaches to a word may be very different from the conventional one. "Cat" may mean any animal with fur and four legs. "Mama" is offered to any adult who might offer assistance. Knowing what a baby intends when it utters a word is a complex question. If the word is "cat", is the baby saying "there is a cat" or "where is the cat?" The adult may recognize the meaning from the context or from their joint past experience. In fact, it may be a mistake to look for a precise meaning in what an infant says. As with earlier non-verbal communication, the point may be more to enter into social exchange than to convey a precise wish. However, increasingly, speech is used for specific effects—a repeated cry of "milk, milk" may not cease until some milk is forthcoming!

Conveying a meaning
Even though the grammatical complexity of what children say does not seem to change for some months, their understanding of words and of social encounters increases steadily. Quite complex verbal instructions such as "Your bottle is on the table" are understood and acted on by the child long before the child says things of similar complexity. However, even with single words and some help from the parents, children can convey most effectively what they want. An object is stuck in the opening of the letter box at the front door; pointing to it is often enough to have it removed. Actions such as this emphasize how much the infant's social understanding has advanced. Soon two words will be combined, and then more to form simple sentences.

Which comes first—thought or language?

There is a long-standing debate among psychologists about whether thought precedes language or vice versa. The answer seems to be that the two go hand in hand. Without thought you cannot speak. At least, without the capacity to hold mental images of the world in your head, speech is impossible. So obviously a child must be beyond Piaget's object permanence stage before speaking. But at the same time the advent of speech seems to allow more complicated thought and the ability to solve problems without acting them out on objects in the world. Imagination only flowers after language acquisition has proceeded some way, or so it appears. But appearances may be a bit deceptive. Watching children at the one-word stage you cannot but be impressed by their understanding of the world. In a familiar environment with familiar people they seem to detect quite subtle changes in mood of those around them and play complicated games.

Time to move on

By 18 months or so, the newborn becomes a toddler and so leaves infancy and enters the next stage of childhood. Never again in a lifetime will the rate of change be so fast or new skills and abilities arrive so quickly. As their child leaves this first phase, parents are likely to have mixed feelings. The newly found expressiveness and autonomy bring new possibilities and rewards in daily life and the endless days and nights of unremitting cleaning and feeding begin to retreat a little as they are relieved by moments of almost adult-like behaviour. But at the same time most of us have some feelings of regret. There is a very deep satisfaction for most parents in being able to hold and (occasionally) comfort an entirely dependent baby. But we have to move on with our own children though the experience of those first weeks and months always stays with us.

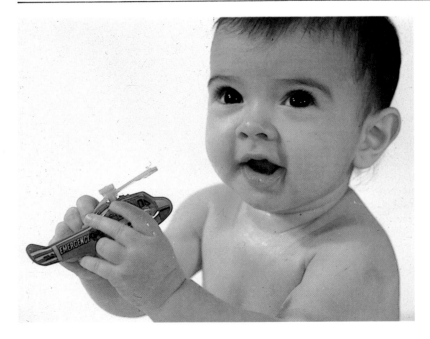

Although unable to convey meaning with words, it is clear that the child's mental capabilities are developing rapidly—by expression alone we can see the wealth of feelings and emotions he is experiencing.

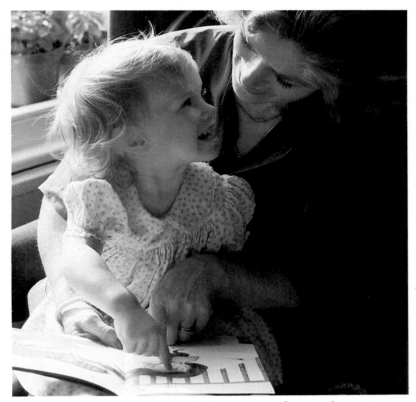

With the mastering of language, a whole new range of means of expression come to the child without resorting to childish babble.

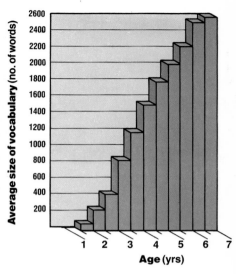

Average vocabulary

A baby's first word has usually been uttered by the end of the first year. For a few months vocabulary is only slowly acquired. But by the end of the second year a rapid and continuous growth rate is established. From the brief, simple phrases of infancy, the child learns to put words together to express specific meanings.

Age	Some highlights in language development
23 weeks	Cooing emerges as well-formed vowel sounds.
24 weeks	Consonants used as a form of "speaking" to toys—*b-b-b*.
32 weeks	Vowels and consonants combined in repeated syllables—*mum-mum, bubbuh, da-da*.
37 weeks	First word, *tick-tick*, repeatedly applied to a clock.
45 weeks	Addresses mother as *mama*, but *nana* if fretful or angry.
49 weeks	Says *dadda* in imitation of mother's speech.
50 weeks	Uses *dadda*, *hello* and *bye* with meaning.
15 months	Recognizes picture of familiar object and names it.
16 months	Uses imitations of words heard—*cuggle (cuddle) me*, *goh* meaning cow. Toy animals all described as *Teddy*.
20 months	Vocabulary of more than 50 words, including imitations. Says *bad* if hurt or scolded for naughtiness.
21 months	First two-word sentences: *shut door*, *daddy go*, *ball red*.
23 months	Three-word sentences: *here you are*, *no want that*. Able to pronounce own name clearly. Makes moral judgement—*me bad*.
24 months	Able to answer simple questions such as name and age. Four-word sentences: *mummy go cake shop*.
26 months	Begins to use verbs in correct tense in simple sentences: *daddy coming home*, *daddy came*. Makes connections between objects and abstractions: a round cushion—*a circle*.

Highlights of language development

There are characteristic trends in the language development of infants, though individual rates of progress can vary considerably. Babies perceive intonation and meaning in the language they hear before their own utterances become specific. As babbled syllables give way to recognizable sounds, infants first apply words to the people and objects closest to them. Generalizations occur—"kitty" may be applied to all animals, but not at first to a picture of a kitten which remains an abstraction. Words are invented through approximate imitations of sounds heard. As two or three words are put together, the precise meaning of a phrase can be interpreted by adults in context.

Health problems in infancy

Illness is described as either acute or chronic. An acute illness is one which is sudden, intense, usually brief and not necessarily serious, e.g. the common cold. A chronic illness is one which lasts for some time without any rapid developments.

Health problems which arise before birth are known as congenital disorders. These include inherited conditions (such as haemophilia and sickle-

ILLNESS Congenital disorders 1. Inherited diseases	SYMPTOMS	TREATMENT/ ACTION	ILLNESS 2. Other problems at birth
Cystic fibrosis	Found in one in 1000 live births. All mucus-secreting glands are malfunctioning. It affects the digestive system by causing diarrhoea and weight loss; and the respiratory system where excessive lung mucus can lead to bronchitis or pneumonia.	Antibiotics used against infection. Breathing can be aided by physiotherapy. Treatment still being developed.	Coeliac disease Cleft palate and hare lip
Haemophilia	Lack of a substance called Factor VIII which promotes blood clotting can lead to internal bleeding or to prolonged bleeding from a slight external injury. Only males suffer from it, and most die prematurely.	Sufferers are given transfusions of plasma containing Factor VIII.	Club foot Down's syndrome (Mongolism)
Muscular dystrophy	Duchenne muscular dystrophy affects the pelvis, shoulders, trunk and later the limbs. It is first noticed when the child begins to walk.	A degenerative disease which cannot be cured. Later, a wheelchair will be necessary.	Heart deformities: hole in the heart, blue babies
Phenylketonuria	An absence of enzymes that metabolize certain toxic phenyls in the bloodstream. If untreated can lead to severe mental retardation.	If detected soon after birth, can be dealt with by diet containing proteins from which phenylalanine is removed. The diet is continued until adulthood and resumed during pregnancy.	Hip dislocation
Sickle-cell anaemia	Red blood cells become sickle-shaped when deprived of oxygen and they impair circulation. Over-exertion leads to severe pain in abdomen and joints.	Blood transfusions may be needed, but this condition is often fatal.	Spina bifida

cell anaemia) and conditions which develop *in utero* (e.g. various heart disorders) or at birth (e.g. brain damage). Rather less serious problems may arise from the baby's eating and sleeping routines.

SYMPTOMS	TREATMENT/ ACTION
Fats cannot be digested. Diarrhoea and weight loss.	The cause of this disease is unknown. A gluten-free diet is necessary.
The two sides of the roof of the mouth fail to join before birth, leaving a gap in the nasal cavity. Usually occurs together with a hare lip—a split between the two halves of the upper lip.	Surgery improves and often cures both conditions. A cleft palate can be operated on at 15 months and a hare lip at three months.
One or both feet are twisted out of position by a malformation of bones or a stretching or shortening of muscles and tendons.	Mild cases will respond to manipulation. Special shoes, exercises and sometimes surgery may be necessary.
A chromosomal disorder which causes mental deficiency and certain physical characteristics.	None available.
A hole in the heart is often due to foetal development stopping too soon. Maldevelopment of the circulatory system leads to deoxygenated blood flowing into vessels that should carry only oxygenated blood (hence the 'blue' appearance).	A hole in the heart often closes of its own accord. Surgery has improved the survival rate for 'blue' babies.
The thigh bone is out of the hip socket at birth. It is more common in girls.	Can be corrected by wearing a special splint. Surgery may be necessary.
One or more vertebrae are open at the back. In severe forms the spinal cord is deformed or damaged before birth, producing paralysis in the lower body. Most mild cases go unnoticed.	For severe cases an operation only sometimes succeeds. Physiotherapy and special treatment are necessary.

COMMON PROBLEMS OF INFANCY
Birthmarks
Many mothers are alarmed by the appearance of birthmarks on newborn infants, but most are temporary. Of the rest, the "strawberry" mark (a red, raised spongy area of skin) may enlarge and then disappear; if not, it can be shrunk by injections or removed surgically. "Port wine" stains (dark red, flat areas on face and neck) can be treated to make them less noticeable and concealed by special cosmetics. Vitiligo (an area of white skin) can be concealed but not treated. "Liver spots", dark patches, come to look like large freckles.

Crying
Crying is the baby's only means of communication and parents soon learn to distinguish between different reasons for crying. Frequent causes of crying are hunger, wind, teething pains, discomfort or loneliness. These situations are easily dealt with but other reasons for crying may be more difficult to resolve, for example colic, a severe abdominal pain which is hard to treat. Or the child may be hypertonic – a condition in which he or she is tense and is disturbed by even the slightest noise. If crying is persistent or in any way unusual, a doctor should be consulted.

Feeding
Feeding problems which occur while the baby is being weaned are usually brought about by his or her reaction to the novelty of the experience. Conscious swallowing has to be learned and this may take time, so do not force or trick the child into eating.

Sleeping
Most children go through a phase of refusing to settle when put to bed. Sometimes this is due to anxiety about being left alone or fear of the dark. This is usually remedied easily by parental reassurance and use of a nightlight or leaving the door ajar. For severe bedtime crying a doctor may prescribe a mild sedative for short term use.

Early waking may be a problem for parents; children can be encouraged to play in their bedrooms in the early morning.

Waking during the night may be caused by disturbance from noise elsewhere, so it is best not to accustom a child to complete silence while he or she sleeps. Alternatively, a child may need less sleep, and a later bedtime or cutting out a daytime nap should adjust the balance.

Nightmares are often a sign that the child has developed the ability to think on a symbolic level and invent imaginary characters. He or she needs to be calmed and reassured before returning to sleep.

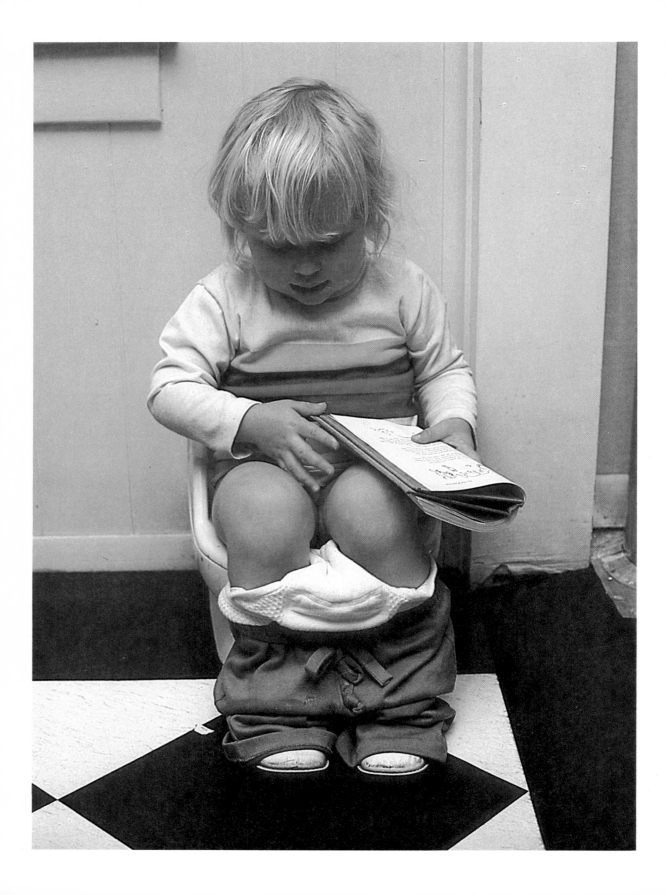

Childhood

If there is anything we wish to change in the child, we should first examine it and see whether it is not something that could be better changed in ourselves.

Carl Jung *Psychological Reflections*

Through many processes of learning and over a period of years, children will make their way towards the world of niches, roles and games that is adult society. How should they travel? What must happen to our two-year-olds to enable them to become inhabitants of that larger world in which adults live? First, they must learn to communicate. Many adults spend their days in a constant process of spoken, written and electronic communication with each other. Initially, this learning process will be haphazard. However, when children enter school, they begin the long, deliberate and challenging task of learning to read and write. We now expect all children to obtain in a few years skills in literacy and numeracy that it took adult society thousands of years to develop. Secondly, children must learn to see the world from an adult viewpoint. The world around us does not appear marked off in inches, miles, hours, Thursdays and Januaries. Adults have developed such sophisticated ways of cutting the world into segments. Thirdly, our children must learn a bewildering variety of social norms and conventions which allow us to relate to each other with varying degrees of intimacy. And they will learn to accept responsibility and impose self-discipline.

Children spend their pre-school years in what more than one commentator has likened to the Garden of Eden. Long sunny days, a big beautiful world to be explored and mastered. But this is a kind of romantic myth-making that some adults like to engage in. The point obscured by the poetry of the Garden of Eden is, of course, that pre-school children experience much less scheduling and conflict of will now than they do in the later years of childhood. It may take 20 years or more to grow up today, to finish training and take a free-standing place in the adult world. Once, not so long ago, it took a dozen years for most children. In modern societies, there are a great variety of ways to be an adult. But all of them require much learning and personal growth.

Left: Every experience is an opportunity to learn

How a child's thinking develops

Piaget's theory of cognitive development

In 1919, Jean Piaget, a young zoologist and naturalist, went to the Paris laboratory of Théophile Simon to work on the then very new business of testing children's mental development. In the years since 1919 until his death in 1983, Piaget and his collaborators produced some 50 books and a multitude of articles about children's thinking processes.

Piaget's early training as a zoologist profoundly influenced the kind of theory he developed about human thinking and his choice of method for the study of cognitive development. Many of his early ideas in fact came from his detailed observations of his own children, from their first days of life. Later, Piaget collected most of his data by devising tasks for children, observing how they carried out each task and questioning them about what they had done. This point will be referred to later, because this "naturalistic" method of studying children is probably one of the keys to the weaknesses of Piagetian theory which have been highlighted by more recent research.

Intelligence as adaptation

The question which concerned Piaget was "How do animals adapt to the environment?" As he noted, human beings have an outstanding capacity for adaptation. Not only do we rapidly change our behaviour in the face of new environments, we change our environments to suit our behaviour. Unlike non-human animals, we can also deal in possibilities and abstractions, and reflect on our own thought processes. Obviously, not all humans can do this. Infants cannot. Piaget was therefore concerned with describing and explaining how these cognitive changes, between infancy and adulthood, come about.

Piaget's theory of cognitive development is very complex and, at times, some would say very loose. This makes it very difficult, even for those who are extremely familiar with the theory, to know exactly what Piaget was saying. However, his theory has been profoundly influential not only in psychology but also in education. Because of this, it is important that those concerned with the education of children, whether parents or teachers, should understand something of the theory and its problems.

Assimilation and accommodation

For Piaget, the process of coming to terms with the environment is an active one. The human organism can deal with the environment by making the latter fit its own existing capabilities. Piaget called this part of the adaptive process *assimilation*. However, the organism also needs to alter its behaviour to deal with the properties of its environment. This process is called *accommodation*. Piaget used the example of the make-believe play of the young child ("this box is really a racing car") as an example of assimilative behaviour. Imitation, on the other hand, is almost totally accommodatory.

The two processes, however, can rarely be separated out. Both go on together. Through them, the organism can achieve both continuity, variability, growth and change. It has been suggested that learning is maximized when the child's environment creates some

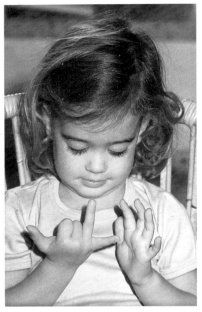

Fingers are so fascinating. At an early stage a child practises counting using objects or pictures before assimilating the more abstract sense of number sequences, addition and subtraction. At the same time, for a young child there is still a self-absorbed interest in physical capabilities. Counting on fingers exercises more than one recently acquired skill.

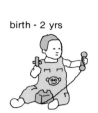

birth - 2 yrs

Sensori-motor Stage
Beginning at birth, the child learns that there are objects independent of himself or herself and that actions have consequences. The child begins to organize experiences and can respond to his or her environment—walking, talking and manipulating objects.

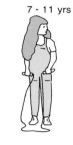

7 - 11 yrs

Concrete Operational Stage
Piaget considered a child to have reached this stage when he or she understood reversibility. The child is gradually able to consider more than one aspect or dimension of an object or problem at a time. And he or she is less egocentric and can see other people's points of view.

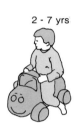

2 - 7 yrs

Pre-operational Stage
At this stage the child, having made some sense of the chaos of stimulation present since birth, begins to use words and images to represent the external world to itself. These symbols enable the child to think about objects and to communicate with others. He or she has a growing ability to remember and to anticipate things, but cannot retrace mental steps to reach a conclusion.

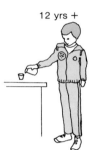

12 yrs +

Formal Operational Stage
The adolescent can perform these same mental acts internally with verbal propositions, rather than externally with concrete objects. He or she is able to formulate and test hypotheses through logic and to think in abstract terms and consider all possibilities. The possibility that adult intelligence develops further is left open.

tension between assimilation and accommodation. A very basic example of this is the use of puréed foods between liquids and solids. They cannot be sucked, but they do not have to be chewed.

Stages of development

Piaget emphasized that development is continuous, but he talked of it occurring in a series of *stages*. Transition from one stage to another indicated that some very fundamental cognitive reorganization was taking place. Piaget's use of the term "stage", and the way in which it has been used by later writers, is very important in understanding the weaknesses of his theory and the problems of applying it to education. This point will be mentioned again later.

The first 18 months or so of life constitute what Piaget called the sensori-motor period. This period was discussed in "Infancy"; in this section we are interested in the stages which span the childhood years. Piaget divided this period into two stages—the concrete operational (spanning roughly 18 months to 11 years) and the formal operational (11 to 15 years). The age boundaries here are, of course, very approximate and Piaget attached no significance to age *per se*. The concrete operational stage is divided into two parts: the first of these lasts until about age seven and is called the pre-operational stage. It is during this period that the "concrete" operations are being prepared for. They are established and consolidated during the concrete operational stage.

During the pre-operational stage, the operations are being "prepared": children are laboriously learning that items can be combined by addition or separated by subtraction, but their understanding of what they are doing is precarious. When children pass into the concrete operational stage, however, they are able to perform

Piaget divided the stages of the development of the thought processes to show how they passed from actions in response to the environment (sensori-motor); to the use of symbols (pre-operational); to the ability to perform mental acts with physical objects; and, finally, to deal with concepts that are detached from the environment.

many mental "acts", but only with actual physical objects (hence the term "concrete" operational period). In the formal operational period, however, children can perform these operations with verbal propositions—they do not require the actual objects to work with. They can deal with propositions and abstractions ("supposing x is equal to twice y . . .").

Piaget attempted to capture the difference between concrete operations and formal operations in the following example: Edith is fairer than Susan. Edith is darker than Lily. Who is the darkest? Many children of 9 or 10 find this problem extremely difficult. If, however, they were asked to work it out using three dolls, they could do it quite easily.

Going back to where you started

For Piaget, one of the most important mental operations which children learn to perform is reversal—understanding that, in principle, every act is reversible: things that have been added can be taken away again, and things that have been taken away can be added, leaving the original state of affairs intact.

Suppose you and a friend are in a pub. Both of you ask for sherry. Yours comes in a long, narrow glass, while your friend's comes in a large, round glass. Your friend's drink will obviously come much less far up the side of the glass than will yours, but he doesn't make a scene and claim that you have more sherry than he. Why? Because he understands that both drinks came from the same measuring glass and that, if poured back, would be shown to be equal.

Very young children, however, have difficulty in coming to grips with reversibility. For Piaget, the ability to make use of this principle was one of the main signs of having reached the concrete operational stage. He devised a number of tasks which he claims tell us whether or not a child understands the principle of reversibility and, thus, whether he or she has reached the concrete operational stage.

These are usually referred to by psychologists as conservation tasks. One of the best-known and simplest involves presenting the child with two sticks of equal length arranged thus ———— . The child agrees with the experimenter that the sticks are of equal length. The experimenter then pushes the sticks out of alignment thus, ———— and repeats the question: "Are the sticks the same length?" Many very young children will now claim that the sticks are unequal. When questioned, they will usually say that one of them (pointing) sticks out more than the other. According to Piaget, such children have not yet reached the concrete operational stage: they cannot carry out the crucial operation—reversal—required in this task. In other words, they do not grasp that the sticks could easily be pushed back into alignment, thus restoring the original state of affairs.

More recent research casts serious doubt on the validity of Piaget's explanation. In one study, the experimenters omitted the first question. The sticks were put in alignment, and pushed out of alignment by the experimenter; only then was the child asked if they were equal in length. Under these conditions, far more children gave the correct answer than in the standard version of the task. In another, ingenious, experiment, the researcher presented the first part of the task in the standard Piagetian way. He then introduced a character called "naughty teddy" who appeared from behind a screen and

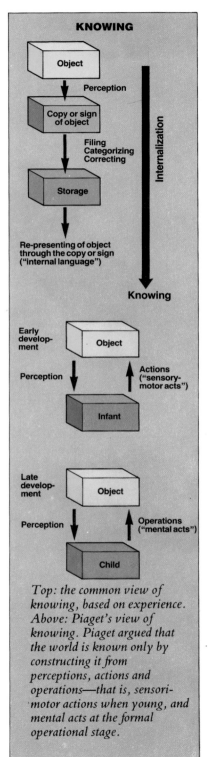

Top: the common view of knowing, based on experience. Above: Piaget's view of knowing. Piaget argued that the world is known only by constructing it from perceptions, actions and operations—that is, sensorimotor actions when young, and mental acts at the formal operational stage.

"messed up" the sticks so that they were out of alignment. The children were then asked again if the sticks were the same length. In this version of the task, significantly more children aged between four and six gave the correct response.

What these findings seem to indicate is that for young children the difficulty is not understanding reversibility, but freeing themselves from the context and cues of the experiment. In order to answer correctly, they must attend solely to the question being asked and nothing else. Imagine how the standard Piagetian task might appear to a very young child. The experimenter arranges things in a certain way and asks the child a question. She then takes the trouble to rearrange things, in front of the child, and asks the *same* question. It seems reasonable to suggest that many children take this as a cue that their answer should be different. If, however, the original question is omitted or the rearrangement made to look accidental, then the children are not misled into thinking that they should change their answer. In other words, some of the children are paying too much attention to the social context of the experiment and not enough to the task itself.

When asked to draw the same subject—the family—children of different ages will nearly always produce pictures typical of their age. In this case, the bodyless, monochrome people and animals of a three-year-old are compared with the more intricate work of a six-year-old.

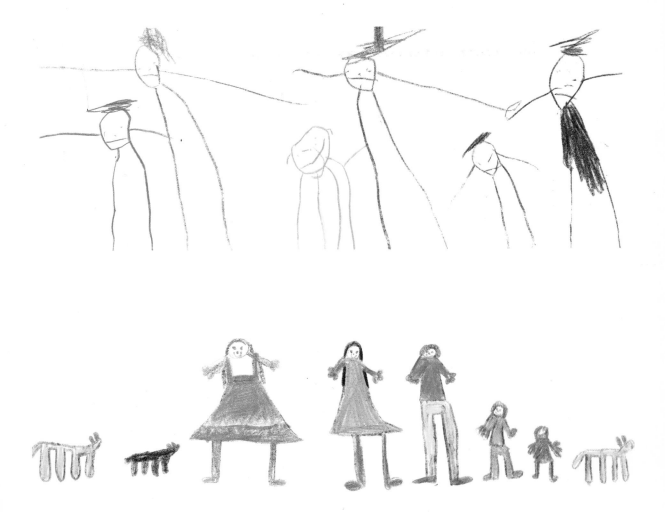

As we saw in "Infancy", all early learning takes place within a social context. Children first start to understand language by observing that certain things are said in certain situations. It should not surprise us that pre-school and early-school-age children pay such close attention to social cues. (This point is also covered on pages 66 and 67.) It seems that one of the goals of school education is, necessarily, to free children's thinking from this dependency and enable them to think about problems in a more abstract manner.

Piaget and education

According to Piaget, children's thinking develops in an invariant sequence of stages. Children are said to be "in" a particular stage if they are able to perform certain tasks and to understand what they are doing. Performance of these tasks is determined, in turn, by the ability to carry out certain mental operations, such as reversal. Piaget further claimed that these skills cannot be "taught" but were learned by the child through "discovery". Thus cognitive development was seen as a sort of "unfolding" process. If children could not perform certain tasks, then it was because they did not yet possess the necessary cognitive structures. What they need is not direct teaching, but more experience with the environment around them, more opportunity to discover things for themselves.

The research that has just been discussed, however, presents very serious problems for this view of cognitive development. If children fail a Piagetian task, it is claimed to be the result of their inability to perform some mental operation. How, then, can they perform this operation quite adequately when the task is presented in a slightly different way? Clearly, Piaget's explanation will not suffice. The children obviously *do* have problems with the standard task, but it seems to have much more to do with the way in which they interpret the experimenter's questions, whether or not they attend to and understand the questions themselves, or whether they are misled by other aspects of the experimental situation to which older children attach less importance.

Adult thinking

Piaget's ideas about cognitive development give the rather misleading idea that children's thinking proceeds in an orderly, rational fashion until it reaches a mature, adult level. Unfortunately, Piaget never actually studied adult thinking. If he had, his views about cognitive development might have been somewhat different.

Studies of adult reasoning show that adults, in many cases, approach problems in a manner apparently as illogical as that of a very young child, in the standard Piagetian tasks, and, like the young child, they are adamant that their erroneous solutions are correct. The fact that many of these studies have been carried out on university students makes the results even more surprising.

To say that these adults have not yet reached the more advanced Piagetian stages is to miss the point that there is no distinctive style or way of approaching problems which characterizes the thinking of young children, older children, adolescents or adults. Perhaps the major debt we owe Piaget is that his theory has led to an increased emphasis on the role of *understanding* in cognitive development. What we still do not know is how best to bring this about.

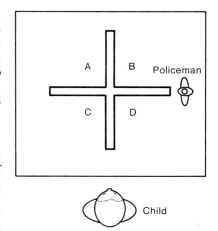

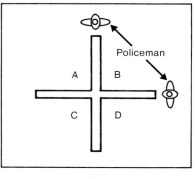

Martin Hughes's test of the child's egocentricity. The large cross represents two walls and the child has to position a doll or "child" so that the "policeman" cannot see it (top). In a more complicated version (above) the "child" has to be out of the viewing range of two "policemen".

Relating to other people

Children's social development can be viewed from many angles. They are learning "social skills"—how to behave in particular situations, how to cooperate in play, how to form friendships. They are also learning about other people and forming judgements of them. Children are absorbing the ways in which others react to them, and forming judgements about themselves. And they are learning to differentiate "right" from "wrong" and to exert self-discipline.

Developing social skills

The foundations of adult skills are laid in childhood, and children who fail to acquire these skills often have real difficulties as adults. It has been shown, for example, that children who were isolated—who did not socialize much with their peers—tend to be over-represented in groups of delinquents and adults with mental health problems.

Several studies have tried to identify differences in the behaviour of popular and less popular children. This is usually done by asking children to indicate which classmates they like to sit beside, play with, work with, and so on. The children are then observed, either during "free play" or in a more structured situation, and their behaviour is recorded. The results of these studies have been quite consistent: popular children tend to give positive feedback to others (compliments, praise, etc.) at a high rate, they smile more (perhaps because they are so popular!), they initiate play with other children, rather than waiting to be approached, and they are helpful to others.

It is interesting to note that popular children are also more able to describe verbally how to go about making friends. Another striking finding is that physical appearance is important for popularity. Attractive children, regardless of their behaviour, are usually judged more positively by both their peers and their teachers. And when children are given descriptions of other children and asked how much they think they would like them, it is children who exhibit aggressive behaviour who are most rejected.

We still lack detailed information on how children learn social skills. The best guess is that it is by a mixture of imitation of adults and direct teaching from them, although the amount of teaching will vary enormously from family to family. From these experiences, children presumably construct "rules"—as in the example of popular children being able to describe how to make friends—which govern their behaviour in social situations.

If this is the case, then we can identify groups of children who may be less likely than others to develop appropriate social skills. The most obvious groups are those whose parents themselves lack social skills and who therefore cannot serve as appropriate models. Parents may also unwittingly teach their children inappropriate social behaviour by, for example, encouraging them to show off to visitors or allowing them to interrupt other people's conversations. It can sometimes be difficult for parents, attached as they are to their children, to appreciate that what seems fetching or cute to them may simply be a nuisance to others. It can then come as a rude awakening to a small child to realize that behaviour which was always rewarded at home is punished by classmates at school.

Parental influence

What can parents do to help? Perhaps they should become more aware of when they are applying a different set of standards to the social behaviour of their own child than to that of other children or adults. They should try to expose their children to a wide range of social situations and encourage them to mix with other children.

Given the importance which children assign to aggressive behaviour in judging other children, parents should be alert for signs of inappropriate aggression in their child. Aggressive behaviour is often resorted to by both children and adults because they know of no other way to deal with a difficult situation. Parents can help their children control aggressive behaviour by, for example, discussing with them alternative strategies for handling such situations and pointing out the negative long-term consequences of aggression. And it goes without saying that parents who themselves handle difficult situations by resorting to verbal or physical aggression will soon find their child behaving in the same way.

Judging others and judging ourselves

If we want to know what children think of themselves or others, then the most obvious thing to do is to ask them. Many researchers adopted this approach by asking children of various ages to describe their friends or other people they knew, using the question: "What kind of person is he/she?"

One very consistent finding from these studies was that very young children rarely used psychological terms to describe others, but instead described them in physical terms or by their possessions. Around the age of eight, however, children began to use a much greater proportion of psychological language. But it would be a mistake to conclude that very young children do not "think" of others in psychological terms. Anyone who has had contact with children can attest to their extreme sensitivity to psychological cues. This seems to be yet another case of researchers failing to make their task real enough or simple enough for young children. When children are asked to watch video-tapes of people behaving in various familiar ways—being angry, helpful, shy, etc.—or are asked to choose between two people described by different psychological terms, then they have far less difficulty in understanding the terms and will use them spontaneously to describe people to a much greater extent. The same trends are still found in older children, who use a higher proportion of psychological terms in their decriptions, but this may well reflect an increasing sophistication of language use rather than a significant change in the attributes used for judging others.

The growth of self-esteem

The attitudes of schoolfellows, as well as feedback from parents, teachers and other adults, contribute in large measure to the child's view of him- or herself. Such a view is often called a "self-concept" and develops gradually through the years of childhood. It has been suggested that children form some idea of their "worth" at a relatively early age and carry this view of themselves, for better or worse, for the rest of their days. This picture is both over-optimistic and over-pessimistic. It also gives the misleading impression that there is one unified view of self. For young children this may well be the case, unless they are unfortunate enough to be treated in drastically different ways by each parent. But we can see development as including the process of taking on a variety of views of self.

A child may be treated differently by his parents than by his teacher and his peers. What is likely to be similar, however, is that all of them will judge him in global terms: "You are a good/bad boy." We seem to find it inordinately difficult to give children feedback in terms of their behaviour (that was a nice/nasty thing which you did). If this general kind of feedback is positive, then this probably does not matter. There is a danger, however, that children who are often criticized in this way will develop the idea that they are generally bad. The parents too, by using global negative feedback, may come to ignore the children's positive behaviours.

Interpreting feedback

We still have very limited information about how the self-concept or, more accurately, concepts, develop in children. What is particularly interesting is that, gradually, our view of our "self" comes to influence the way in which we interpret feedback from others. Young children may form an image of themselves which is directly related to the way in which others respond to them. Adults, however, often interpret others' responses to them in such a way as to maintain their existing self-image. Depressed people, for example, may generalize wildly from one piece of feedback (This woman won't go out with me, therefore I am a total failure). On the other hand, it seems that non-depressed people have a slightly rosier image of themselves than is warranted by others' opinion of them!

Putting the differences into perspective is all part of social integration. From very early on, children are curious about differences between the sexes (this fades between the ages of five and puberty) but they cannot relate to adult sexual features.

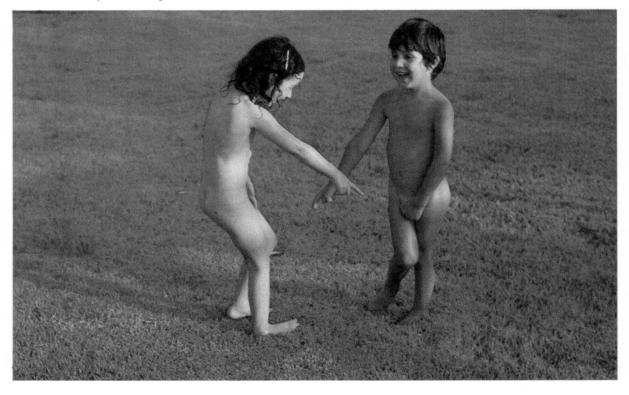

Making sense of the social context

Children's knowledge of social institutions and conventions increases rapidly in the school years. If five- or six-year-old children are asked what things such as schools, stores, money or governments are supposed to do, they offer very idiosyncratic ideas. At about 9 or 10, they begin to articulate ideas about what a store, any store, ought to do. From the age of about 11, they show the first faint sense that things such as stores and money and government are linked together in a working society.

Eliot Turiel at the University of California asked children to talk about social conventions such as whether people address each other formally or by their first name, correct dress, conventional living arrangements, stereotyped male and female activities and polite ways of eating. At six or seven, children are quite familiar with most social conventions. They regard them, for the most part, as arbitrary. This is the way things are. By 9 or 10, children sense that some pressure or force keeps things in order. Someone, some authority perhaps, will disapprove if conventions are violated. The meaning of some conventions becomes clear early on—for instance, if you eat with utensils, your hands stay clean. However, others do not make sense. Why do people dress formally at some times and not others? By about 14, children begin to see social conventions as part of a larger design. Knowing a little about other societies, they come to understand that conventions of politeness operate everywhere, but the particular forms that manners take vary from one society to another. Only by obeying these conventions is the individual fully accepted by society in adult life.

Social scripts

In coming to understand social situations, children first develop a sense of what generally happens over time. Faced with a shop, the entrance into church on a Sunday morning, a bowling alley, the sight of two friends approaching each other on a street, children can generate something like a movie, a *script* that allows them to anticipate what is likely to happen. But knowing what happens precedes knowing *why* it happens (indeed, many adults would find it difficult to describe the "whys" of social situations).

Social events are more complicated and harder to predict than physical events—at least, the kinds of physical events schools deal with and psychologists study. Faced with a balance beam, a pendulum or a set of gears, a child of eight or nine can often make exact predictions about how they will behave. However, social events unfold in a sequence that is only roughly regular. One Sunday in church is only roughly like the next. Time sequences are related in complex ways: the minister does not deliver the sermon just because the congregation has finished singing the hymns. And, unfortunately, adults seem less concerned with directly teaching children about social situations and social behaviour than about physical events. Children must discover the veiled regularities of social behaviour by gradually connecting various aspects of the social system. Social understanding takes place more slowly than physical understanding and follows different paths. However, there are certain patterns of development that have been identified as common to most children, during this phase of social adjustment.

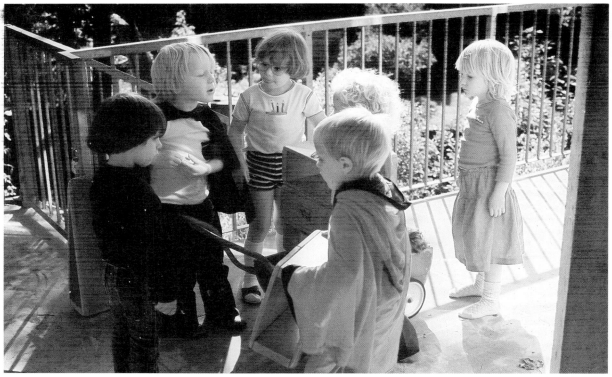

Notions of right and wrong

One important aspect of social understanding involves the assignment of responsibility or blame, either to oneself or to others. Lawrence Kohlberg of the University of Chicago has argued that there are six stages of moral reasoning in children, one stage following the next in a fixed sequence. Kohlberg derived his ideas from Piaget and sees these six stages as moving in parallel with the stages of cognitive development postulated by Piaget.

In the first two stages, right and wrong are defined externally: actions are judged by their consequences and children seek to avoid punishment while satisfying their own needs. In Kohlberg's next two stages, between 10 and 13, right and wrong are judged in terms of conventional morality. Society has rules and laws, and individuals are good or bad depending on their ability to conform to them. Children are motivated by desire for social approval and respect for consensus values. Intention, rather than outcome, is what counts in judging an action. In the last two stages, which may be found in some children at 13, but in others much later or not at all, right and wrong are seen in a broader context as expressions of a social contract, a legal system or universal ethical principles. Children act in accordance with the values they have worked out for themselves.

Like Piaget, Kohlberg derived his theory about the growth of moral reasoning by giving a relatively small sample of children a series of tasks and noting their responses. The children were presented with a set of moral dilemmas, in story form (should a man steal to obtain the money he needs to pay for medical treatment which will save his wife's life?). Their responses, in terms of the *reasoning* they used to

The way we interact with each other as adults has its foundation in our early years—the tendencies to be gregarious or solitary, domineering or shy become obvious as soon as the child mixes with others of the same age, and probably before. How easy to imagine the dominant child as a thrusting business executive in later years!

reach a decision, were the data on which the theory is based.

There are a number of problems, however, with the way in which Kohlberg collected his data and therefore with his account of the development of moral reasoning. Thus, it is often very difficult to assign a child's response to the moral dilemmas to one stage or another. The standards by which this is done have never been objectively defined by Kohlberg.

It has also proved very difficult to demonstrate any relationship between the stage of moral reasoning, as defined by responses to the stories, and actual behaviour. In one study, for example, both delinquents and non-delinquents clustered around stage 3.

Another way of approaching the development of morality is to study how children actually behave in situations which would be considered by adults as involving moral judgements of one sort or another. Walter Mischel of Stanford University has made an extensive study of how young children learn to "resist temptation". One of the most striking findings has been that it is impossible to categorize children as either "resisters" or "non-resisters" or as honest or dishonest. Instead, it seems that a host of situational factors must be taken into account in predicting whether a child will, for example, cheat if given the opportunity. A child who refrains from cheating under one set of circumstances will cheat readily under another.

Mischel views moral development as involving processes of self-control, where immediate gratification is delayed in favour of some longer-term goal. The scheme takes account of both positive (altruistic) acts and negative acts (for instance, not using office telephones for personal calls). From his study of children, Mischel suggests that each situation will be assessed in terms of possible outcomes (Will I get caught? Will I feel bad?) and in terms of the standards which have been set by significant others—in the young child's case, usually the parents—for that particular situation. It has been shown that young children will usually abide by the standards which they have observed in other people. Thus, children will follow what their parents actually *do* rather than standards they impose verbally. Many parents make life extremely difficult for their children by saying one thing and doing another. One important aspect of moral development is the shift from parents to peers as important standard-setters.

Internal or external control?

The outcome of "moral transgressions" for any individual can be seen as external—getting caught or getting away with it—or internal—feeling guilt or anxiety. What most parents would like is to see their children develop internal standards of morality, where they avoid wrongdoing—as defined by the parents or society—because it violates these internal standards and not because they are afraid of being caught and punished.

Martin Hoffman, a psychologist at the University of Michigan, has found that there are two basic patterns of parental discipline that have different effects on moral development. He calls them *power-assertive* and *non-power-assertive*. The second pattern can be divided into two main sub-types: *love-withdrawal techniques* and *induction* (in which the parent provides explanations or reasons for requiring certain behaviours from the child).

In power-assertive techniques, the parent does not rely on the

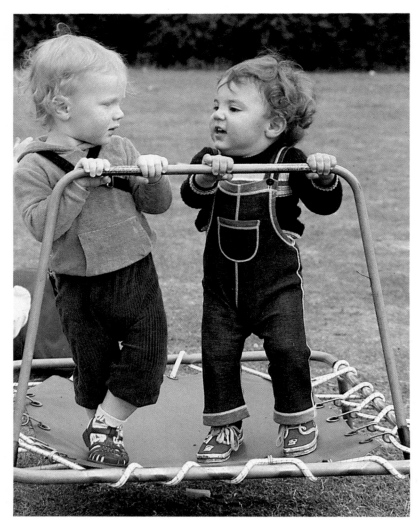

Childhood play and discussion is a rehearsal for adult social interaction, though necessarily operating within different limits and expectations. Children early acquire the ability to mix co-operation and competition in establishing codes of behaviour among peers.

child's own inner resources—such as guilt, shame, dependency, love or respect—or provide the child with the relevant information needed to develop such resources in order to influence his or her behaviour. Instead, the parent seeks to accomplish this by punishing the child physically or materially or by relying on fear of punishment. The child is then less likely to act on the basis of his or her own internalized norms—that is, conscience—and more likely to continue to be influenced by external rewards and punishments. The probability of being caught thus becomes an important determinant of the child's behaviour. Not surprisingly, a pattern of "power assertion" is frequently found among the parents of some kinds of delinquents.

Parents who employ love-withdrawal techniques do not physically punish or deprive the child. Instead, they react to undesirable behaviour by such things as conspicuously ignoring the child, refusing to speak to it, expressing dislike, or even in some cases by threatening to leave it. The message the child gets is clear: "If you behave this way, I won't love you."

In fact, the implication is likely to be that the child is unlovable. As Professor Hoffman observes, although love withdrawal does not involve physical or material threats, "it may be more devastating emotionally because it poses the ultimate threat of abandonment or separation". Love withdrawal also contributes little to the development of positive, mature moral standards, although the child, motivated largely by anxiety, is more likely than the child of power-assertive parents to confess to violations and to accept blame.

The third approach to parental discipline—induction—does encourage the development of a mature conscience based on internalized moral standards. In this approach, the parent treats the child as a potentially responsible, capable individual. Such a parent explains to the child the reasons for requiring certain behaviours, pointing out the practical realities of a situation or how inappropriate behaviour may be harmful to the child or to others.

Parents do not need to be saints to use inductive techniques. For example, a mother can explain to her child that if he persists in some undesirable behaviour, it will worry her or wear her out and therefore make her more irritable or cross with the child—and she does not want that to happen. She can label the behaviour as "unlovable". But that is a far cry from labelling the child as unlovable.

Personal values and standards

Look, for a moment, through a child's eyes at the early years of school life. Suddenly, all around, shadowy, somewhat unfathomable judgements are being made. At school, children are prodded by standards, goals, rules and rituals. The adults around them, the teachers and parents, are more serious about things now. Why? The larger logic of this new pattern eludes small children. It will be many years before they can explain to themselves why children ought to go to school. Now they go because that is what they are supposed to do.

Children are placed in school at a time when, on the whole, we expect them to begin to take responsibility and to be guided by standards within themselves. Where do these come from? It seems that children form conceptions of who they would like to be: they see and admire certain adults around them, some real, some fictional. They *identify*—act like these admired figures, imagine themselves in their place (as, indeed, do adults). This looks like imitation and play, but children are in fact, incorporating the values, standards and principles embodied in the actions of these figures.

Children starting school meet the new rules and expectations as best they can. From many studies we know that they generally enter school with optimism and anticipation, but that in many cases this positivity turns into a fairly deep negativity within the first six years or so. We may feel this is a problem in the way schools are set up, but this may also be children's first experience of the inescapable bittersweetness of a more mature life. Either way, children cope with school through an idiosyncratic mixture of compliance, inertia and defiance. However, children need a larger meaning to their efforts, both inside and outside school, some sense of why they are doing things beyond the fact that adults say they must be done. During the school years, children will gradually form their own set of motives and goals. They will bring to the enterprise all the varied elements of the self-image they are beginning to form.

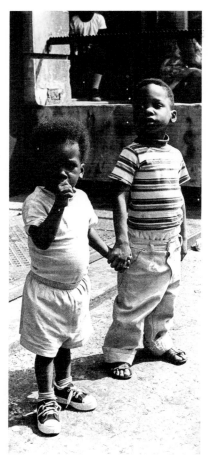

Despite the interruptions of sibling rivalry, instincts for friendship and protection assert themselves, especially in the greater world outside the safety of home. Learning to share and trust emotions is a crucial part of training for life.

Child Prodigies

While the controversy about IQ testing as an accurate assessment of ability at any age continues, there is no doubt that some children excel in certain subjects, such as music or mathematics, from a very early age. Each generation has its share of exceptionally gifted children, but how can we distinguish bright children from the potential geniuses? Until recently most research was designed to demonstrate that such children exist and to distinguish characteristics they had in common. It has been found that such children are generally very alert at birth and need little sleep during the first few months; they are lively and curious, usually walking and talking before their contemporaries; they ask a lot of questions and are easily bored. But it should not be assumed that a child who walks early is otherwise gifted, and this takes us back to intelligence testing. Research findings suggest that gifted children make up from five per cent to 0.05 per cent of the population depending on the criteria used.

The gifted child often faces problems at school, and many in fact are educated by their own parents (including Ruth Jayne Laurence; see the picture below). Education specialists are divided over the best way to help such children. Some consider that dwindling resources should not be used to benefit a tiny minority and that they should be forced to conform to the system like other children; others feel that gifted children should get all the help they need. Segregated schools—as distinct from schools specializing in music or ballet, for example—exist in Russia and in America, but not in Britain.

The exceptionally bright child may not always shine at school and his or her abilities may not become apparent until much later. There are many cases of classroom 'misfits' who conceal their intelligence in order to be like other children, or who find an outlet for their talents by disruption. Bright children may do badly in examinations and realize their talents only later in life.

The names of famous child prodigies are familiar to us all: Yehudi Menuhin who studied the violin seriously at three and was admitted to the Vienna Conservatory at seven; Prokofiev, who composed an opera, *The Giant*, at seven; Mozart; John Stuart Mill; Macaulay; and Francis Galton who himself tested the mental and physical characteristics of children.

On the other hand, we have examples of people whose talents were not discovered in childhood, although they subsequently rose to fame; such as Winston Churchill who did badly at school; Picasso and Monet who were both unruly pupils; Albert Einstein who was considered by both his teachers and parents to be "dull"; and Thomas Edison who was diagnosed as mentally ill by his teacher.

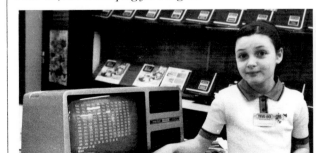

Ruth Jayne Laurence, of Britain, never attended school but was educated by her father, a computer consultant. Now 12, she is studying for a degree.

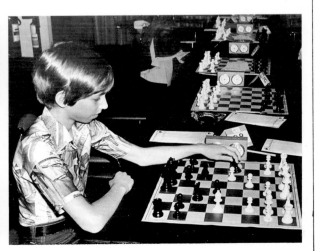

Joel Benjamin of New York, top 14-year-old chess player of 1978 is a future contender for the world title.

Going to school

Both non-industrialized and industrialized societies assume that children change between the ages of five and seven. By seven, so the received wisdom goes, they have minds, can reason, will remember what you tell them, know right from wrong, should be held accountable for what they do, should be taught courtesy and respect, have lost a certain innocence and magic and have become faintly sexual.

However, whereas from this age onwards a child in a non-industrialized society begins to work in a limited way at adult tasks, a child in an industrialized society begins schoolwork. In the former, children move towards adult life and company; in the latter, if anything, children move away from it, spending their days and much of their spare time among their peers.

Early care and education

Early child care through nursery schools, day-care centres and kindergartens is growing everywhere, though no country yet authorizes and provides early care for *all* its children. A child usually attends one of these facilities from three, or three-and-a-half, until school age. Child care before the age of three is expensive and, where it is available, not all parents find it acceptable. In no country do more than 10–15 per cent of all children attend such facilities.

Care for the under-threes: loss or gain

It has been argued, notably by the British psychoanalyst John Bowlby, that infants under three who are cared for outside the home

Nursery school children are sometimes introduced to the more formal skills that will provide the basis of later education, but activities are usually arranged within a broad understanding of educational value. Creativity of thought and action is encouraged in these formative years.

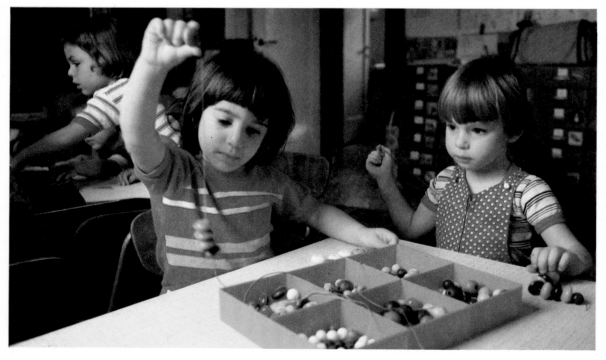

may suffer because of the separation from their mothers. Not surprisingly, some people have concluded from Bowlby's work that children should not be subjected to day care before the age of three because of the parental separation it entails. There are several arguments against such a conclusion.

Firstly, Bowlby's theory about the effects of early separation was based on observation of delinquents, many of whom had apparently suffered early "maternal deprivation". They had also, however, suffered other deprivations to which Bowlby paid less attention. Bowlby, of course, did not see those children who had been separated from their mothers, for long or short periods, and who had emerged unscathed from the experience.

Secondly, common sense tells us that day care would not be so widespread today if parents, caretakers or paediatricians found that children had problems with it. Thirdly, in the last decade, there have been a number of careful American studies of children in day care. They have uniformly reported that the experience has a neutral or slightly positive effect on children's development.

Whatever the long-term effects, parents sometimes find the immediate effects difficult to deal with. Children under three are likely to protest at leaving their parents and show unhappiness. At the age of three-and-a-half, almost all children find the transition to nursery school easy, and this is undoubtedly why more and more parents make use of child care at this time.

The pre-school experience

The most common reason for the use of nursery schools is to provide social support for the parents and the child. With families living in cities and with women working, nursery schools provide an attractive environment for children during the day.

A very secondary reason until now for putting children into nursery school has been to provide them with formal training or education. In the broadest sense of the term, of course, *any* absorbing experience the child has—with other children, with games, toys, clay or paints—is educational. All nursery schools provide an informal educational environment, and most of them stress the need to give breadth to a child's experience.

Formal pre-school education may be said to exist when specific and stated changes in children are sought through training. In the United States, the nursery school has traditionally been a place where children engage in free play in an environment that is friendly and undemanding, but encouraging. The Soviet Union has a formal kindergarten curriculum, but there are probably wide variations in the extent to which it is followed in different parts of the country. Other countries (Belgium, France, the Netherlands, Sweden) have nationally organized systems, but not national curricula. West Germany specifies goals nationally, and the regions are responsible for their implementation. Italy and the United Kingdom do not have centrally directed systems. There is, in short, no international consensus that formal pre-school education ought to exist, that children's development ought to be turned or modified in specified directions before they enter formal schooling.

This is quite in contrast with elementary school education, of which all modern countries have similar expectations. Everyone

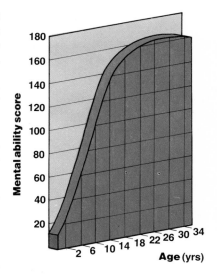

The growth curve of intelligence based on a large-scale longitudinal study which followed the same individuals from birth to age 36. Mental ability increased up to age 26, then it levelled off and remained unchanged. It should be remembered that this is an average so some people may well show an increase after 26.

agrees that children in primary schools should learn how to read, write and do arithmetic. Any debate is about *means*, not ends, or else it is about what the elementary grades should include over and above the basics.

When it comes to pre-school education, there are no generally accepted "basics". Debates are about *ends*, not means. Should pre-school education be formal? Who is to have it? What kind of changes in a child should one try to bring about? Formal pre-school education could aim at one or more of the goals outlined below.

Speeding up the development of thought

Whether or not Piaget's ideas are used as a basis for activities, the assumptions embedded in this approach are that there is one main line of development for children, that it is useful to think of differences among children as due to their having reached different points along that line and that it is beneficial to accelerate children's progress. At the High/Scope Foundation in Ypsilanti, Michigan, the curriculum put together by David Weikart and his associates is an example of a plan specifically designed to speed up the course of a child's cognitive development.

Teaching specific skills

Two psychologists, Carl Bereiter and Siegfried Engelmann, developed in the early 1960s a curriculum for nursery-school children. It focused specifically on the skills needed for successful performance in later school work. Their approach, which was based on the belief that nursery schools cannot offer the disadvantaged child the varied stimulation of a middle-class home, achieved some success.

Raising IQ

It is questionable whether any nursery school has ever accepted raising IQ as its basic purpose. Nevertheless, in the United States this goal has been much discussed for educational pre-schools as a group. In the early 1960s, when a child's IQ score was taken as an index of his or her destiny, two writers, J. McV. Hunt and Benjamin Bloom, argued that IQ is modifiable in infancy and "hardens" later. A pre-school, it seemed, might perhaps change a child's destiny. But since then there has been growing scepticism as to whether the IQ score is a fair statement of children's intelligence, much less their destiny.

Increasing attention and self-directedness

In 1907 in Italy, Maria Montessori established her "children's houses" for three- to seven-year-old children from slum tenements in Rome. Her curriculum was carefully organized and skill-oriented, not unlike that of Bereiter and Engelmann. Montessori's children did sensory exercises, carried out practical activities such as sewing or table-setting and received training in reading and writing. Montessori was shrewd at observing children and inventive at devising techniques. But her greatest strength, probably, was that she saw the social design of her children's houses as a form of curriculum. Children lived in a free and mobile environment. With their training routines, teachers helped children to sustain their own attention and action.

The modern approach that most resembles that of Montessori is that of the American Bank Street College of Education. The Bank

---

The development of children's art
Rhoda Kellogg in 1970 identified four distinct stages—placement, shape, design and pictorial—in the development of children's art.
Placement *(up to 2½):
experiment with placing and organizing scribbles.* **Shape** *(2½–3): circles, rectangles, etc.*
Design *(3–4): combined lines and shapes.* **Pictorial** *(4–5): houses, animals and people.*

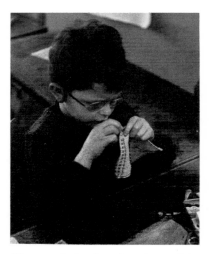

The practical value of sewing and the mental and manual organization it requires are often overlooked in the traditional notion that it is an activity for girls, not for boys. Though many educationalists recognize the need to ignore or combat such social stereotyping, it usually becomes reinforced at a later stage by differentiation at school, college and work.

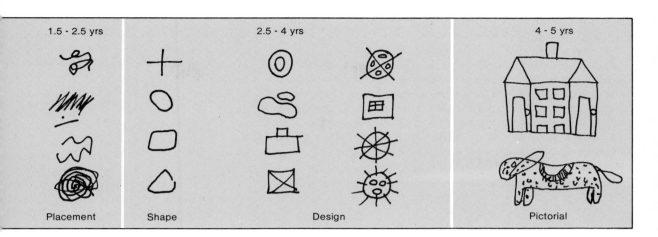

1.5 - 2.5 yrs	2.5 - 4 yrs	4 - 5 yrs
Placement	Shape	Design	Pictorial

Street teacher allows the children to select their own activities. She then moves in with highly structured training routines intended to support the children in elaborating their own activities. Bank Street uses very different teaching and psychological concepts from Montessori. Nevertheless, it sustains her important idea that the medium is part of the message of early education.

Ready for school?

Industrialized societies know how old a child is and put him or her in school promptly at the legal age. Non-industrialized societies often do not know how old a child is. When the British set up schools in colonial Africa, one of the methods used to judge whether children were ready for school was to ask them to reach their right arm over their head and touch their left ear. If the children could reach their ears, they were old enough for school. The method depends on the fact that very young children's heads are large in relation to their bodies and the bodies catch up as the children grow.

Testing "readiness"

American schools today often use what are called "readiness tests" to decide whether a child is fit for conventional schooling. However, the tests pose certain serious problems. Firstly, they are not very good at predicting how a child will perform in the future. Secondly, they constitute one of those instances, all too common in the case of children, where adults make a "diagnosis" without being sure they have a treatment. Reading tests generally assume that schooling ought to be slowed down for immature children. Yet schooling today is rather strictly paced. Standardized national achievement tests, standardized curricula in elementary schools, parents' expectations, slowly built up around tests and curricula—all these act to determine far too strictly what to expect from children year by year. If children get off the train and walk for a while, they have real trouble catching up again.

A third problem with readiness tests is that they are developed to detect a hypothetical maturity whose form is unknown. It is not too hard to guess that a child who is visibly growing on the outside must be changing on the inside. It is quite another thing to estimate what

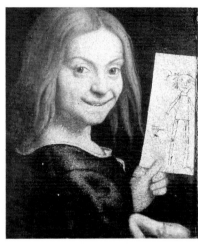

Children's art has not changed over the centuries. This lively portrait of a small boy showing off his handiwork was painted by the sixteenth-century Italian painter G. F. Caroto.

those internal changes are and what they imply for the child's learning.

Current tests are generally based on the assumption that "reading readiness" depends on perceptual and intellectual skills. But they do not all test the same range of abilities. Each test is divided into subtests, and each subtest tests a specific ability (for example, auditory discrimination, following directions, copying or giving the names of letters). These subtests are even poorer than the tests as a whole at predicting ability, so that extreme caution should be exercised in making judgements based on them.

Biological changes

Children's mental development goes hand-in-hand with the biological process of *maturation*. It would be an oversimplification to say that these biological changes *cause* the changes we can observe in children's cognitive skills. There is good reason to believe that the amount of environmental stimulation which children receive, the challenges they face, can affect the nature and amount of biological change, which in turn allows further behavioural development.

Brain structure

One index of physical maturation is *myelinization*, the process whereby certain nerve fibres become sheathed in myelin, a grey, fatty substance. The study of myelinization in the brains of deceased children has made it possible to estimate how fast different areas of a child's brain develop. Myelinization is important because myelin, which covers only the nerves of the human "higher" brain centres, is known to speed up the rate at which messages are transmitted along these nerves. At birth, myelinization is incomplete. It advances rapidly during the first few months of life, but is still taking place in several areas of the brain at the age of 10 and may even be detectable as late as 30. What is interesting is where in the brain myelinization is found.

In the years 6 to 10, myelinization of the corpus callosum is completed. The corpus callosum is a major bridge of nerve fibres connecting the right hemisphere of the brain with the left. In the 1970s, many claims were made about the different functions of the left and right hemispheres of the brain. The left hemisphere was claimed to be responsible for logical and analytical thinking and for any ability, including language, which depends on linear sequences. The right hemisphere was claimed to govern spatial and geometric abilities—anything which deals with patterns rather than an orderly succession of items. In fact, the evidence for this differentiation of functions between left and right hemispheres is much weaker than many over-enthusiastic writers would have us believe. It is still impossible for us to draw any conclusions about what changes in children's behaviour we would expect from the myelinization of the corpus callosum.

Between the ages of 6 and 10, myelinization is generally also completed in the parietal and frontal areas of a child's cortex (outer layer of the brain). If you look at a child's right ear and imagine a line running straight north, and another north-west, then the right parietal lobe is the area of the surface of the brain between those lines. The left is the equivalent area on the other side. The frontal cortex is the area situated between the north lines and the forehead. It appears to be implicated in the planning and execution of behaviour sequences and in the control of extraneous behaviour.

David Rose of Tufts University believes there is a link between the frontal cortex and the hippocampus in children which is completed at the age of about four-and-a-half. The hippocampus is part of the limbic system, which seems to be connected with the feeling and expression of emotion. Studies of the hippocampus in animals have suggested that its maturation plays a role in bringing an end to "juvenility", the free and frisky behaviour generally found in young animals and in ushering in the more sober, staid behaviour of the adult. We have no way of knowing if the same is true of humans. But it may be that the link between the frontal cortex and the hippocampus which David Rose has studied is involved in the changes in young children's memories and in their increasing ability to control their impulses.

Brain waves

Brain waves are detected from the electrical activity on the scalp and are measured in frequencies (cycles per second). Frequencies vary according to the activity being undertaken. For instance, people will have much faster (higher frequency) brain waves when they are solving a problem than when they are asleep. What interests us is that the faster frequencies appear more and more often in children up to adolescence and are probably associated with the characteristic speeding-up of their reactions. Some theorists believe that when it comes to

The problem of learning to throw a ball accurately is neatly sidestepped when the ball is almost as big as oneself. But this illustrates the different stages of physical competence. A young child will grasp with the arm and whole hand while an older child gains control of smaller muscles in the wrist and fingers.

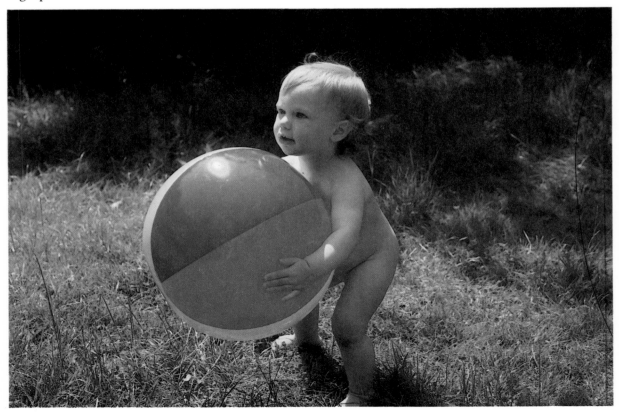

children's thinking processes, speed equals power—that is, the ability to calculate rapidly determines the complexity of the problems they can deal with.

Control of fine muscles

One particular maturational feature is more conspicuous than those we have dealt with so far. Nursery-school children as a group are slightly awkward in their movements, which is one reason why they tend to be accident-prone. Children of elementary school age are much more competent with their bodies. This change in physical competence has been attributed to the fact that neuromuscular development progresses from the trunk outwards to the limbs and finally to the hands and feet. Most nursery-school children do not throw a ball very well, because they use only the large arm and shoulder muscle, and do not involve the smaller muscles controlling the wrist and fingers. School-age children are able to coordinate their musculature more completely and may take an active part in sports. They improve all the way to adolescence, becoming quicker and better coordinated as well as stronger.

Reading and writing call for many precise movements of fine muscles, including those of the eye. In recognition of their limited abilities, children are given small quantities of large type to read in their first years at school, and when they write they print in large letters.

Soft signs

The term "soft sign" comes to us from neurology. It refers to an odd behaviour or reaction pattern that is not quite clear enough to point to a recognizable neurological disorder—in which case it would be a "hard sign"—but which may indicate trouble somewhere. All children show a high incidence of soft signs in the nursery-school years, because of the immaturity of their nervous systems.

Ask a nursery-school child to hold both hands in front, palms down, and to spread the third and fourth fingers of his left hand away from the rest, and he will often spread the fingers of his right hand as well. Ask a child to bend her ankles and walk on the outer edges of her feet, and she will often arch her wrists and hold her hands in imitation of her feet as she does so. These are "associated" or "reflected" movements, a kind of soft sign. The children do something on the left side and unconsciously echo it on the right side or they echo with the upper part of their bodies something they are doing with their lower limbs. All young children exhibit soft signs, the incidence of which declines as they grow older. But a high incidence may be associated with learning problems in the early years at school.

Early learning disability

An enormous amount has been written about the problem of "learning disability" in the early school years, and the reviews express severe scholarly frustration. How common is the problem? Reasonably informed sources have estimated the incidence as anywhere between 2 per cent and 40 per cent. Standards adopted in applying the label vary, although it is usually applied when children have obvious problems in making headway in the lower classes. Some authorities apply the label only when there are some soft signs of neurological

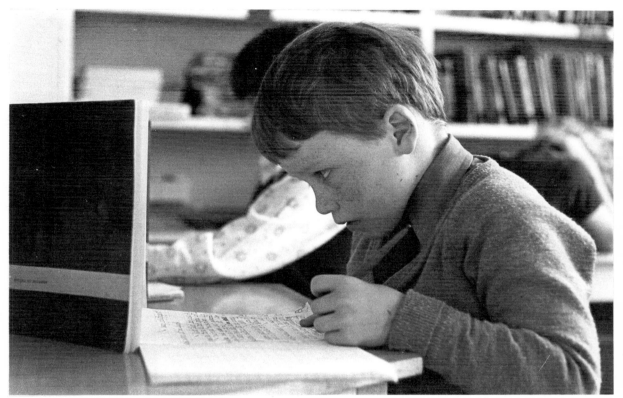

problems—clumsiness or uncoordination, tremors, twitchiness, pathological reflexes or brainwave abnormalities—any of which may be linked with reading difficulties. The incidence goes downwards, towards 2 per cent, when this kind of standard is applied.

However, one cannot draw a line separating the children whose reading problems are neurologically based from those whose problems are clearly not neurological. Recognizing this, some have argued that learning disability should be defined simply as poor reading. If one approaches the problem this way, the incidence rockets towards 40 per cent.

Rapid acquisition of the skills of reading and writing is the major goal of education in all industrial societies. For some children the task is easily mastered; for others, learning to recognize and form the words and letters is an obstacle that limits their communicative powers.

What's in a name?

If the estimates of the incidence of learning problems vary, so too do the labels used—learning disability, reading disability, educational handicap, hyperactivity, minimal brain damage, minimal brain dysfunction, perceptual disability, attention deficit syndrome, dyslexia and many others. These labels tend to give a spurious impression of being informative, when in fact some of them are simply statements of the problem and other unvalidated inferences—the term minimal brain damage, for example, is applied to children who show no real evidence of brain damage, the term "minimal" signifying that the hypothetical damage cannot be detected. And since various school systems and treatment services couch their regulations in different terms, a child may have to be labelled "educationally handicapped" in one place or "minimally brain damaged" in another before he or she can qualify for help.

The first day at school

To enter the adult world, children have first to learn simple forms of conventions and routines which, as adults, they will have to live within. The first day at school is a step into a life in which demands will be placed and responsibilities incurred, and in which others will be competing for attention and consideration. Of course, pre-school children experience discipline within the family—but the scheduling is likely to be less rigid, more tailored to their individual needs than the school environment—however open.

With the first day at school, too, comes the beginning of a lifelong process of being classified and labelled. Children become aware of the differences between themselves and others of the same age. Like the adults around them, children find themselves judging their own behaviour and abilities. They become aware that other children are more, or less, skilled than themselves at different tasks expected of them. These first experiences of self-awareness, judgement of oneself and others, and of conflicting priorities, form a pattern for the increasingly complex and subtle experiences to come.

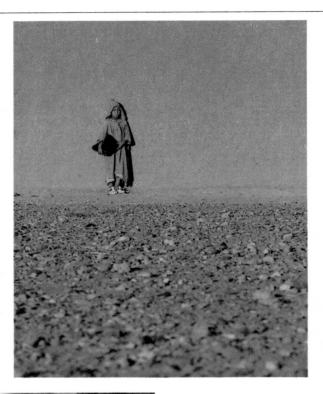

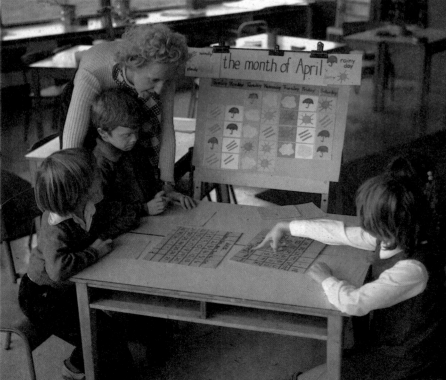

A Moroccan schoolboy faces a different routine from that prepared for his English counterpart—but for either, is going to school likely to be a challenging adventure or an occasion for anxiety and isolation?

Attention and sympathy are the expectations of many children still accustomed to full-time parental care. They must learn to share a teacher's attention and to make reasonable demands. Later, as lessons become more impersonal, some children suffer from being unable to make their needs properly understood.

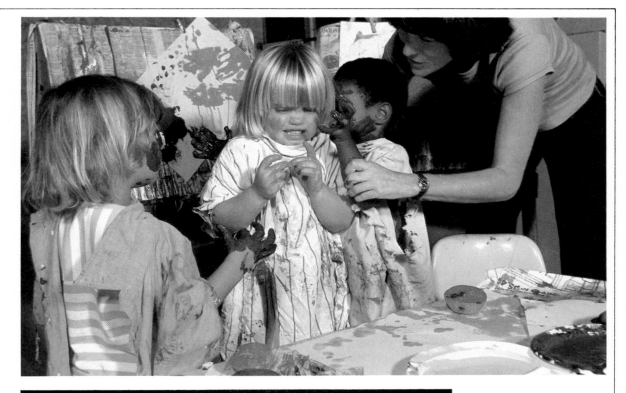

Painting is fun—or is it? For some children school is their first encounter with group activities, with the idea of performing a task in front of an audience, and with concepts of success or failure.

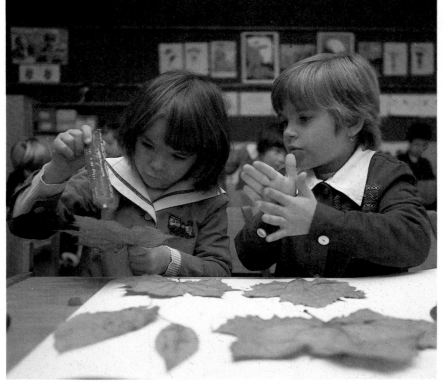

Some childhood interests seem common to societies and cultures. In Budapest, as elsewhere, leaves are a decorative natural resource for educational play.

Who has learning problems?

Firstly, some children have severe neurological problems of a kind that may lead them to have chronic problems with reading and writing for the rest of their lives. The incidence of such children is probably low, of the order of one to two per cent. Secondly, most children with learning problems have probably not yet learned a number of prerequisite skills—their language development may be poor, their attention span very short, their motor coordination very poor. Thirdly, children with sensory deficits, especially if these are undetected, may have learning problems. Finally, a school may uncritically pronounce, say, a Spanish-speaking or West Indian child as having a "learning disability" because he or she gets swept into the category by some test. Or it may knowingly pronounce them so, realizing that they need individual teaching and that this label entitles them to special resources.

The structure of schooling

It is notable that all the labels applied to children who have learning problems in their early school years locate the source of the problem within the child. And yet if we take the figure of 40 per cent of children being "learning disabled" as having some validity, then we are faced with the conclusion that almost half the early school population have something "wrong" with them which requires special "treatment". Can this really be the case? Perhaps we should turn the problem on its head and ask not whether this child is ready for school, or reading, or whatever, but "Is the school ready for the child?"

Margaret Donaldson, a developmental psychologist from Edinburgh University, relates the following story from the British writer Laurie Lee:

> I spent that first day picking holes in paper, then went home in a smouldering temper.
>> "What's the matter, love, didn't he like it at school, then?"
>> "They never gave me the present."
>> "Present? What present?"
>> "They said they'd give me a present."
>> "Well, now, I'm sure they didn't."
>> "They did. They said: 'You're Laurie Lee, aren't you? Well just you sit there for the present.' I sat there all day but I never got it. I ain't going back there again."

We find this and similar tales amusing, but, as Donaldson points out, they have more serious undertones. The teacher was behaving in a manner which Piaget had led us to expect only of young children—she was being egocentric.

It was emphasized in "Infancy" that children's learning of cognitive skills, of language, occurs within a social context. The school environment can in part be seen as the removal of this social context. To be an educational success, the child must learn to turn language and thought in upon themselves, to think about words and mathematical symbols quite independently of the context in which they occur. This reflecting on words as words, rather than as vocalizations in social contexts, is not a feature of most children's experience. It has, in fact, been shown that many five-year-olds have

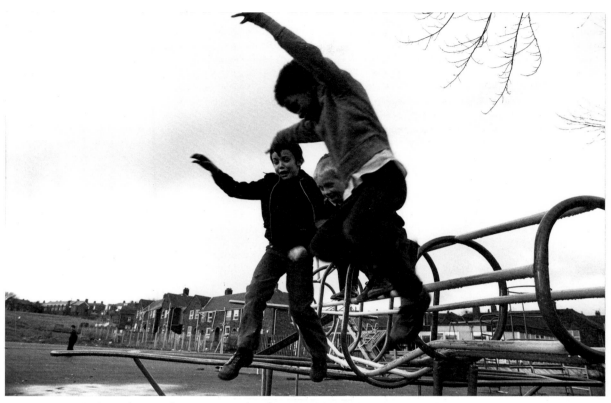

very confused ideas about what is meant by the word "word". And yet, at school, children are suddenly confronted with the necessity of dealing with words as abstract entities.

Worse, no one may explain to children exactly why they are having to perform this mammoth task. The advantages of reading and mathematical skills are so obvious to adults that, in our egocentrism, we may fail to inform children of them. They are left to find out for themselves—perhaps when reading is no longer part of the curriculum.

How many adults would happily take on an extremely difficult learning task with no idea of what they were doing it *for*? One study showed that some children, even after three or four months in school, cannot say how the postman knows which house to bring a letter to, or how their mothers know which bus to take.

Another way in which school curricula may fail to take the child's perspective into account is in the adoption of certain teaching schemes or methods based on unproven assumptions about children's abilities, or lack of them. We have seen that the adoption of some of Piaget's ideas by educationalists is an example of this. Other examples are provided by the introduction of certain methods of teaching reading.

One of these, commonly called the "look and say" method, involves getting children to repeat words printed on large flashcards. When they can do this proficiently, it is believed they can then read the words in sentences from their reading books. This method is based on the assumption that children read by recognizing the shape of a word. There is, in fact, no evidence for this: the assumption was made because *adults* can easily recognize words from their shape. This

As children become accustomed to working and playing in groups, the mutual encouragement can lead to more adventurousness and confidence. Quite naturally, simple pleasures are more fun when someone else watches and joins in.

scheme further assumes that children find it very difficult to make fine discriminations between different written words, so that children should be presented initially with words which differ widely in shape. Thus, a five-year-old might quickly be able to read the sentence, "The hippopotamus stole my umbrella," but not "The cat, the bat and the rat sat on the mat."

However, not only is there no evidence that children find it very difficult to make fine discriminations, there *is* evidence that the use of words widely different in shape actually discourages children from developing true reading skills, which require the close analysis of individual letters.

Another example of a scheme no longer used in schools which made *a priori* assumptions about children's abilities was that based on the Initial Teaching Alphabet (ITA). This scheme assumed that the complicated phonetic structure of the English language creates difficulties for children learning to read. It therefore presented children with a simplified and elaborated alphabet, where each phoneme had its own written symbol. It was claimed that children learned to read very quickly using this method. They could, of course, read only specialized books and nothing else. They also had to unlearn what they had learned and cope eventually with the complexity of written English. It is not surprising that some children found this transition very difficult (did anyone tell them *why* they had to unlearn what they had learned?).

Adult misconceptions about learning

Both of these approaches are based on the superficially valid assumption that the tasks facing the new schoolchildren should be made as simple as possible and that errors should be reduced to a minimum. There are two problems with these assumptions. One is that "simplicity" is defined from an adult point of view and, as we have seen, may be based on false ideas of children's abilities. The second is that the idea that errors are a "bad thing" is also an adult notion. Indeed, it is not unreasonable to suggest, at least as far as early school learning is concerned, that errors are only a bad thing for a child because adults say they are and make a fuss about them.

Margaret Donaldson has suggested, contrary to this view, that error can play a highly constructive role in the development of cognitive skills. She points out the widely held belief that children must not be told the complexities of, for example, the phonetic system, to begin with, because they could not cope with such complexities. She suggests that what underlies this mistaken assumption is the failure to distinguish between understanding the nature of a system and mastering all the individual patterns of relationship. Children will obviously take many years to master the intricacies of the system. The question is simply whether they will do this more successfully if they are correctly informed of what to expect.

In practice, many teachers will use a variety of schemes to help children learn to read and, when failures occur, will explore any possibility which seems to work. This would seem to be the best approach, as it is extremely unlikely that any one scheme will suit the needs of all children. The point here, however, is that educational, even non-traditional educational *theories* are still largely adult-centred. Is it then fair to regard children as having a problem when they cannot cope?

There are two possible solutions to this problem. One is for educators and psychologists to become more aware of the extent to which educational methods are based on assumptions, as yet unproven, about how children learn. On the other hand, there is now a voluminous literature on the psychology of learning which has never been widely applied in the classroom. Programmed instruction, for example, is based on tried and tested principles of learning, but it has not found favour in many classrooms partly because of the (unproven) belief that it might damage the relationship between teacher and child.

A second solution, of more relevance to the day-to-day business of home and classroom, is for parents and teachers to encourage a child to state how he sees the problem, to say what he does *not* know or understand, rather than, as usual, what he does know. It has been shown that pre-school children rarely ask for clarifying information when they are given an inadequate message. However, it is only by finding out how the problem looks from where the child (and not the adult) is standing, what difficulties it presents to him or her, that we can begin to build up an educational system that is truly child-centred that is of true benefit to the child.

Refusing to go to school

At one time or another, most schoolchildren invent excuses which will keep them away from school, or exaggerate small illnesses to get an extra few days at home. A small number of children, however, do this so often that they miss large amounts of schooling or, finally, do not attend at all. It may be some time before parents realize what is going on; indeed the idea that there are certain children who could be called "school refusers" or "school phobic" is itself a relatively recent one.

One of the first writers about school refusal described the problem in these terms:

> The child is absent from school for periods varying from several months to a year. The absence is consistent. At all times the parents know where the child is. It is with the mother or near the home. The reason for the truancy is incomprehensible to the parents and the school. The child may say that it is afraid to go to school, afraid of the teacher or say that it does not know why it will not go to school. When at home it is happy and apparently carefree. When dragged to school it is miserable, fearful and at the first opportunity runs home despite the certainty of corporal punishment. The onset is generally sudden. The previous school work and conduct had been fair.

In the last 30 years, some of the details of this problem have been filled out, but the broad outline described above remains valid. It is difficult to determine the scope of the problem, but the Isle of Wight study described on page 88 estimated it to be present in about three per cent of all children with some kind of psychological problem. Several American studies have noted that black children rarely figure among school refusers and a British study noted the same about West Indian children living in London. It is still not clear why this should be the case.

In order for a child to establish a pattern of school refusal and remain at home, it is obvious that the mother or father, usually the

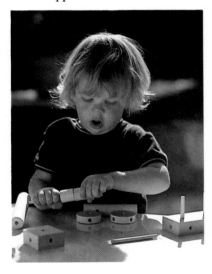

An enjoyable game can also provide a means of measuring dexterity and perceptual skills, but too often tests assume a particular 'correct' method of problem-solving that inhibits understanding of an individual child's mental approach.

mother, must cooperate. This may be done actively—by rewarding the child for staying at home with play, attention and so on, by reassuring the child that he does not have to return to school until he is "ready", or even by making arrangements for home tuition. Or the cooperation may be passive, as in the mother who is genuinely concerned about the problem, who attempts to take the child to school or tries to persuade him to go but who, in the end, gives way and allows him to stay at home. The child, of course, may be able to bring considerable pressure to bear and it is often difficult for a mother to resist her child's obvious distress.

Help for school refusers

Successful intervention must also involve the home and school. It is important to establish, first of all, what factors in the school might make the child reluctant to attend and secondly, what factors in the home are encouraging non-attendance. In different children, the balance between these two elements will vary. Information about the school can be obtained from the teacher, the parents, the children themselves or even classmates. Problems which often come to light include difficulties with schoolwork, lack of friends among class-mates, teasing or bullying. These last are related. Children who are teased or bullied are also likely to lack friends. Whether they remain friendless or become victims of bullying will depend on factors connected with the school rather than with the children. It may be that problems at school can be alleviated by cooperation between teachers and parents; it may be that the children need help in learning the skills of making friends, or it may be that a change of school is necessary.

Even if these factors can be dealt with, it is usually still necessary to help such children overcome the considerable amount of anxiety which will now be connected with attending school. This may be done by teaching the children to relax, by encouraging them to rehearse in their mind what will happen at school until they can do this without fear, or by gradually re-exposing them to the school situation by, for example, travelling increasingly close to the school each day, standing at the school gates or attending school for longer and longer periods of time each day. In any case, the class teacher will have the major responsibility of coping with a child's reappearance in the classroom. Some therapists introduce external rewards for school attendance (or gradual approximations to it), such as outings, books or toys, but these are usually withdrawn as soon as the child has settled down at school, although verbal praise and encouragement will continue. All therapists emphasize, however, that an important part of the intervention is to convey to the children that, in the end, they simply must reattend school. This may be particularly difficult to do if, for example, a mother has been in the habit of taking her child to school, but allowing him to return home in the middle of the day.

The function of school is not only an educative one in the academic sense, important though this is. It is also where most children make their friends and learn other skills such as sport, drama or music which they are unlikely to learn at home. Children who are afraid to attend school, and spend most of their time at home with their mothers, will miss all this and will also develop a negative attitude to dealing with life's problems—which is likely to cause them further difficulties as they grow up.

Measuring IQ

At some point in their school career, many children will find themselves at the receiving end of an "intelligence test". Some of the basic ideas in IQ testing come out of a "measuring scale of intelligence" put together by Frenchmen Alfred Binet, a psychologist, and Théophile Simon, a psychiatrist, in 1905. Their test has had a large influence, for better or worse, on the way in which we now think about human intelligence (although, in fairness, we do not know that the two authors would have wholeheartedly endorsed many of the ideas that were built up around their measuring scale).

Binet and Simon designed their test at the behest of the French Government to provide a uniform and objective method for screening out poor learners ("subnormals") in schools. From that day to this, many people have identified intelligence, ability or merit in children solely with the ability to perform well at school.

What is IQ?

IQ, or intelligence quotient, is derived from the following:

$$IQ = \frac{\text{mental age}}{\text{chronological age}} \times 100$$

Consistency of performance

There is much evidence that IQ depends a good deal on what is going on around him or her. When the environment changes, the IQ is likely to change too. Often if we look at the lives of children whose IQs have shown a change, we can find events that may account for it.

What's wrong with IQ tests?

In the last decade, some American states and cities have placed formal restrictions on the use of IQ tests. They claim, for example, that the tests are not even-handed in their assignment of IQ scores to children of different cultural backgrounds. This is because the sample on which the test was standardized (on which the average performance was worked out) may be very different from that on which the test is used. And because performance on the test may be influenced by familiarity with certain things and ideas which may be commonplace in one culture but not in another, the tests cannot be applied outside the range of their standardization sample.

The many faces of intelligence

Paradoxically, IQ tests have contributed evidence against one of the assumptions that launched them: that there is one generalized human talent determining how well a child does in a range of tasks. It now seems likely that human "intelligence", even that restricted portion of it that applies to performance at school, is not one grand talent. On IQ tests, certain items tend to cluster together: a child who does well on one item of the cluster will tend to do well on the others.

A number of educational reformers have argued forcefully that traditional mental tests and school practices favour the verbally gifted child. Children with visual and spatial skills are passed over in schools, it is said, and all children are somewhat deprived of opportunities to develop visually-based forms of reasoning which might greatly benefit them as individuals and society as a whole.

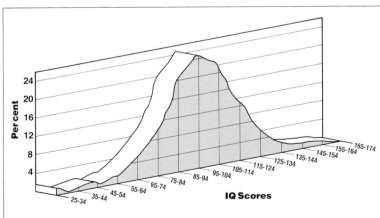

Distribution of IQs

IQ (intelligence quotient) tests have been the subject of increasing doubts in recent years. But children are still likely to meet them during their school careers. The tests are devised so that the average IQ score for any age is 100. A higher IQ indicates that a child is able to answer questions that on average only older children answer correctly.

Coping with children's problems

Social progress

Part of the historical development of modern societies, an admirable part, has been the growth of a humane attitude towards children, accompanied by the growth of facilities to help children in trouble. Yet we tend to take our modern state of affairs for granted and even to complain about how difficult it is to feel secure in raising children nowadays. A glance at recent history affords a certain perspective and optimism.

In 1918, an American committee reviewed what it regarded as the most important things that had been accomplished on behalf of children in the nineteenth century. With minor variations, this list of achievements would serve for most modern countries. In the last century, institutions were set up for groups of disadvantaged children—orphans, the deaf, the physically or mentally handicapped—who at the beginning of the century would have been found in the poorhouse, in jail or on the street. These children were now brought under the care of statutory bodies. The legal system acknowledged juveniles' need for special legal provisions, including probation and separate detention facilities from adults. Societies were established for the prevention of cruelty to children. School attendance began to be made compulsory, and legislation governing child labour made its first appearance.

No cause for complacency

We have done much, then, to prevent the lives of many children from being thown away. But it would be a mistake to believe that the risks to children pinpointed during the nineteenth century have now all been dealt with adequately. Today, children do not starve or roam the streets homeless. Private or public agencies offer children who have no family an institutional home, adoption or foster care. Abuse and neglect are still significant problems, however. In the United States, about 64 000 cases of child abuse are reported per year, of which 30 000 are cases of incest or other sexual abuse. The damage to a child may be considerable—or lethal—by the time it is reported. Until very recently, an official response could be triggered only *after* a child was reported battered, misused or starved, and it is probable that many cases were and are not reported.

Handicap: the English experience

In 1970, British researchers Michael Rutter, Jack Tizard and Kingsley Whitmore reported on an unusually well conducted survey of treated and untreated children's handicaps on the Isle of Wight, a small island off southern England. At the time the Isle of Wight had a population just short of 100 000 and a social composition reasonably representative of that of England as a whole. All the eight-, nine- and ten-year-old children on the island were canvassed: 3468 in all.

The study revealed an incidence of 7.9 per cent for educational handicap, 2.6 per cent for intellectual retardation, 5.5 per cent for chronic physical handicap and 5.4 per cent for serious psychological problems. A total of 16.1 per cent of the children surveyed were found to have problems in one or more of these areas. Although the Isle of

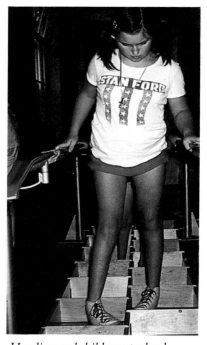

Handicapped children at school. Special educational units have been set up in many schools so that children with mental and physical problems can be taught in the same kind of environment as most other children. Dividing off all children with one specific problem into 'special' schools is a system which is now seen to lack many important factors necessary for the children's development, particularly their social integration. Much still remains to be done to ease the difficulties faced by handicapped children and their parents.

Wight was comparatively well endowed with facilities for assistance to children, the survey provided evidence that these services did not reach all the children in need of them. Two-thirds of those with intellectual or educational handicaps were receiving no remedial help at school. Nine-tenths of those with psychological problems were receiving no professional help. All children with physical handicaps were receiving medical treatment, but 29 per cent of those with physical problems had clear educational and psychological problems associated with their disorder. Help for these secondary problems was not available to the children or their families.

Institutions are not enough

The institutions of nineteenth-century London fulfilled a basic need in the community as places of peace and order for orphans—to save lives that were otherwise doomed. Nowadays, merely keeping infants safe and alive in an institution is not enough. Without stimulation, children show poor perceptual and cognitive development. Without close human relationships, they show a distressing tendency to turn into disturbed, unhappy or anti-social adults.

In the nineteenth century, people could point with justifiable pride to the many new institutions. Those institutions had a positive function when they first came into being, singling out children's problems—deafness, blindness, retardation—and trying to deal with each of them appropriately. Now modern societies are moving a step further. Still committed to recognizing and treating each child as an individual, they are trying as far as possible to keep the child in the everyday world that all children experience. Efforts are made to keep children in ordinary, rather than special, classes at school for as much of the day as possible. In England and Wales, the Education Act of 1981 obliges ordinary schools to take in some handicapped pupils if facilities are available. Foster homes and adoption are used in preference to orphanages. Physically or mentally handicapped children are helped at home, if possible.

Why this kind of doubling back on a historical trend, from putting children in institutions to keeping them out? Having begun by tending to children's physical needs and their need of special training, societies have become more and more sensitive to their psychological needs.

Freud's theory of development

At the end of the last century, Freud presented society with a view of childhood quite at variance with traditional conceptions. He depicted children as confronting a central dilemma of human psychology—that of finding harmony between competing inner wishes and drives. Freud pictured the eternal antagonists of psychic life as the biological drives (the id) versus knowledge of practical necessity (the ego) versus the person's perception of what society/authority asks of him or her (the superego). For Freud, the most important biological drive was sexual. The main sources of sexual gratification, he claimed, changed throughout infancy and childhood from the mouth (the oral stage) to the anus (anal stage) to the genitals (genital stage). "Traumatic" experiences at any of these stages would leave a person "fixated" so that his or her behaviour in adulthood could be accounted for in terms of his or her experiences at this point. Thus people who were

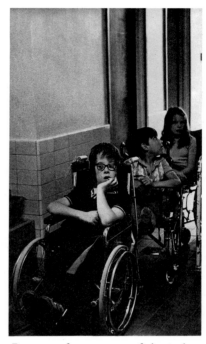

Resources for treatment of physical problems vary from one region to another. This child benefits from the facilities at an orthopaedic centre.

Trend	Examples of behaviour
Problems declining with age	Incontinence, speech problems, fears, thumb-sucking, overeating, tantrums, destructiveness
Problems increasing with age	Nail-biting
Problems declining and then increasing with age	Restless sleep, disturbing dreams, timidity, irritability, attention-seeking, dependence, jealousy, food fastidiousness (boys), sombreness
Problems increasing and then declining with age	Poor appetite, lying
Problems unrelated to age	Oversensitivity

Despite Freud's theories about the effects of childhood traumas on the adult, it seems that most childhood behaviour problems are not carried into adulthood. Each stage has its characteristic problems and the preoccupations of adolescence sooner or later replace those of childhood. This table shows five "developmental trends" in the expression of behavioural disorders in children, together with examples of behaviour typical of each trend.

excessively tidy would be said to be fixated at the anal stage, with its concerns for cleanliness through toilet training.

Freud saw both the infant and the child as being in danger of being overwhelmed by the anxiety generated by the conflict between id impulses and the forces of the superego. This anxiety was dealt with, he claimed, by an elaborate array of defence mechanisms which operated unconsciously. The mechanism to which Freud paid most attention was that of repression, whereby traumatic experiences, centring around id impulses, were made inaccessible to the conscious mind, but still retained the power to influence adult behaviour. Indeed, Freud saw *all* adult behaviour as being traceable to these early conflicts.

The weakness of Freud's theory
We owe a debt to Freud for calling attention to hitherto neglected psychological aspects of childhood and for his at times remarkable insights into the mental acrobatics which both children and adults perform in order to deal with anxiety. His theory, however, has many weaknesses which make it of questionable value. For the most part, Freud based his theory on the recollections (or his interpretations of the recollections) of adults. We now know that such recollections are unreliable.

Research studies have not produced convincing evidence of any relationship between the kinds of childhood experience to which Freud attached importance and adult behaviour. The importance of early experience seems to have been overplayed by Freud, which is probably just as well. Most of us would not like to think of ourselves as being at the mercy of far-off childhood experiences and unable to "grow" until we have come to terms with them. Freud underestimated the crucial role of a person's *present* environment in maintaining behaviour, whether adaptive or maladaptive.

The medical model
Freud was a physician, and throughout the time he was developing his theory he clung to the belief that, sometime or somehow, he would be

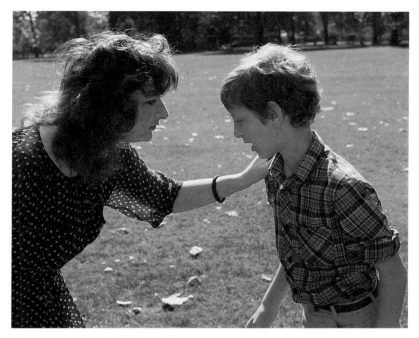

It may be difficult to deal with a persistently aggressive child, since such behaviour ultimately tends to elicit a response in kind. Parents and teachers face the problem of trying not to aggravate the child's aggression while at the same time restraining the adverse effects.

able to categorize all psychological problems within the kind of cause-and-effect framework that works so well for physical diseases. Problems would be found, on analysis, to fall into a finite number of distinct patterns of symptoms. Each unique cluster of symptoms, each *syndrome*, would be found to arise from a unique psychological source. A *taxonomy*, or classification of psychological disorders, would exist, with a cure for each disorder rationally related to its known cause.

Not only Freud, but many psychiatrists and psychologists after him, pursued this expectation. And so our terminology for children's (and adults') problems today still expresses a basic and unfounded assumption that they are like physical diseases or, indeed, that they *are*

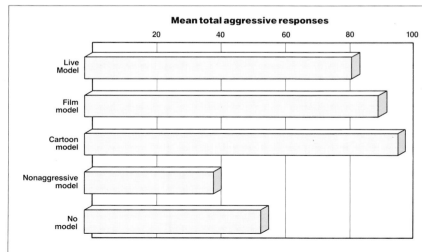

Mean total aggressive responses

Imitation of aggression
A series of experiments by Bandwa in 1973 has shown that children display more aggressive behaviour after observing aggressive models—either live or on film—as compared to nonaggressive models or no models at all. The film models (real-life and cartoon) elicited more aggressive responses, whereas the live model provoked more imitative aggressive acts.

How things can go wrong: case histories

Even children in a generally secure and happy environment are liable to suffer from psychological problems of one kind or another. Some of these problems, if not dealt with, may threaten the psychological health of the child, and, eventually, that of the adult.

In most cases, a child's psychological uneasiness can be dispelled by the adults surrounding him or her, such as parents or teachers. If they take a calm and sensitive approach to discovering the cause of the problem.

Tommy

Take the case of nine-year-old Tommy. He has been a consistently good student and happy among his classmates, but suddenly he turns listless and his work drops off. He is sullen and aggressive towards other children. Circumspect enquiry by the teacher reveals that his parents have agreed to get a divorce. The atmosphere in the home is extremely tense, with frequent rows between Tommy's parents. He is unsure about the future and scared that he will lose one of his parents. Underlying his stress is a suspicion that the break-up of his parents' marriage is somehow his fault.

Tommy's parents handle the situation reasonably well. They talk to him and tell him that he is in no way responsible for the divorce; they keep their arguments out of his hearing. They convince him that they will both continue to be an important part of his life. Tommy's teacher, on her part, adopts a policy of patience and discreet management. She does not pressure Tommy about his schoolwork. She arranges for him to work alone or in a peaceful atmosphere. Within three or four months, Tommy comes back to something like his old self in the classroom.

Carl

Carl is four years old. He is bitten by a dog and from then on shows a general fear of dogs. Not only is he afraid whenever there is a dog within sight, he is reluctant to go anywhere he thinks he might encounter a dog. He won't go with his parents to the supermarket, because there might be a dog in a car park and the dog might bark at him. He won't go to his grandmother's, because a large dog runs about in her neighbour's back garden. To try to counteract his fear, his parents buy a small, attractive puppy, which they put in a cage in the corner of Carl's playroom. At first he is a little nervous of going into the room, but eventually, drawn by his toys, he goes in and plays in the presence of the dog. In a day or so he seems reasonably calm and content and his parents bring the puppy, still in its cage, a little closer to where he plays. Within a week, Carl is happily playing with the puppy and, over the course of the next few months, his fear of dogs in general completely disappears.

Edna

Edna, who is in her first year at school, suddenly seems to be in capricious health. One day she complains of feeling sick and can't go to school. Next day she has a headache. Then she dawdles, finally getting out of the house 20 minutes late for school. Her mother starts a casual discussion and discovers that Edna is upset about school. She thinks that the teacher thinks she is stupid. *All* the other children in the class have been assigned a day to take care of the hamsters, Karen *twice*, and she hasn't even been asked *once*. A telephone conversation between her mother and the teacher soon sorts out the problem. Edna is given *her* day to look after the hamsters, and she quickly regains her good health.

These three problems are representative of the psychological problems all parents—and teachers—have to face with their children from time to time.

The psychologists' approach

Tommy's teacher, having become aware of his stress, set out to establish its cause. Once this had been done, his parents dealt with his concern about their divorce by addressing his specific fears, and his "fantasies" about the divorce itself and the part he might have played in it. They tried to change his perception of the situation which they knew he must face and adapt to.

Carl's parents dealt with his fear of dogs through a systematic training procedure that seemed to tackle the core of his growing fear of dogs. They used an approach known as counterconditioning, where mild experiences of fear were, in effect, progressively dampened by competition of stronger feelings of pleasure Carl felt as he played with his toys.

Edna's mother dealt with her daughter's problem by locating and correcting an environmental source of stress. The "situation" that had to be pinpointed in Edna's case was probably imperceptible to the adults around her—an oversight in her teacher's assignment of hamster care, strongly over-interpreted in the little girl's mind.

physical diseases. Words such as "diagnosis", "treatment", "psycho-pathology" and "psychotherapy" carry these assumptions into every-day discourse. Freud never found his taxonomy, nor has any later official body of psychologists or psychiatrists ever come up with a rigorous, universally acceptable classification of psychological dis-orders, although the search continues.

Calling in outside help

If parents routinely engage in successful psychotherapeutic activities, why does a child ever need a professional therapist? There are times when a child's difficulties exceed the resources and the time of the parents. Carl might have come to resemble a severely phobic child, beset by a hundred anxieties, virtually unable to leave the house. Tommy might have settled into a habitual posture of bitter antagon-ism towards school and classmates. Edna's early resistance to going to school might have crystallized into a classic "learning problem", a baffling inability to make any headway at school.

It is unfortunate but true that many of the problems seen by professionals are in part made worse by the parents themselves, sometimes with the best of intentions. It can seem cruel to expect a small and very distressed boy to confront something he is afraid of. And in the distress surrounding divorce, it can be difficult for the parents to step outside their own emotions and imagine how it all must seem to a child. If your child wets the bed every night, it can be difficult to remain calm and reasonable in the face of mountains of wet sheets, even if you know that getting angry only makes things worse. It is also interesting to note that parents seem more likely to seek professional help for their children at times when *they* are feeling depressed and unable to cope with what at another time might be seen as just a normal part of childhood.

And, on a hopeful note—studies of groups followed up over some years show that the majority of children who have problems of one sort or another do not carry them with them into adulthood.

The dilemma of growth

Fictional treatments may paint a picture of the beautiful child happily ensconced in the arms of a loving family. However, life for a child or a family is always marked by more light and shade than these mythical formulations. It is one function of the media to normalize, to set forth ideals, to picture things happening the way one would like them to happen just once. These images help keep things going. If we mix the truths of the happy stories with those of the unrelentingly catastrophic soap operas, we get a little closer to life as children and their families experience it. As Erik Erikson remarked, "Children 'fall apart' repeatedly and, unlike Humpty Dumpty, grow together again."

Finding harmony

Very early on in the process of development, a child starts to experience what an adult continually experiences. Life provides values and goals, standards and possibilities, which the child is moved to pursue. But life comes at the child not once, but several times, not from one direction, but many. The child confronts competing goals and purposes which pull in opposing directions, and must repeatedly find ways to harmonize them.

A custom in writing about children is to try to keep things direct and uncomplicated. To say that children are inevitably pulled by different value systems as they grow up is a little distressing. It makes development complicated. It says that there are problems that cannot be nicely and neatly "solved". It does not lead to a unitary list of goals and standards for the guidance of children. And it says to a parent or a teacher that his or her influence on a child will depend on the work or influence of others.

Yet this kind of view of children's development is realistic and does not have to be depressing. Adults manage competing demands on their time and attention all day long. Indeed, they may welcome them. The amount of time and attention we give to one thing always depends on how much we have to spare. We move from home to work to friends. We listen to competing political speeches. We are subjected to a barrage of major and minor exhortations from the media. Sympathetic to many of the claims upon us, we find our own balance between what we want to do and what various others would have us do.

The challenge of time-sharing

Watch a nine-year-old boy sitting in a classroom. Officially, of course, he is doing schoolwork. If he is not, he is being "inattentive". But children are attentive to something most of the time. Even a very able and motivated student will be found to be doing schoolwork only about 80 per cent of the time. Assigned a set of problems, children plough right into them. They pause after a while, rest and revive. Back to the problems. A few minutes later, one of their friends catches their eye. A little signalling and whispering about what to do after school. Back to the problems. A child across the room is asking the teacher something. They watch for a while, interested in the interchange. These children are doing something which in a modern computer we would call "time-sharing". They work back and forth among a number of concurrent plans or interests. Everyone does. The childrens' problem is to balance their intellectual interests, their social interests and their personal needs in the classroom. More gifted students seem able to strike that balance and take care of the business in hand. Less able students can be seen to devote large amounts of their time to social business, daydreaming, private diversions. Perhaps this is a cause, perhaps an effect of their problems with schoolwork.

Finding a reasonable harmony between the several interests that a child must necessarily pursue while continuing to grow and develop is inherently a bumpy process. As the child approaches adolescence, yet another set of interests and preoccupations enters the scene. Whether this inevitably leads to conflict with family, peers or society in general, we will explore in the next section.

Health problems in childhood

Many childhood diseases are now comparatively rare in industrialized countries; for example, rickets, a vitamin deficiency. Widespread vaccination against smallpox, diphtheria and tuberculosis has saved thousands of lives. However, there are links between whooping-cough vaccines and encephalitis (inflammation of the brain) and this has greatly worried some parents and doctors. Some of the symptoms of childhood illnesses can seem alarming, but many have trivial causes.

ILLNESS	SYMPTOMS	TREATMENT/ACTION
Asthma	A chronic disorder of the bronchial tubes, causing breathing difficulties. It may be due to infection, or inherited. Allergic asthma is stress related.	Antibiotics are used against infection; injections can control allergic reactions; an attack can be controlled with an inhaler. Breathing exercises are helpful.
Chicken pox	An infectious viral disease accompanied by aching and shivering and a rash of dark red pimples on which blisters develop. Spots are found on face, scalp and chest. Scars can result from scratching.	Rest; a lotion to soothe the itching.
Infantile convulsions (unrelated to epilepsy)	Febrile convulsions lasting a few minutes, followed by sleep.	Child must not be left because of the risk of inhaling vomit. Call a doctor after he or she has fallen asleep.
Leukaemia	Diseases characterized by the proliferation of abnormal white cells, leading to anaemia, infection and bleeding.	No known cure. Drugs, including steroids, are used to try to prevent the white cells from reproducing.
Measles	Begins with fever, a cough and conjunctivitis. After five days a rash merging into blotches appears behind the ears and spreads to the trunk.	Rest, cough syrup, light diet and protection from cold, damp and bright light.
Mumps	Chill and fever, headache, swollen glands.	Rest, light diet, aspirin.
Parasites 1. fleas, body lice, head lice, mites 2. threadworms, roundworms, tapeworms, hookworms	1. Fleas cause severe irritation; some animal fleas also live on humans. Body lice live and lay eggs in clothing—bites may spread infection. Head lice live on the scalp. Mites cause scabies, infectious groups of scabbed pimples. 2. Threadworms are common in children, causing stomach pains, nausea and itching. Roundworms invade the liver, lungs and intestine. No symptoms until a large number blocks the bile duct. Tapeworms attach themselves to the intestine. Hookworms suck blood; symptoms are anaemia, malnutrition, constipation and diarrhoea.	1. Fleas and body lice can be controlled by strict cleanliness. Head lice can be banished by the frequent use of a special shampoo and a fine-toothed comb. Scabies require medical treatment. 2. Threadworms and roundworms: treatment is straightforward, but consult your doctor. Tapeworm: drugs are needed to clear it. Hookworm: drugs, high protein diet and extra iron.
Urinary tract problems	Infections anywhere in the urinary tract are common in young children.	Resulting fevers are treated with antibiotics. See a doctor early.
Whooping cough	Convulsive cough with typical whooping breathing. Vomiting.	Hospitalization for serious cases. Antibiotics, mild sedatives, rest, fresh air.

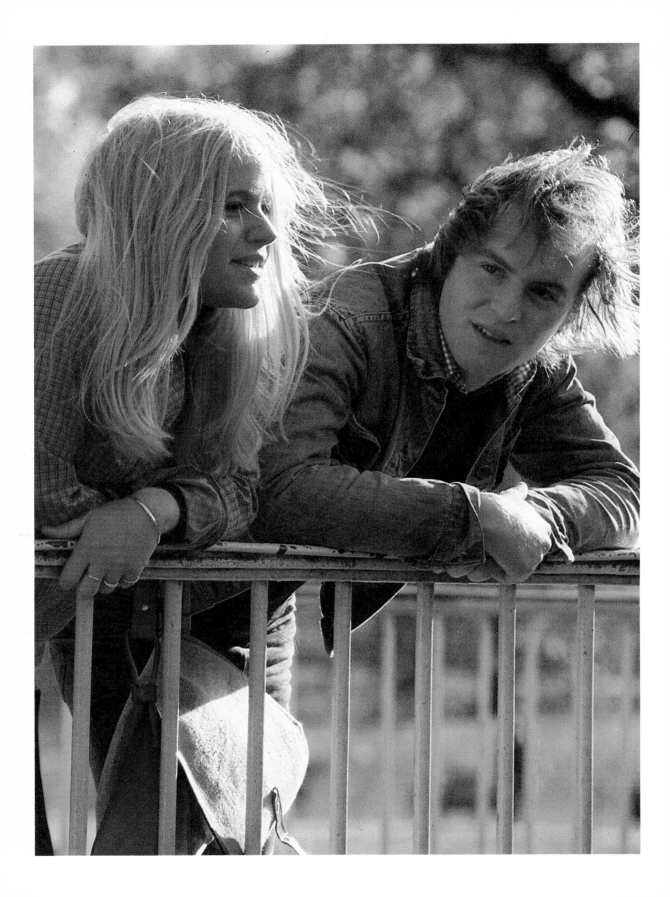

Adolescence

Rejoice, O young man, in thy youth; and let thy heart cheer thee in the days of thy youth.

Ecclesiastes

Over the centuries, no period in life has been more celebrated—and condemned—than adolescence, by poets, philosophers and politicians. It is easy to recognize some contemporary views in those irritably stated by Aristotle, 23 centuries ago: the young, he said,

> are passionate, irascible, and apt to be carried away by their impulses, especially sexual impulses . . . in regard to which they exercise no self-restraint. They are changeful, too, and fickle in their desires, which are as transitory as they are vehement . . . If the young commit a fault, it is always on the side of excess and exaggeration . . . They carry everything too far, whether it be their love or hatred or anything else. They regard themselves as omniscient . . .

However, there is a more favourable view of youth, for which poets have had memorable kind words and on which old people look back with regret and loss. Somewhere between the excess and the ecstasy lies the real human experience. That same experience was characterized by Samuel Butler in *The Way of All Flesh* as being "like a spring, an over-praised season—delightful if if it happens to be a favoured one, but in practice very rarely favoured and more remarkable, as a general rule, for biting east winds than genial breezes." Yes, it is not all fun.

What *does* lie behind this long-standing fascination with adolescence? In part it is a recognition that young people are our links with the future, our guarantee of continuity for our species, our own vicarious triumph over death and failure. But there is also a more personal side to our preoccupation with youth. For most of us, adolescence is remembered as the time when our identities began to crystallize, when our potential was at its height; when, whatever the pains, we lived most intensely.

Left: The search for self begins, and with it the joys and conflicts of youth

A time for becoming

Adolescence can be a time of irrepressible joy and seemingly inconsolable sadness and loss, of gregariousness and loneliness, of altruism and self-centredness, of insatiable curiosity and boredom, of confidence and self-doubt. But, above all, adolescence is a time of rapid change—physical and emotional changes within adolescents, and environmental changes in the nature of external demands placed by society on its developing members.

At no other time, from the age of two onwards, does the individual undergo as many changes as during the period surrounding puberty. Small wonder that so many adolescents, faced with an ever-changing physical image in the mirror, conscious of new—and sometimes strange—feelings and thoughts, ask themselves "What is that person all about?"

Developmental "tasks" of adolescence

The changes of puberty are much the same everywhere, but the developmental "tasks" young people are expected to master may vary widely from one society to another, both in kind and degree of difficulty.

In non-industrialized societies, the tasks to be mastered may be relatively simple and few in number, and represent only a gradual emergence from earlier stages of development. Unlike youth in many Western countries, there is usually no societal or familial expectation that a boy will leave home and obtain an unfamiliar job, if necessary in

Adolescence is a time of change from within and without—physical and psychological changes in the individual are accompanied by changes in what society expects of him or her.

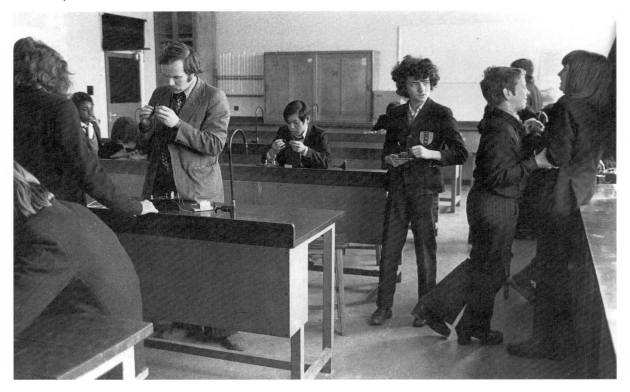

DEVELOPMENTAL TASKS OF ADOLESCENCE

Goals	Tasks
Personal matters	To identify with adults and recognize maturity among peers; to learn co-operation, tolerance and appropriate leadership qualities when collaborating towards common goals.
Social and sexual confidence	To learn about oneself and adjust to social expectations; to acquire a social role as a man or woman.
Acceptance of the physical	To take pride in one's body or tolerate its defects; to use and enjoy the body while protecting its health and safety.
Personal independence	To develop respect and affection for parents while breaking away from childish dependence; to have friendship and respect for other adults without developing emotional dependence; to nurture and trust one's own judgement.
Realizing responsibility	To take a responsible attitude towards partnership and parenthood; to learn basic skills for managing a home or rearing children.
To make ready to take up a job or career	To put energy and planning into organizing a future career; to feel equipped to take up a job and earn a living.
Discovery of social and personal values	To take a social and political role based on personal ethics.
Assessing civic responsibility	To participate as an active citizen in local and national affairs; to take a responsible adult role, recognizing collective social values and the effects of personal behaviour.

a strange community. By the time a girl reaches puberty, she may already have been chosen as a wife by her future husband's parents and will have gradually learned to assume the daily responsibilities of a household. Although her partner may not be the man of her choosing, she will have been prepared by the older women for the changes that she is about to experience, and will have been able to adjust to them over a long period of time.

In modern industrialized societies such as our own, however, adolescents are expected to master far more complex developmental tasks, and there is a much more rapid shift from childhood dependence, with its relative lack of responsibility. In the years between puberty and nominal adulthood, adolescents may be expected to achieve independence from their parents, to establish new kinds of social and working relationships with peers of both sexes and with adults, and to adjust to increasing sexual maturity and changing roles. This will include a consideration of the possibilities and demands of marriage and parenthood, or alternative relationships. In addition, adolescents will be under pressure to decide on personal education and their job future, and to prepare for the responsibilities of active citizenship.

The developmental tasks of adolescence. Puberty is accompanied by no less dramatic adjustments which have to be made with regard to society, family and friends. The shifts from, for example, childhood dependence to adult responsibility, and from schoolchild to wage earner require considerable mental adjustment.

Who do you think you are?

We are familiar with the expression "adolescent identity crisis", but we tend, misleadingly, to use the term "identity" as if it denoted something a person has. In fact, the use of the term as a psychological concept is a peculiarly Western idea. Were we to pose the question "Who are you?" to a member of, say, a New Guinea tribe, the answer would be quite straightforward: "I am X, son of Y of tribe Z". The question "Who am I?" would be met with incomprehension or taken as indicating that the speaker was suffering from amnesia.

Rather than looking at identity as a quality of the individual, it is perhaps more useful to examine the way the term is used in Western societies and see if this helps explain why it should so consistently surface whenever adolescence is mentioned.

People use the term "identity" in a variety of ways. First of all, it is used to denote the separateness of individual people, that they are defined in terms of their own personal attributes and not just as "a schoolgirl" or in relation to someone else. The period of adolescence may mark an individual's first experience of this kind of anonymity: the move from a small elementary school where everyone knew everyone else to a large secondary or high school where teachers and pupils may just be faces in the crowd. The rest of society does not help, with its tendency to lump young people together under negative labels such as "rebels" or "troublemakers", rather than treating them as the individuals they are.

How a boy grows into a man

The prepubertal growth spurt usually begins in boys at about the age of 12—a little later than in girls. During the following few years the physical changes are more rapid than at any time since infancy. But the rate of growth varies enormously. Some boys display the physical characteristics of manhood by the age of 15, while others are only beginning to show the effects of puberty. At the same time, significant behavioural changes occur. Young boys are typically most interested in the companionship of other boys. Willingness to become involved in romantic or sexual relationships increases after puberty as sexual self-awareness grows. As the relationship with his peer group changes, the boy may briefly seem to need a closer relationship with parents. This is soon replaced by the desire for independence and control of his own life. He might even want to leave home altogether. Economic independence is therefore an important goal.

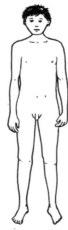

11–12 years
The prepubertal period marks the beginning of a stage of rapid growth. The boy's shoulders and chest start to broaden and the penis lengthens and thickens. The voice may deepen, but not yet break.

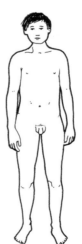

13–14 years
At puberty the growth spurt causes a sudden gain in height. The penis and testes enlarge and the ability to ejaculate is acquired. Pubic hair begins to grow. The voice breaks unevenly.

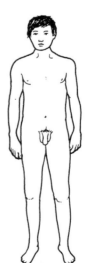

15–16 years
The changes of puberty are consolidated in physical shape and a more even, adult tone of voice. Skin texture changes at puberty and enlarged pores may contribute to the problem of acne.

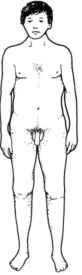

17–18 years
All the major physical changes are complete but body hair becomes more apparent. Facial hair requires infrequent but regular shaving. Behaviour is more independent and geared to adults.

The term "identity" is also used to refer to our perception of ourselves as consistent, both physically and psychologically, from one day to the next. We do not, of course, expect total consistency. We can be happy one day, sad the next. We can gain or lose weight, change our hair colour without feeling that we have changed our identity. It is abrupt and major changes in these areas that are likely to have us feeling like a different person. Adolescence, as we shall see later in this chapter, is a time of exceptionally rapid, and major, physical chang°.

The way we think of ourselves psychologically is strongly related to the way in which people react towards us. Not only do people's reactions to an adolescent differ from their reactions to a child ("You're a man now"), they also tend to fluctuate from moment to moment. Adolescents may be expected to take responsibility, to "act their age" but still, in many ways, be treated as children.

Adolescents are also expected to make major choices which may affect them for the rest of their lives. To leave school or stay on? To take this subject or that? To "go steady" or date lots of people? To start smoking or not? In some ways, this range of choices and opportunities is beneficial, but it can be very problematic—not because of the number of choices, but because we still expect these choices, once made, to be irrevocable. If you do not believe this, try telling your friends (or your future spouse) that you do not expect your marriage to last more than a few years. Or tell an interviewing

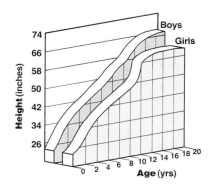

Average heights

During childhood, boys and girls follow a steady, relatively slow rate of increase in height. In both sexes there is a growth spurt in adolescence, usually lasting for about two years. Girls typically reach this phase earlier than boys. Boys, on average, grow taller and their full period of growth may last longer.

How a girl grows into a woman

Girls commence puberty earlier than do boys and, in general, mature more quickly. For this reason they become interested in relationships with the opposite sex at an earlier age—and a girl of 13 or 14 will typically have a boyfriend about two or more years older than herself. In early adolescence close friendships with girls of the same age are important, and a girl may have one best friend and constant companion in the first few years of her teens. The physical changes that a girl goes through at puberty are likely to be more obvious than those occurring in a boy of the same age. And it is generally true that girls take more interest in their personal appearance, and at an earlier age. With menstruation a visible sign of potential motherhood, many girls look forward to marriage, homemaking and having babies while still in their teens. But educational and economic opportunities are also looked for, all as signs of growing independence.

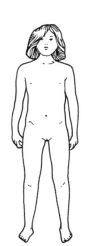 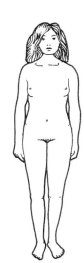 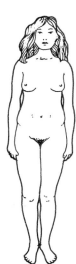 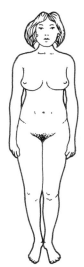

11–12 years
A girl is entering upon puberty at this age and for some it is the time when menstruation starts. The face and body acquire more fullness with development of breasts, hips and pubic hair.

13–14 years
More commonly it is at this age that girls start to menstruate. The swelling of hips and breasts is more pronounced. But the rate of general growth has passed its peak and slows down.

15–16 years
As the evidence of physical maturation increases, behaviour becomes more adult. Physical development continues; but growth in terms of height may have finished completely by 16.

17–18 years
Physical maturation is complete; adjusting to adulthood is focused on social and emotional factors; in dealing with education; work; or preparation for partnership and motherhood.

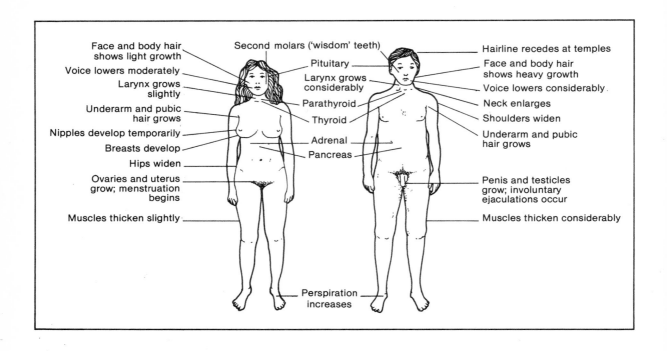

Face and body hair shows light growth
Voice lowers moderately
Larynx grows slightly
Underarm and pubic hair grows
Nipples develop temporarily
Breasts develop
Hips widen
Ovaries and uterus grow; menstruation begins
Muscles thicken slightly

Second molars ('wisdom' teeth)
Pituitary
Larynx grows considerably
Parathyroid
Thyroid
Adrenal
Pancreas

Hairline recedes at temples
Face and body hair shows heavy growth
Voice lowers considerably
Neck enlarges
Shoulders widen
Underarm and pubic hair grows
Penis and testicles grow; involuntary ejaculations occur
Muscles thicken considerably

Perspiration increases

Gland	Hormone	Main effect
Pituitary		
Anterior lobe	Adrenocorticotropic hormone (ACTH)	Stimulates adrenal cortex, the gland producing steroids.
	Growth hormone	Stimulates growth generally.
	Thyroitropin	Stimulates thyroid producing thyroxin.
	Follicle-stimulating hormone (FSH)	Originates production of ova and sperm.
	Luteinizing hormone (LH)	Fosters maturation of ova and sperm and encourages ovulation.
	Prolactin	Stimulates milk production.
Posterior lobe	Antidiuretic hormone	Regulates urination to prevent excessive loss of fluids.
	Oxytocin	Controls uterine contractions and flow of milk in nursing.
Adrenal		
Cortex	Steroids (such as cortisol)	Increases blood glucose and keeps up mineral levels.
Medulla	Epinephrin (adrenalin)	Stimulates ACTH; increases heart rate, blood pressure; blood glucose and perspiration.
	Norepinephrin (noradrenalin)	Stimulates ACTH; slows heart rate, increases blood pressure.
Thyroid	Thyroxin	Increases metabolic rate.
Pancreas		
Alpha cells	Glucagon	Increases blood glucose.
Beta cells	Insulin	Decreases blood glucose.
Parathyroid	Parathormone	Controls blood calcium.
Ovaries (female)	Oestrogens	Develop female sex characteristics.
	Progesterone	Develops uterus lining and fosters development in pregnancy.
Testes (male)	Androgens (such as testosterone)	Develops male sex characteristics; may influence male and female sex drives.

Major endocrine glands and their hormones

The endocrine glands secrete their hormones directly into the bloodstream, to be carried throughout the body. They are also known as ductless glands. The pituitary, located within the skull, below the brain, is mainly responsible for the growth changes of adolescence. Its frontal lobe emits hormones that control the functioning of many other glands—including the gonadotrophins FSH and LH, which stimulate the activity of the gonad, the internal organ which produces sex cells.

panel that you intend to take up a quite different profession in five years' time. Adolescents, confronted with the necessity to choose, may say "I need time to find myself" when they simply mean that they do not want to make an irrevocable choice at such an early age (or, indeed, at any age). Many of the identity problems of which adolescents complain may be created by a society which expects them to take up a role and carry it with them for the rest of their lives. Looked at in this way, we can see that identity problems are by no means confined to adolescence.

Sexual identity

An important part of our sense of identity is the awareness and acceptance of our basic biological nature as a man or a woman. Because one's sex is a biological fact about which little can be done, sexual identity conflicts are likely to create significant problems for adolescents who experience them.

It is important to distinguish between *sexual identity*, in the sense of biological sex, and sex role *behaviour*. People who complain of sexual identity problems are often confusing the two. Appropriate behaviour as a man or a woman need not mean rigidly conforming to sex-role stereotypes such as that of the ambitious, self-reliant, assertive but not very sensitive male and the affectionate, gentle, sensitive but not very assertive female. There is no biological reason why men and women should not be capable of both independence and a reasonable kind of assertiveness, as well as sensitivity. Indeed, the findings of recent scientific investigations suggest that young men and

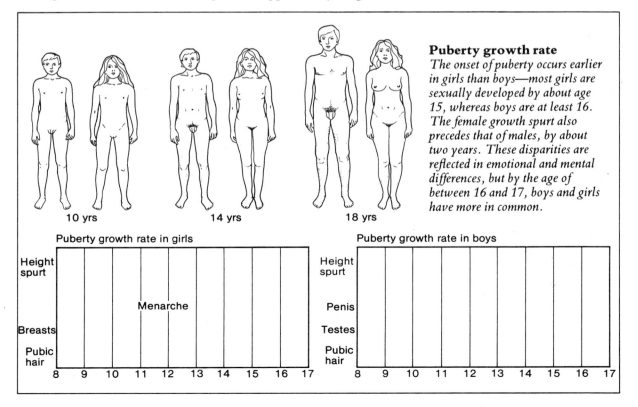

10 yrs   14 yrs   18 yrs

Puberty growth rate

The onset of puberty occurs earlier in girls than boys—most girls are sexually developed by about age 15, whereas boys are at least 16. The female growth spurt also precedes that of males, by about two years. These disparities are reflected in emotional and mental differences, but by the age of between 16 and 17, boys and girls have more in common.

Puberty growth rate in girls

Height spurt									
			Menarche						
Breasts									
Pubic hair									
8	9	10	11	12	13	14	15	16	17

Puberty growth rate in boys

Height spurt									
Penis									
Testes									
Pubic hair									
8	9	10	11	12	13	14	15	16	17

women who are androgynous (that is, who display both "masculine" and "feminine" behaviours) score higher on measures of self-esteem, do better in their academic work in school and college, have better relations with the opposite sex and are more self-reliant and independent and less conforming than more purely masculine or feminine types.

Although this "mix" is probably a very desirable state of affairs, it is perhaps important, in our enthusiasm for women's—and men's—liberation, to avoid imposing a new set of stereotypes, even some "ideal" androgynous balance, on all boys and girls, men and women. The ultimate aim of any process of socialization should be to permit each adolescent to develop his or her unique potential as an individual, consistent with the rights of others.

Growing up: the body

Unlike younger children, whose physical growth is gradual and orderly, adolescents are likely, over a short period, to find that they feel strangers to the self with which they have been familiar since early childhood. The process of integrating these dramatic physical changes successfully into an emerging sense of a stable, self-confident personal identity may be a prolonged and difficult one. There is no doubt that it could often be made considerably easier if young people (and their parents) had a clearer idea of the true nature of the physical changes of their puberty and later adolescence.

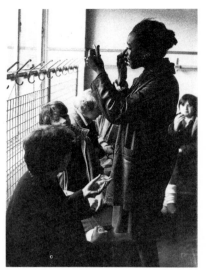

Adolescence brings dramatic biological and physiological changes, and changes in the individual's awareness of his or her body.

Hormones and the biological clock

The term "puberty" derives from the Latin word *pubertas*, meaning "age of manhood or womanhood". It refers to the first phase of adolescence, when sexual maturation becomes evident. The onset of puberty becomes most readily apparent with the initial appearance of pubic hair and, in girls, the first signs of elevation of the breasts (the "bud" stage). In fact, by this stage, the process has already been going on for some time internally, with an increase in the size of the testes in boys and of the ovaries in girls.

The intricate sequence of events producing physical growth and sexual maturation is controlled by hormones secreted by the endocrine glands. These hormones are triggered by signals originating in the hypothalamus, an important coordinating centre in the brain. This can only occur when the hypothalamus is sufficiently mature. The signal stimulates the pituitary gland, which lies immediately below the base of the brain, to release hormones which themselves have stimulating effects on other endocrine glands in the body. It is from these that more hormones finally come—they will affect physical growth and sexual development. Among them are thyroxin from the thyroid gland, cortisol from the adrenal gland, and sex hormones, including androgens (the masculine hormones) and progestins or gestagens (the pregnancy hormones). By means of a complex feedback system, these and other hormones stimulate and accelerate the many physical and physiological developments of puberty and adolescence.

The growth spurt

The term "adolescent growth spurt" refers to the accelerated rate of increase in height and weight that accompanies puberty. The age at which the growth spurt (and puberty generally) begins varies widely even among perfectly normal children. In boys, the growth spurt may

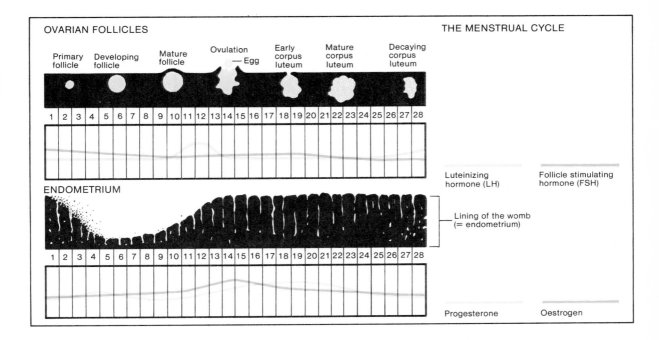

OVARIAN FOLLICLES

THE MENSTRUAL CYCLE

| Primary follicle | Developing follicle | Mature follicle | Ovulation — Egg | Early corpus luteum | Mature corpus luteum | Decaying corpus luteum |

1 2 3 4 5 6 7 8 9 10 11 12 13 14 15 16 17 18 19 20 21 22 23 24 25 26 27 28

Luteinizing hormone (LH)

Follicle stimulating hormone (FSH)

ENDOMETRIUM

1 2 3 4 5 6 7 8 9 10 11 12 13 14 15 16 17 18 19 20 21 22 23 24 25 26 27 28

Lining of the womb (= endometrium)

Progesterone

Oestrogen

begin as early as 10½ or as late as 16; some boys may have almost completed their physical development before it begins in others, without any implications that either one or the other is abnormal. For the average boy, however, rapid acceleration in growth begins at about 12½, reaches its fastest rate at 14 and then declines to pre-growth rates around the age of 14. The growth spurt begins on average two years earlier in girls.

Changes in height and weight are accompanied by changes in body proportions in both boys and girls. The head, hands and feet reach adult size first. In turn, the arms and legs grow faster than trunk length, which is completed last.

These differences in rates of growth of different parts of the body account for the temporary feelings of awkwardness felt by some adolescents, especially those who are growing fastest. For brief periods, some young people may feel that their hands and feet are too big, or that "they are all legs". Thoughtless comments by adults will not help.

Sex differences

Sex differences in body shape are also magnified during early adolescence. Although girls have wider hips than boys even in childhood, the difference becomes pronounced at the onset of puberty. Conversely, boys develop thicker as well as larger bones, more muscle tissue and broader shoulders. Partly because of this, boys become and remain much stronger than girls as adolescence proceeds. There are, however, other reasons for the boys' relatively greater strength. Relative to their size, boys develop larger hearts and lungs, a higher systolic blood pressure, a greater capacity for carrying oxygen in the blood and a lower heart rate while resting. They are also chemically more resistant to fatigue.

The menstrual cycle

*Blood flow occurs as the uterus sheds its lining and blood supply to begin a new cycle of egg production. First the pituitary gland secretes follicle-stimulating hormone (FSH) causing the ovary to make a **follicle**— an ovum (egg) surrounded by cells. The cells secrete oestrogen to prepare a uterus lining. At 14 days oestrogen levels inhibit FSH, and the pituitary secretes luteinizing hormone (LH). This releases the ovum from the ovary and converts the follicle cells into a **corpus luteum**, which produces progesterone to help prepare the uterus for the fertilized ovum. At 14 days, if no fertilization occurs, the corpus luteum degenerates and menstruation begins again.*

Below: The pathway of an unfertilized egg, from ovary to vagina.

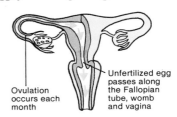

Ovulation occurs each month

Unfertilized egg passes along the Fallopian tube, womb and vagina

Nutritional needs

Many discouraged parents, with a wary eye on the ever-rising cost of food, have the feeling that rapidly growing adolescents, particularly boys, are "eating us out of house and home". As can be seen in the accompanying table, on average boys need more calories at every age than girls. However, a very large, very active girl will obviously have greater nutritional needs than a small, inactive boy. (The problems of adolescents who eat too much or too little will be discussed in a later chapter.)

Recommended daily dietary allowances (calories)

	Age	Weight (pounds)	Height (inches)	Calories
Boys	11–14	97	63	2800
	15–18	134	69	3000
	19–22	147	69	3000
Girls	11–14	97	62	2100
	15–18	119	65	2100
	19–22	128	65	2000

Anxieties

A number of normal characteristics of sexual maturation may be a source of embarrassment or anxiety to a male adolescent. During the process of voice change (which can be abrupt or gradual), the larynx (Adam's apple) grows larger and the vocal cords virtually double in length. As a result, the boy's voice drops about an octave in tone. It takes at least two years for the average boy to gain full control of this change, during which there may be sudden jumps from a deep bass to a high-pitched squeak.

In all adolescent boys, there are increases in the size of the areola (the area surrounding the nipple): in some, perhaps 20 to 30 per cent. There is also a distinct enlargement of the breasts themselves about midway through adolescence, which usually appears in about a year. This enlargement may cause some boys anxiety about their masculinity, and it is a good idea to reassure them that this is normal and will pass. They are not going to turn into girls. Likewise, the prepubescent boy may show a tendency to rounded hips, which may reinforce the anxiety, but in all normal circumstances this too disappears after the onset of the growth spurt.

Like boys, adolescent girls frequently harbour a number of anxieties about their bodies during this period of rapid physical change. They may worry, but usually less these days than formerly, whether their breasts will be "too big" or "too small". Breast size, in fact, has nothing to do with capacity for either breast-feeding or sexual arousal.

A few girls who are worried about aspects of their maturation may develop a reactive sexuality, as, indeed, may boys. They may pursue sexual experience, not so much for its own sake, but to reassure themselves about sexual normality. Adolescent girls may also be concerned about such things as the size of their hips, and many may be anxious about the physical, psychological and social aspects of

Menstruation

Nowadays, more and more girls seem to accept the onset of menstruation calmly. Some look forward to it. But many other girls look on this normal—and inevitable—development negatively as "something women just have to put up with".

One common reason for these negative attitudes is how other women present this experience. If a girl's parents and friends act as though she requires sympathy for her "plight", the girl herself is likely to react in a similar fashion.

Also, if she resents growing up, or if she has been unable to establish a satisfactory feminine identification, the adolescent girl may be disturbed by the unmistakable signs of approaching womanhood. A wise and understanding approach by parents, who show pride in their daughter's maturity, may help to alleviate these problems.

Menstrual problems

Negative reactions to menstruation may also stem from physical discomfort during the early years of puberty. A number of girls experience headaches, backache, cramps, abdominal pain and feelings of fullness. In many cases these disturbances disappear or lessen in time.

The female hormones oestrogen and progesterone play their part in the menstrual cycle. They have also been implicated in menstrual pain and in the physical and psychological changes labelled "premenstrual tension" (PMT). Different theories of the causes of menstrual problems have their own, often fierce support. The difficulty is that no one theory seems to apply to all cases.

menstruation. Accurate and freely given information about normal development and its many possible variations can help to dispel much unnecessary distress.

Being different

As adolescents stop being dependent mainly on the family and more on the peer group as a major source of security and social status, they need to conform to peer group standards more, not only in social behaviour, but in appearance and physical skills. If they deviate from the idealized peer group norms in body build, facial features, physical abilities—even, at times, in such seemingly irrelevant matters as whether one's hair is straight or curly—this may be a source of great distress to adolescents.

Many adolescents, however, find themselves faced with very real problems about their appearance. At a time when it seems vitally important to them that they look their best, their lives are made unhappy or miserable by acne. While it is nice to think that it is what you are and not what you look like which is important, there is quite overwhelming evidence that physical appearance plays a crucial role in the judgements which we make about each other. The problem of acne therefore deserves to be taken as seriously by adults as by adolescents themselves. In fact, even severe acne can be significantly controlled or abolished by specialist medical treatment.

Early and late maturers

In general, early or late maturing appears to have a greater effect on boys than on girls. Adults and other adolescents tend to think of the 14- or 15-year-old boy who looks 17 or 18 as older than he actually is and therefore to expect more mature behaviour from him. Because there is less of a physical discrepancy between an early-maturing boy and most girls of this age (because of the earlier growth spurt in girls), he may become involved sooner, and with more self-confidence, in boy–girl relationships. He may also have an advantage in athletics and in other activities. So although an early-maturing boy may feel different from his peers, he is not likely to feel insecure about the difference.

By contrast, a late-maturing boy is more likely to be treated "as a child", which may infuriate him, even while he continues to behave maturely. He will probably have a harder time achieving recognition in athletic and other physical activities as well as in his relations with girls.

Much can be done by parents, teachers and others to minimize the anxiety and other negative psychological effects of late maturing. They can make a conscious effort to avoid the trap of treating the later maturer as younger than he is. They can help him to realize that his slower maturation is perfectly normal—that he will indeed "grow up" and be just as physically and sexually masculine as his peers.

Among girls, the effects of early and late maturing are generally fewer and more variable. Although early-maturing girls tend to be somewhat more relaxed, more self-confident and secure, the differences are not large. Why the differences should be greater among boys is something of a mystery. One reason, however, may be that our society's expectations for adolescent boys are less ambiguous than for girls, but whether they are greater in general is open to dispute.

Erection, ejaculation and nocturnal emission

A boy's capacity for erection of the penis and for pleasurable genital stimulation is present from infancy, but only with the onset of puberty and the associated increases in testosterone (male hormone) levels do sexual urges become strong and insistent. Erections become far more frequent and are likely to be aroused by a wide variety of stimuli, some of which are patently sexual but others much less obviously so. Boys may be proud of their capacity for erection as a symbol of emerging virility, but its uncontrollability can be a source of social and even moral anxiety.

The adolescent boy's first ejaculation is likely to happen within a year of the onset of the growth spurt and may happen as a result of masturbation or during sleep (the so-called "wet dream") or of spontaneous waking orgasm. A boy who has previously masturbated, with accompanying pleasant sensations but without ejaculation, may indeed be taken by surprise by his initial ejaculation of seminal fluid and wonder whether it is harmful.

Anxieties

The "wet dream" experience common to almost all males may produce anxieties in adolescent boys, to the point where they may be afraid to sleep or to sleep in strange beds or even their own if they think their parents disapprove of sexuality. Nocturnal emission occurs more frequently among youths without other sexual outlets, such as masturbation, petting to orgasm or intercourse and may or may not be accompanied by overtly erotic dreams.

Sexual behaviour

In early adolescence, at least, the problem of sex is likely to be greater for boys than for girls. For reasons that we do not entirely understand—although physiological (including hormonal) and psychological factors are probably both involved—boys seem more conscious of specifically sexual impulses than girls and find them harder to deny. Sexual drive among girls is likely to be more diffuse and ambiguous. Many younger adolescent girls may choose to deny their sexual impulses for a time.

However, boys and girls also have much in common in their concerns about sexuality. Both want to feel liked, loved and wanted, and not just be treated as sex objects. They want to know about practical matters such as masturbation, sexual intercourse, conception, pregnancy and birth control. They also want to know how to fit sex into their overall values and how to have mutually rewarding, constructive relations with others, both of the same and the opposite sex. On these matters, most young people receive little help from the inconsistent, conflict-ridden and sometimes hypocritical world in which they live.

Sex education

A good many adults in Western society remain adamantly opposed to adequate sex education. Some parents believe that sex education, even at high-school level, is dangerously premature for "impressionable" adolescents and likely to lead them into promiscuity. Others maintain that information about sex should be taught only by parents in the privacy of their homes. Still others have apparently reached the conclusion that today's adolescents have nothing left to learn about sex—certainly nothing their parents could teach them. None of these views will stand up to scrutiny.

In the light of current statistics on premarital intercourse and pregnancy, it is difficult to see how sex education for adolescents could be in any way "premature". Whether or not parents should be educating their young about sex, the fact is that the great majority are still not doing so. When adolescents in a recent national survey in the United States were asked whether their parents talked "pretty freely" about sex, over 70 per cent reported that they did not. When asked specifically if their parents had ever discussed such topics as masturbation, contraceptive methods or venereal disease, two-thirds or more said they had not.

The notion that adolescents have nothing left to learn about sex is equally shaky. Myths about sex are widespread. More than a quarter of adolescents aged 16 and over expressed the belief that "if a girl doesn't want to get pregnant she won't have a baby, even if she fails to use any contraceptive measure". Nevertheless, only about a third of high schools in the United States provide comprehensive sex education.

Changing values and sexual behaviour

One of the more prominent aspects of the youth culture of the 1960s—and clearly one of the more enduring—was the development of a new sexual morality. This brought a greater openness and honesty about sex, and an increasing tendency to see decisions about individual

---

**Mixed messages:
adolescents and masturbation**

Although there has been a marked liberalization of views in recent years among professionals, parents and young people themselves, masturbation is still a source of concern for a significant number of adolescents. And there are still doctors who assert that masturbation among children and adolescents is likely to make it difficult for them to transfer to heterosexual intercourse.

What are the facts? Obviously, early predictions that masturbation would severely impair physical and psychological health are wrong. Furthermore, in the absence of previously acquired guilt and anxiety, masturbation may be enjoyable and reduce tension. There is no indication that it increases the difficulty of later adjustment to heterosexual relations—indeed, available evidence suggests the opposite.

In the case of women who have difficulty in achieving orgasm, sex therapists have found that practice in masturbation can often be of help in learning sexual arousal during sex with a partner.

It is sometimes argued that masturbation, though not physically harmful, may lead to a preoccupation with sex. It seems more reasonable to suppose that such preoccupation is likely to result from continuing, anxiety-ridden efforts to avoid masturbation. Nevertheless, in some instances, it may reflect some adolescent problems. Young people who use masturbation not just as a sexual outlet when "real" sex is unavailable, but as a substitute for other activities in which they feel inadequate, have a problem—not masturbation, although its availability may delay seeking a solution to the real social problem.

sexual behaviour as a purely private concern of the person or people involved. This trend appears to reflect in part a growing disenchantment with established social institutions, together with a shift in values among many young people in the direction of self-discovery and self-expression. In a recent study, most adolescents in the sample agreed that "it's right that people should make their own moral code", but only a minority (a quarter of 16 to 19-year-olds) agreed that "so far as sex is concerned, I wouldn't do anything that society would disapprove of".

The growing emphasis on openness and honesty is not evidence of an increased preoccupation with sex, as many parents and other adults seem to think. Indeed, it may well be that today's average adolescent, accepting sex as a natural part of life, is less preoccupied with sex than his or her counterparts in earlier generations, with their atmosphere of secrecy, guilt and suppression.

How are these changing attitudes about sex among adolescents reflected in their behaviour? Although almost all adolescent boys already engaged in masturbation before the so-called "youth revolution" of the 1960s (and indeed did so as far back as human records go), there is some evidence that masturbation among boys is currently

Sexual development in adolescents is undeniable, and it is difficult to argue that they should not be given information on sexual topics.

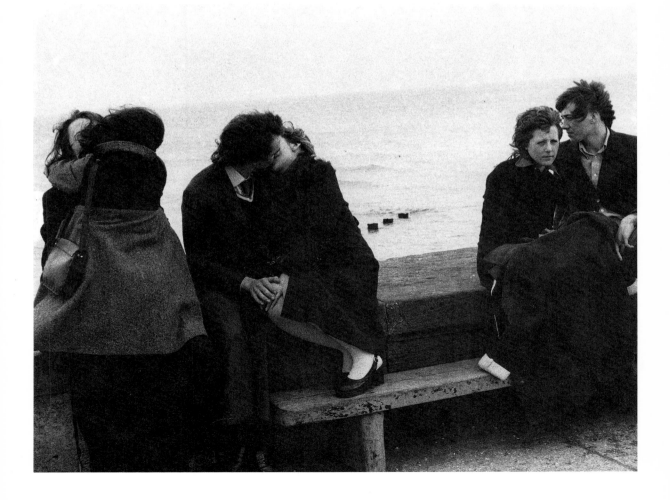

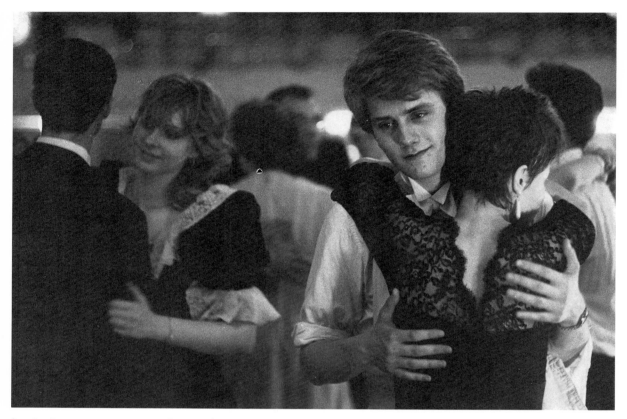

beginning at younger ages than in the past, and is accompanied by less guilt and anxiety than previously. Among girls, recent data indicate that there has been a significant increase in the incidence (or, at least, the reported incidence) of masturbation at all ages between 12 and 20. However, girls generally appear to engage in masturbation—or admit to it—only about half as often as boys. Interestingly, it occurs three times as frequently among those with experience of sexual intercourse or petting to orgasm as among the sexually inexperienced.

Petting appears to have increased somewhat in the past few decades and to occur earlier. The major change, however, has been in the frequency of petting, the degree of intimacy involved, the frequency with which petting leads to erotic arousal or orgasm and, certainly, frankness about this activity.

These manifestations of sexuality are something most societies and parents have become used to dealing with. Currently, however, the greatest amount of concern from parents and society is focused on the dramatic increase in actual sexual intercourse among young people.

This trend has been found in the United States and other Western countries, although there are clear national differences in the total incidence of premarital intercourse. For both males and females, England, West Germany and the Scandinavian countries (in that order) show a higher incidence than the United States and Canada, while some other countries, such as Ireland, show a lower incidence.

However, there are wide individual differences within each country, with the lowest incidence generally occurring amongst

Sexuality, for adolescents as for others, incorporates the need to be liked and cherished.

adolescents who are younger, female, highly religious and politically conservative. More adolescent virgins than non-virgins have "a lot of respect" for their parents' ideas and opinions, feel close to and liked by their parents, believe that their parents understand what they want out of life and find it relatively easy to communicate with them. By contrast, nearly three times as many non-virgins as virgins agree that "I've pretty much given up on ever being able to get along with my parents". Compared with the parents of non-virgins, the parents of virgins are more likely to have discussed topics such as masturbation, birth control and venereal disease with their children.

These findings are echoed in an investigation of American high-school youth, where another important finding was that the degree of influence the mother had was related to the amount of maternal affection she exhibited.

Effects of the "new morality"

In today's more open social climate, many experienced adolescents seem able to handle sexual involvement without undue stress. Four out of five non-virgins in the United States report getting "a lot of satisfaction" out of their sex lives.

However, significant minorities report feelings of guilt, find themselves exploited or rejected, or discover belatedly that they cannot cope emotionally with full sexual relationships. Especially after their first experience of sexual intercourse, girls are far more likely than boys to experience negative feelings: whereas boys are most likely to report being excited, happy and satisfied, girls often report being guilty, afraid, worried or embarrassed after their initiation. As one 16-year-old girl expressed it, "I felt really guilty. I wondered if my mother really knew. When I came in after it had happened, I felt I had guilt written all over my face."

On the other hand, another 16-year-old girl who had been going with her boyfriend for several years had a very different experience: "What were my feelings? . . . They were warm feelings, physically close feelings . . . The only thing I could think of is the wanting each other, a sharing each other. I still feel that way." There are obvious dangers in the assumption that sexual involvement is OK "as long as you're in love". Encouraged by such a philosophy among peers, a girl or boy may become more emotionally and physically involved than

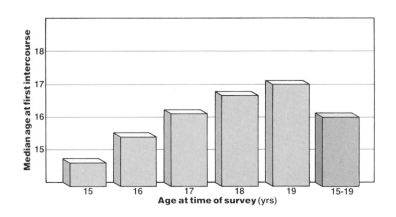

Sexual intercourse among American teenagers
In their 1976 survey of 15–19-year-olds, Zelnik and Kantner observed that the median age was 16.2 years for first intercourse in sexually active females. This suggests a strong case for earlier sex education than is currently practised in some schools, certainly before senior school age.

he or she can handle. An adolescent may also think that his or her attitudes are more "liberal" than they really are, and involvement may lead to unanticipated feelings of guilt, anxiety or depression.

Adolescents, like adults, may become involved in sexual relations for a variety of reasons which have little to do with liking the other person or seeking sexual satisfaction. Often, it may be to gain peer approval, to escape from or to rebel against parents, to gain affection denied by parents or others or as a "cry for help".

Pregnancy and contraception

Family planning workers often adopt the simplistic view that the answer to unwanted pregnancy is to make effective birth control devices freely available. Noble as these sentiments may be, the fact is that less than a third of unmarried girls having intercourse have used the contraceptive pill to prevent pregnancy, and a disturbingly high percentage—between 55 and 75 per cent—have used no contraceptive device whatsoever, at least in their first experience. Only a minority consistently use such a device thereafter. Even among those in steady relationships, only two-thirds reported always using contraceptive devices.

This widespread failure to take contraceptive precautions, together with the continuing increase in premarital intercourse among adolescents, has resulted in more than a million 15 to 19-year-old girls in the United States alone (10 per cent of this entire age group) becoming pregnant each year; two-thirds of these pregnancies happen outside marriage. In addition, annually some 30 000 girls under the age of 15 become pregnant.

The consequences of this "epidemic" of adolescent pregnancies are serious indeed. More than a quarter are terminated by induced abortion; 10 per cent result in marital births that were conceived premaritally; over one-fifth result in out-of-wedlock births. Fourteen per cent miscarry.

In recent surveys, the main reasons given for not using contraceptives were that the teenagers thought (usually mistakenly) that they could not get pregnant because of the time of the month, age, or frequency of intercourse, or that contraceptives were not available when they needed them. Planned Parenthood in America noted that "the first set of reasons could be remedied by better education, the second with more adequate service programs". Yet only one in three high schools currently teach about birth control methods, despite the fact that 8 out of 10 American adults old enough to have adolescent children favour such teaching.

However, we must be careful about assuming that more education and widely available contraception are the whole answer. It is easy to lose sight of the fact that, compared with 10 or 13 years ago, the availability and acceptability of contraception has increased dramatically. Those who wish to see more education about birth control certainly have a point: ignorance about the mechanisms of conception is widespread among adolescents (and some adults).

What these changes do not deal with are the complex psychological factors which underlie the decision to have sex and to use or not use contraception. The immediate consequences of sexual activity are (usually) pleasurable. The negative consequences (pregnancy, venereal disease) are significantly delayed. Likewise, the immediate consequences of using effective contraception may be negative

Homosexual behaviour

Many adolescents worry at one time or another that they may be homosexual. But at least half of all boys and one third of girls have engaged in some form of sex-play with other members of the same sex during pre-adolescence. Most of these young people go on to lead heterosexual lives.

Kinsey found that most adults are more or less exclusively heterosexual. A small minority are exclusively homosexual. But a quarter of adults fall in between these two groups. They may be mainly heterosexual, but with some homosexual involvement or the reverse. The most important factor in predicting whether an adolescent will become primarily or exclusively homosexual in orientation is not whether the young person is capable of arousal with members of the same sex, but whether he or she is incapable, for whatever reason or reasons, of attraction to the opposite sex.

What about "true" homosexuality?

In some instances, disturbed parent–child relations seem to play a part. Homosexuality seems to occur more frequently among boys with overly intrusive, dominating mothers and detached or rejecting fathers.

Among girls, a number of factors may contribute to a homosexual orientation: a sexual education that encourages girls to view men as dangerous, threatening or dirty or, conversely, as weak and inadequate, or in the situation in which the father, while outwardly puritanical, is subtly seductive, encouraging a too-close relationship with himself, but discouraging relationships with boys who are the girl's own age.

(medical examination, unwanted side-effects, mess, interference with spontaneity), while the positive consequences (avoiding pregnancy) are delayed.

Psychologists have long been aware of the importance of immediate consequences in controlling behaviour. The use of contraception requires the setting aside of these immediate consequences and engaging in long-term planning and foresight. Specifically, it requires the conscious acknowledgement that sexual activity will take place and must be prepared for. A girl may know all there is to know mechanically about birth control, but if the reaction of her family, friends and teachers to planned sexual activity is somewhat negative (and in spite of the sexual revolution this is often the case, particularly for girls), then we should not be surprised if she "chooses" to be erratic in her use of a contraceptive or in her expectation that one will be used by her partner.

It seems likely that premarital intercourse will continue to become accepted practice, and steady relationships will still be viewed as the most frequent and the most socially approved pattern among sexually experienced adolescents. What we must hope is that those who do enter sexual relationships can be helped to become sufficiently mature, informed, responsible, sure of their own value systems and sufficiently concerned about the welfare of others, for the inevitable casualties of sexual activity to be reduced to a minimum which, of course, depends on the attitudes of adults towards the adolescent.

Homosexual experiences are not at all uncommon among adolescents, but most of those who have them later become exclusively heterosexual. The parents of those who eventually develop a fully homosexual life style can be distressed by it—these parents in New York are looking for ways of accepting the situation.

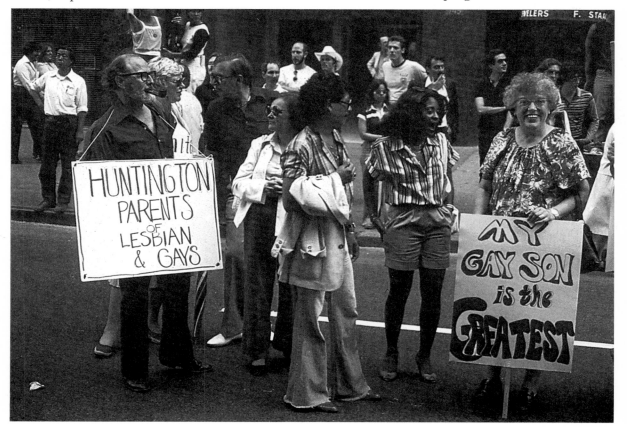

Adolescents and their parents

This is a time when parents and their adolescent sons and daughters must learn to establish new kinds of relationships with each other. Parents must be able to recognize—and encourage—adolescents' need for greater independence. Continuing to think of their adolescent young as "our darling baby" or "our little boy" and treating them accordingly is a prescription for disaster, whether this takes the form of explosive rebellion, or continued and increasingly inappropriate dependence.

At the same time, however, it is vital to recognize that true independence is not created in a day. Partly because so many things are changing in an adolescent's world, he or she very much needs a base of security and stability in home and parents—something to take for granted while more urgent concerns are worked out. Along with the increasing independence comes an inevitable shift in the emotional relationships between parent and child. If the young person is eventually going to achieve emotional, social and sexual maturity, he or she must gradually begin shifting to peers—to "best friends" and boyfriends and girlfriends—some of the intimate personal attachment previously reserved largely for parents.

Even under the most favourable circumstances, the adjustment to a young person's emotional separation from the family is bound to have its painful moments for both parents and children. Inevitably, and quite properly, there will be occasional feelings of loss and longing for a simpler time when there was "just the family".

The family at war

The popular view of adolescence is as a period of great storm and stress. Yet more broadly representative studies indicate that while this is certainly the case with some young people, including some of the most gifted as well as some of the most maladjusted, it is not true of the majority of adolescents.

Some conflicts with parents, however, are natural and to be expected, particularly during the earlier years of adolescence. For one thing, as their horizons expand, adolescents begin to see that the family's values and way of life are not the only possible ones. Younger children usually have the conviction that "how we do it at our house" is the right, the only possible way. Not so adolescents, who perceive not only that there is room for alternative values, beliefs or ways of doing things, but that the style of other parents might actually be superior to that of their own. It may take a long time but, ultimately, young people are likely to conclude that, while parents do not have all the answers their opinions and knowledge—gained from sometimes bitter experience—can still be helpful and are at least familiar. And sometimes the "new" people whose style one takes to admiring turn out to be a good deal more odd than one wants or can cope with.

Another common reason for parent–adolescent conflicts is the "tyranny of habit". It is often difficult for parents to realize that their little boy or girl is no longer a child, and that rules and regulations that may have been appropriate when the children were younger are no longer so. Even when parents do recognize this, it is often difficult to break old habits.

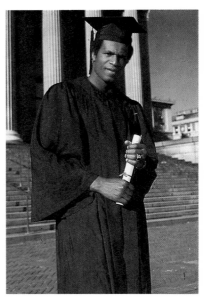

In universities the awarding of degrees is marked by a ceremony—by no means attended by all students—which includes formality and ritual. For the graduate in his or her twenties it marks the end of several years of study and examinations lived almost exclusively in the company of his or her peers. In the eighties, university places are fewer as departments and subjects are cut back, but the degree ceremony remains unchanged.

The problem may be compounded by inconsistencies on the part of the adolescent. As we have noted, adolescents typically have mixed feelings about independence and dependence. The prospect of independence may be both appealing and frightening. Adolescents may be surprisingly mature, independent and responsible one moment and childlike and undependable the next.

Rites of passage

Another reason for some of the conflicts between adolescents and their parents is the lack of clearcut guidelines about what behaviour is appropriate.

In many non-industrialized societies, the privileges and obligations of each age group are clearly spelt out. There also tends to be a more clearly defined boundary between adolescence and adulthood, marked by a rite of passage, or initiation ceremony. Completion of this means that the boy or girl is accepted as an adult, though junior, member of society, with the appropriate freedoms and responsibilities granted and expected by the society, not just the parents.

However, adolescents' impending or achieved maturity is not clearly recognized or marked in industrialized societies today. All we have is a hotchpotch of inconsistent and loosely enforced rules, which may vary from community to community, about when a young person may drink, drive a car, leave school, marry, or own property.

The problem in modern society has been complicated by the speed of social, moral and political change in recent years. So swift has this change been that today's adolescents have grown up in a markedly different world from their parents, whose own experience as children and adolescents may consequently be virtually useless as guidance in understanding their children's needs, problems and goals.

Adolescents need, and want, to make independent choices about their futures, but the views and attitudes of parents are still very important to them.

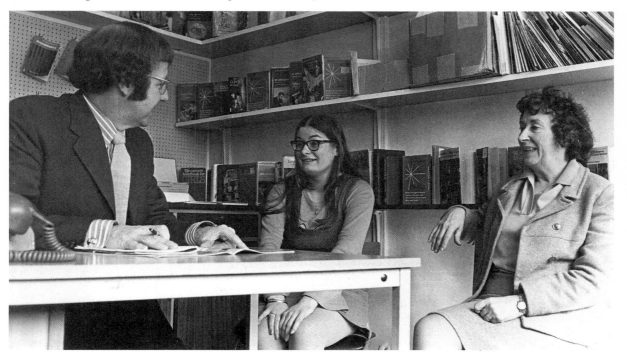

The "generation gap"

Despite the increased difficulty of raising children and adolescents in today's world, most parents and young people manage to succeed, not without some ups and downs, but without unresolvable conflicts and alienation.

There is, as one might reasonably expect for persons at different stages of the life cycle, a generation gap. But it is neither as wide nor as novel as we have been led to believe. Even at the height of the youth culture of the late 1960s, the great majority of both parents and adolescents in the United States expressed the view that, while a generation gap existed, it had clearly been exaggerated.

Current studies give much the same picture. In a recent survey of American adolescents aged 13–19, most of the sample (87 per cent of boys and 89 per cent of girls) stated that they had a lot of respect for their parents' ideas and opinions. Only a small minority stated that they did not feel any strong affection for their parents. And only 6 per cent felt that "My parents don't really like me". Indeed, two-thirds of young Americans aged 16–25 consider the family "a very important value", and a similar proportion would "welcome more emphasis on traditional family ties".

The fact is that, while they may seem earthshaking at the time, most parent–adolescent conflicts are about relatively minor matters. These include getting to bed by a certain time, being able to go to parties or on trips with friends, using the family car, doing chores, spending allowance money, choosing clothes or hairstyles, seeing "too much" of some member of the opposite sex and the like.

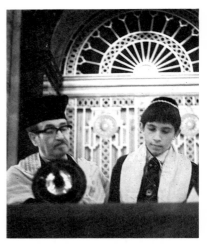

In some cultures, "rites of passage" form a helpful boundary between adolescence and adulthood. Though the Jewish bar mitzvah has something of the same significance, in industrialized societies generally the point of transition is not well defined.

Parents: very important people

Why do some adolescents grow into adulthood confident, competent, caring and secure in their relations with their families, while others emerge from adolescence directionless, insecure, lacking in independence, low in self-esteem, ineffective, angry or alienated? Obviously, there is no simple answer. Many factors may play a part: social disorder, disruptive peer influences, discrimination, poverty, poor schooling.

Nevertheless, an impressive body of research suggests that the single most important influence in helping or hindering the average adolescent to cope with the demands of adolescence in today's world is his or her parents. But what kind of parents? Parents may be loving or rejecting, calm or anxious, relaxed or inflexible, involved or uninvolved, but two dimensions of parental behaviour seem of particular importance.

Love versus hostility

The first of these dimensions may be labelled love–hostility or acceptance–rejection. Without strong and clear manifestations of parental love, a child or adolescent has little chance of developing self-esteem and constructive and rewarding relationships with others.

"I have tried to talk to my father, but it seems that he doesn't want to listen. I don't know why. I guess he thinks my problems aren't important. Anyway, he's pretty busy . . ." (15-year-old boy).

"I can't pick out a future. I ran away because our step-dad beat us all the time . . . I can't see any adult I dream to be like . . . I've never seen the good life . . . I am lonely all the time" (14-year-old girl).

With real parental warmth and caring, however, young people are often able to overcome many seemingly insuperable obstacles.

Parental hostility, rejection and neglect consistently occur more often than acceptance, love and trust in the backgrounds of children with a very wide variety of problems.

Control versus freedom

To cope effectively with today's and tomorrow's world, adolescents need discipline (ultimately self-discipline). However, they also need independence, self-reliance, adaptability and a strong sense of their own values. Research has shown that these qualities are fostered best by parents who show respect for their children, involve them in family affairs and decision-making and encourage the development of age-appropriate independence—but who also retain ultimate responsibility with confidence.

"Because I said so": authoritarian parents

In contrast to the authoritative parent is the authoritarian (or, in more extreme form, autocratic) parent who just tells a child or adolescent what to do and feels no obligation to explain why. Such parents favour obedience as an absolute virtue and tend to deal with an attempt at protest with punitive, forceful measures. Any sort of free discussion between parents and child is discouraged, in the conviction that the young person should unquestioningly accept the parent's word for what is right.

Many children of autocratic or authoritarian parents—because they are not given a chance to test out their own ideas or take independent responsibility, and because their opinions are not treated as worthy of consideration—emerge from adolescence lacking in self-confidence and self-esteem, or unable to be self-reliant, act independently or think for themselves. They are more likely than the children of authoritative parents to say that they felt unwanted by both fathers and mothers.

Laissez-faire and egalitarian parents

Parents who are *laissez-faire* or who assume a false and exaggerated egalitarianism also fail to provide the kind of support that their adolescent young need in today's world. In several recent studies of middle-class adolescents, high-risk drug taking and other forms of socially deviant behaviour were found to occur most frequently among the children of parents who outwardly expressed such values as individuality, self-understanding and the need for egalitarianism within the family, but actually used these proclaimed values to avoid assuming parental responsibility.

By setting up the family as a pseudo-democracy, these parents are able to abdicate from decision-making powers, responsibility and unequal status. But by placing themselves on the footing of peers, they end up leaving their children to drift essentially rudderless in an uncharted sea.

Parents in contemporary society therefore face the problem of steering a delicate course between authoritarianism on the one hand and over-permissiveness or neglect on the other. For those able to achieve this balance, the rewards can be great for both parent and child, although usually some trial and error is involved before reaching this situation.

AREAS OF FRICTION IN THE FAMILY

Manners and morals
An adolescent may feel that parental standards are outdated and unnecessary.

Discipline at home
When parents continue such discipline as was applied to childhood, the adolescent feels insulted or unfairly treated.

Personal sensitivities
An adolescent can become very critical of family life in general and individual ways, causing hostility in the family.

Family rules
An increased desire for independence brings clashes with parents over rules.

Immature attitudes
A child may wish to be credited with more responsibility for his or her own behaviour. But if homework or domestic chores are neglected, parents may want to take stronger control.

Sibling rivalry
A younger sibling's activities may be treated with contempt, while the adolescent is resentful of privileges awarded to older children.

Family responsibilities
An adolescent may regard family gatherings as an unwelcome duty or a bore.

Feeling resentment
Having less money, possessions or opportunities than their peers can cause resentment. Emotional crises such as their parents' divorce are particular danger areas.

Taking drugs

Although there may be significant differences between generations in their patterns of drug use (and drug abuse is no modern phenomenon), the broader society of which adolescents are a part has been developing into a "drug culture" for many years. For example, one-quarter to one-third of all prescriptions currently being written in the United States are for pep or diet pills (amphetamines) or tranquillizers. Between 1964 and 1977, prescriptions for Valium and Librium, the two most widely used tranquillizers, increased from 40 to 73 million a year in the United States alone.

Television and radio bombard viewers with insistent messages that relief for almost anything—anxiety, depression, restlessness—is "just a swallow away". Adolescents who have adopted this view of how life is to be coped with may only be reflecting societal and parental models.

Research has shown that young people whose parents make significant use of such drugs as alcohol, tranquillizers, tobacco, sedatives and amphetamines are more likely than other adolescents to use marijuana, alcohol and other drugs themselves. In the case of alcohol, however, adolescents whose parents do not drink at all are also more at risk from heavy drinking than are those whose parents drink in moderation.

It is also true that while too many adolescents are becoming serious, high-risk drug users, the majority are not. Despite dire predictions in the late 1960s about the imminence of an "epidemic" of adolescent drug use, nothing of the kind has materialized.

Nevertheless, there is no room for complacency. Although it is accurate, for example, to state that "only" 3–5 per cent of junior and high-school students in the United States have ever tried heroin, this still adds up to over a million young people. In addition, use of traditional (i.e. adult) drugs, particularly alcohol, has increased in recent years.

Alcohol

A common refrain among many parents of adolescents today is: "I'm becoming concerned about his drinking, but at least it's better than drugs." In fact, alcohol is just as much a psychoactive drug as, say, marijuana and its dangers have been far more clearly established. Furthermore, the use of alcohol is more common among users of marijuana and other drugs—especially tobacco—than among non-users.

Most adolescents have tried alcoholic drinks at some time, although the frequency of use varies with age, sex, religion, social class, place of residence and country of origin. In non-Muslim countries alcohol is the most frequently used of all psychoactive drugs, including marijuana. It is estimated that in the United States between 71 and 92 per cent of adolescents have tried alcohol by the end of the teenage years. One phenomenon of the 1970s has been the equalization of the rate of alcohol use amongst teenage boys and girls: both groups show an increase over the last 20 years or so, with the rate for girls increasing much faster than that for boys. It should be noted, however, that most adolescents who have engaged in drinking are temperate in their use of alcohol and are likely to remain so.

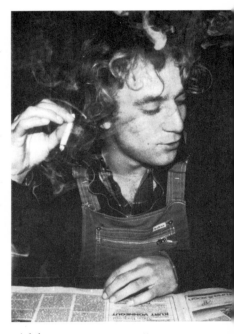

Adolescents may use marijuana to relax while their parents are using alcohol, tobacco or tranquillizers for exactly the same purpose.

Nevertheless, if one uses getting high or drunk once a week or more as a criterion of problem drinking, about 5 per cent of United States teenagers at high school are already problem drinkers. And these figures only include students still at school. Surveys of college students find a much higher figure, at least among males.

Marijuana
Among adolescents who have experimented with one or other illicit drugs, marijuana users account for by far the greatest percentage. In the United States currently more than half of all young people have at least experimented with marijuana. But it is only among chronic heavy users (as is the case with alcohol) that there are fairly consistent indications of real psychological and social disturbance. However, as heavy, chronic marijuana use is typically associated with multiple use of drugs, a direct cause-effect relationship between heavy use and emotional disturbance is difficult to establish.

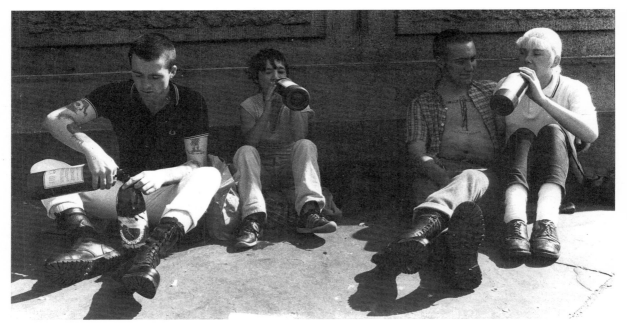

Furthermore, studies of multiple drug users suggest that their use is a result of psychological or social disturbance, rather than its cause. Obviously, once such drug use has begun, a vicious circle may be initiated, with mutual reinforcement of both disturbance and drug need.

Most adolescents experiment with alcohol, and its use has increased in recent years, but the adolescent problem drinker is not common.

Why do adolescents take drugs?
One reason why adolescents may try a drug is simply because it is there. Unlike the average young person of 50 years ago, whose opportunities for drug use were limited in most countries to alcohol and tobacco (and even alcohol was then much less freely available), today's adolescents face a cornucopia of drugs from which to choose, both those sold in pharmacies and those available only on the street. Adolescents are characteristically curious about their expanding world

and far more inclined than most adults to take risks. This is probably partly to prove their boldness, their sense of adventure, and partly because they do not believe, at least initially, that anything disastrous can happen to them.

Young people may also try drugs because of a need to be accepted by a group of peers who are already involved with drugs. In recent research, it has been found that one of the best predictors of whether an adolescent will become involved with a drug is the use of that drug by friends, especially best friends. Adolescents themselves acknowledge the importance of peer group influences.

Parental influence

For the child of democratic, authoritative, loving parents who allow their children gradually increasing, age-appropriate opportunities to "test their wings", the risk of serious drug involvement is generally lower than that for children whose parents have not been loving and who are neglectful, overly permissive or—in contrast—authoritarian

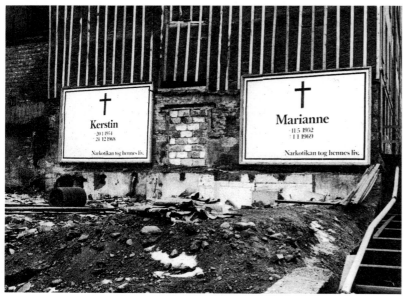

These graphic reminders of the dangers of drug abuse appeared all over Stockholm in 1969. The names and dates of birth and death were fictitious.

and hostile. It is the authoritative parent who is most likely to use the induction techniques, described in "Childhood", that foster the kind of mature morality which to some extent immunizes the young person against the sometimes superficial rewards and punishments which may be exerted by peer groups for using or not using drugs.

Another reason for drug use, often given by the adolescents themselves, is to escape from the tension and pressures of life and from boredom. Ironically, this is also a major reason why adults resort to drugs. One of the greatest dangers of drug use by adolescents is that it can become a substitute for learning to deal with the daily problems and inevitable frustrations of living. And if this learning is never achieved, then drugs may continue to be the answer to life's problems.

What can parents do?

Even the most enlightened, sensible parents cannot guarantee that their children will not become involved with some drug experimentation. There are, however, a number of steps that parents can take to minimize the possibility.

★ Try to keep the lines of communication open with your children.

★ Help your children to become more independent and to take increasing responsibility for their own actions long before the onset of adolescence.

★ Remember that you are role models for your children. What you *do* is often more important than what you *say*.

★ Take an interest in your children's activities—young people need to know that their parents really care.

What if parents discover drug use?

First try to find out just how serious the matter is. The average person who has smoked a few joints or had a few drinks is not in imminent danger.

Assuming that the use of drugs is not, at least yet, out of hand, parents should attempt to discover what lies behind it: curiosity, adventure, a simple desire to share in peer group activities, or resentment against parents, fear of school failure, feelings of inadequacy, and low self-esteem, depression or acute anxiety? Parents should attempt not only to talk to their child, but to look at the young person's life as a whole—and at themselves. Are they part of the problem, as well as part of the solution?

If honest efforts to explore these issues fail, if it becomes obvious that the adolescent's drug use has already become a serious problem, professional help should be sought promptly.

How drugs can affect you

Anyone who regularly uses a drug—from caffeine to heroine—and finds it an impossible habit to break, is an addict. It was previously thought that drug dependence was due to biological changes, resulting in withdrawal. If this were the case, we would expect the intensity of withdrawal to be related to the strength of the habit. On the contrary, cigarette smoking can be just as difficult a habit to kick as heroine addiction—the desire for immediate pleasurable effects acts as a positive reinforcer.

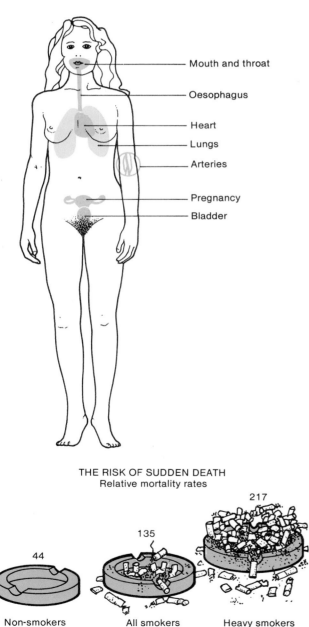

Mouth and throat

Oesophagus

Heart

Lungs

Arteries

Pregnancy

Bladder

THE RISK OF SUDDEN DEATH
Relative mortality rates

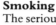

217

135

44

Non-smokers   All smokers   Heavy smokers

Smoking

The serious health risks of smoking are by now well-known, especially the association with lung cancer and heart disease. It is calculated that regular smokers lose 5½ minutes of life expectancy with every cigarette.

The dangerous chemicals in tobacco smoke are tar, a mixture of substances that sits in the lungs as a sticky syrup; nicotine, an addictive drug that acts on the nervous system when absorbed through the lungs; and carbon monoxide, which decreases the efficiency of red blood cells that carry oxygen around the body. It is known that cigarette smoke is carcinogenic, a direct cause of cancers. Lung cancer is not the only risk—a smoker is also 14 times more likely to develop cancer of the mouth or throat. Some tobacco smoke is swallowed rather than inhaled, putting the oesophagus, digestive system and bladder at risk. Carcinogenic chemicals absorbed through the bloodstream may attack other organs of the body. There is a higher incidence among smokers of lung diseases other than cancer, such as chronic bronchitis and emphysema. Sinusitis and influenza are also aggravated by smoking. Tobacco smoke destroys the lungs' inbuilt cleaning system. This leads to the persistent smoker's cough, characterized by a greater secretion of phlegm than is normal.

Heart attacks suffered by smokers are twice as likely to be fatal as those of non-smokers. Diseases of the heart and circulatory system are more common and more serious among smokers. High blood pressure is not caused by smoking, but heart damage is encouraged by the stimulant effects of nicotine.

Women are exposed to particular risks. The slight chance of dangerous side effects from taking the Pill is increased for smokers. In pregnancy, women on 15–20 cigarettes a day miscarry more often and more premature babies are born to smokers. The infant mortality rate is 50 per cent higher in the period following birth, even in full-term babies.

Tobacco smoke increases health risks for non-smokers who spend a lot of time in a smoky atmosphere. This anti-social aspect is one reason why smoking is on the decline. Fewer adolescents smoke than formerly; teenagers cited the health risks, the waste of money and the unpleasant smell of burning tobacco as reasons for not smoking. However, of those adolescents who do take up the habit, about 85 per cent become regular smokers.

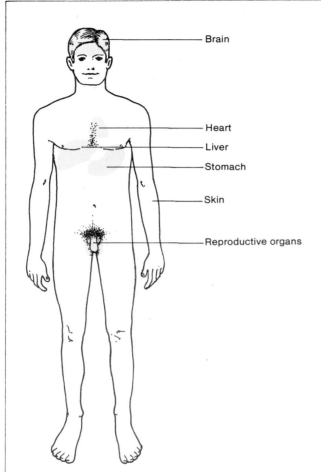

- Brain
- Heart
- Liver
- Stomach
- Skin
- Reproductive organs

Alcohol

Alcohol is the most socially acceptable of drugs used in western society, and the large part it plays in adult social life masks its dangers and less acceptable effects. A small amount relaxes the drinker, producing feelings of warmth, confidence and wellbeing. Regular or heavy drinking results not only in a lack of behaviour control, but gradually does immense harm to the body, some of which is irreversible.

Alcohol is a vasodilator; that is, it makes blood vessels in the skin expand. The greater quantity of blood passing under the skin causes flushing and a rush of warmth. However, vasodilation also increases the rate of heat loss, so that a drunken person is vulnerable to cold and, in extreme cases, may suffer from hypothermia.

Alcohol also acts as a diuretic—by which the body loses water more quickly in heavy and frequent urination. As alcoholic drinks are high in calories but low in nutrients, they cause weight gain but with no nutritional benefit. Nutritional cardiomyopathy is a disease caused by high alcohol intake in which the muscular tissues of the heart are severely weakened.

A stomach upset commonly follows an evening's heavy drinking, but in the long term a drinker may develop chronic gastritis (inflammation of the stomach). More serious are the effects of alcohol on the liver. Cirrhosis of the liver is common and has been increasingly a cause of death over the past 20 years. The liver is unable to perform its function in the digestive process and is ineffective in breaking down drugs, such as antibiotics. Noticeable symptoms of cirrhosis include jaundice and swelling due to fluid retention.

A heavily drunk man may lose the ability to get an erection and impotence is a long-term result of high alcohol consumption. Pregnant women who drink heavily risk damaging the foetus.

Brain functions are also impaired. Alcohol is involved in about one-third of all road accidents. It is often a direct cause of serious injury or death, and a high proportion of domestic and industrial accidents are the result of drinking too much. The adjacent chart shows how the immediate effects of alcohol impair judgement and performance in a way that leads to accidents— such risks increase dramatically with each time the alcohol intake is doubled.

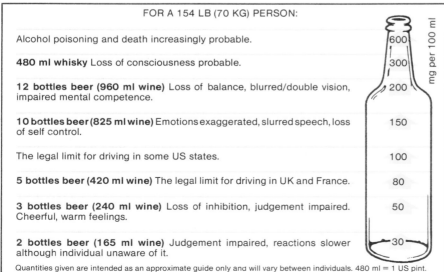

FOR A 154 LB (70 KG) PERSON:

mg per 100 ml

Alcohol poisoning and death increasingly probable. — 600 / 300

480 ml whisky Loss of consciousness probable. — 300 / 200

12 bottles beer (960 ml wine) Loss of balance, blurred/double vision, impaired mental competence. — 200

10 bottles beer (825 ml wine) Emotions exaggerated, slurred speech, loss of self control. — 150

The legal limit for driving in some US states. — 100

5 bottles beer (420 ml wine) The legal limit for driving in UK and France. — 80

3 bottles beer (240 ml wine) Loss of inhibition, judgement impaired. Cheerful, warm feelings. — 50

2 bottles beer (165 ml wine) Judgement impaired, reactions slower although individual unaware of it. — 30

Quantities given are intended as an approximate guide only and will vary between individuals. 480 ml = 1 US pint.

Abused psychoactive drugs

Psychoactive drugs induce an altered state of mind—the user may be seeking euphoria or calmness, an easier night's sleep or hallucinatory effects. The popular image of street junkies and social dropouts is only part of the story of drug abuse. The dangers of illegal drugs are increased because there is no control over the quality of the supply. But any drug or chemical that can be ingested, inhaled or injected is potentially dangerous.

In recent years attention has been drawn to the heavy use of pills obtained on prescription or over the counter. Inadvertent drug abuse has occurred through unforeseen dependency and severe withdrawal symptoms.

Name/common name	Effects sought	Long term dangers/problems
Sedatives		
Barbiturates—Nembutal, Seconal, Tuinal (barbs, candy, phennies, blue heaven, blue devils)	Sleep, relaxation, lessening of anxiety, intoxication.	Dependence or physical addiction; withdrawal symptoms include increased anxiety and insomnia; high dose may cause toxic effects, convulsions.
Tranquillizers—Valium, Librium, Miltown, Tranxene	Release of tension and anxiety, relaxation and mental calmness.	Increased tolerance leads to higher dosage—dependence or addiction occurs with distressing and severe withdrawal symptoms.
Stimulants		
Amphetamines—Benzedrine, Dexedrine, Methedrine (bennies, dexies, speed)	Increased alertness, alleviation of fatigue, reduced appetite, greater capacity for work, feelings of euphoria.	Habit forming, possible psychological dependence; loss of appetite may cause malnutrition, greater susceptibility to infections; persistent use leads to sleeplessness, fever, hallucinations; withdrawal causes apathy and depression.
Cocaine (coke, snow, stardust)	Feelings of euphoria, excitement, sense of power.	Craving develops, leading to psychological dependence; depression, listlessness and difficulty in being sociable.
Narcotics		
Codeine	Feelings of euphoria and relaxation.	Excessive use causes drowsiness, respiratory problems, nausea.
Heroin (H, horse, smack, junk) Morphine Methadone	Permanent "high", euphoria, evasion of stress, avoidance of unpleasant states including withdrawal symptoms.	Craving leads to physical addiction, tolerance develops requiring higher dosage; effects include loss of appetite, weight and sex drive, memory failure, liver disease; danger of infection from injecting or overdose from poor quality drug.
Relaxants		
Marijuana (pot, grass, dope, joint)	Heightened perception, feelings of relaxation.	Loss of drive, impairment of mental functions; association with smoking increases danger of smoking-related diseases.
Hallucinogens		
LSD (acid, sugar, big D) Mescaline Psilocybin	Enhancement and alteration of perceptions, exhilaration, sense of gaining insight and extraordinary abilities.	Anxiety, psychological trauma, paranoia; danger of accident through altered perceptions of time and distance; "flashbacks", temporary effects or hallucinations even without the drug.

Caffeine

Caffeine is a drug found in ordinary coffee, chocolate, tea, cola drinks and some tablets, such as aspirin compounds. It is a stimulant that increases pulse rate and blood pressure. Too much can cause dependency, with symptoms of dizziness, irregular heartbeat, breathlessness and anxiety. Withdrawal causes headaches, restlessness and irritability.

Glue-sniffing

A short period of intoxication comes from a few deep breaths of vapour from glue or solvent. Glue-sniffing is usually a short-lived adolescent craze. There is no evidence that it is addictive, but there is an immediate risk of unconsciousness or even death. Most teenagers recover quickly from the effects on giving it up, but some may be in danger of long-term brain damage.

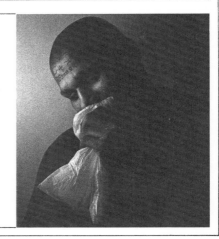

The importance of the peer group

Peers—the contemporaries or age-mates with whom a young person spends much of his or her time—play a crucial role in the psychological and social development of most adolescents.

Adolescents are more dependent on peer relationships than are younger children, simply because ties to parents become progressively looser as greater independence is gained. In addition, relations with family members are likely to become charged by conflicting emotions in the early years of adolescence—dependent yearning existing alongside the desire to be independent, hostility mixed with love.

In adolescence, perhaps more than at any other time in their lives, people need to be able to share strong and often confusing emotions, doubts and dreams with others. Adolescence is a time of intense sociability, but it is also often a time of intense loneliness. Merely being with others does not solve the problem: frequently, a young person may feel most alone in the midst of a crowd, at a party or a dance. This means that acceptance by peers generally and especially having one or more close friends is of crucial importance in a young person's life.

Conformity with peers
Not surprisingly, the heightened importance of the peer group during adolescence leads to heightened needs to conform to its standards, behaviour, fads and fashions. Parents may wonder why it seems so important to their adolescent sons and daughters to have a specific brand of jeans, or why only certain kinds of music, hairstyle, dance, recreational activity, sports or hobbies—the list goes on and on—are

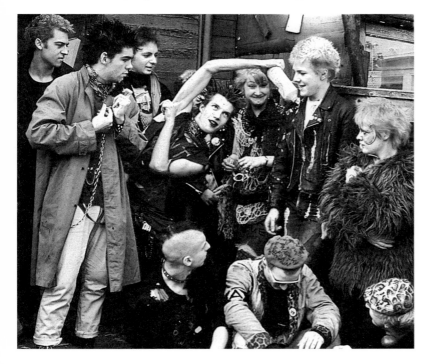

Adolescents want not only to be like each other but also to be different from adults. The result is an adolescent culture in which the "badges" of belonging are all-important. The fads and fashions vary with time and place, but the need to fit in with the crowd is the same.

acceptable. To the parents, these passionate addictions and the rapid shifts they undergo may seem bewildering. But to the adolescents, for whom they serve as badges of belonging, they are anything but trivial.

Parents should perhaps take comfort from these relatively harmless manifestations of difference. For if adolescents can satisfy their striving for independence in these relatively superficial ways, they are less likely to express it in more fundamental matters, such as basic moral values and beliefs. Research has shown that where parents have a basically good relationship with their children, they usually have a stronger influence on a young person's basic values, beliefs and life goals than do peers. Peers, on the other hand, play a stronger role in influencing current modes of social interaction and taste in dress, music and other fashions.

Crowds and cliques

Peer relationships generally fall within one of three categories: the "crowd", the smaller, more intimate "clique" and individual friendships.

The crowd serves as the reservoir for larger, more organized social activities, while the more intimate and cohesive clique provides a source of security and companionship. In this small group, based on mutual attraction, members can exchange information, discuss plans for crowd activities and share some of their dreams, hopes and worries. Girls' cliques tend to be relatively small and concerned with interpersonal relationships; boys' cliques, or "gangs", tend to be somewhat larger, less intimate and more focused on shared activities such as sports and hobbies.

Friendships

Among the peer relationships of adolescence, friendships hold a special place. They are more intimate, involve more intense feelings and are more honest and open than other relationships. There is less defensiveness and less need for self-conscious attempts at role playing in order to gain greater popularity and acceptance.

Adolescents want friends to be loyal, trustworthy and a reliable source of support in an emotional crisis. In the words of one 14-year-old urban girl, "A friend don't talk behind your back. If they are a true friend they help you get out of trouble and they will always be right behind you. That's what a friend is."

At their best, friendships can serve as a kind of therapy by allowing the freer expression of otherwise suppressed feelings·of anger and anxiety. They can also provide the priceless evidence that what one is going through as an adolescent is not unique.

Unfortunately, the course of adolescent friendship does not always run smoothly. By virtue of their very intensity, such friendships may flounder more easily than those of adulthood (which usually involve more modest demands, but also yield more modest rewards). Young people with the greatest number of personal problems may have the greatest need for close friendships, but the least ability to sustain them. And even the most stable and rewarding of adolescent friendships is likely to blow hot and cold, if only because each of the parties to it is in a period of rapidly changing needs, feelings and problems, which in the nature of things will not always coincide. With the approach of the middle years of adolescence, friendships typically become more intimate, more emotionally interdependent and more centred on the personal qualities of the participants.

During this period, the opportunity for shared thoughts and feelings may help to ease the gradual transition to heterosexual relationships. It is also at this time that adolescent friendships are more vulnerable to disruption. By contrast, in late adolescence, friendships, even strong friendships, tend to be calmer, more equable, less exclusive and more tolerant.

Social acceptance, neglect and rejection

Because peers play such an important role in the lives of most adolescents, social acceptance is likely to be an urgent concern for most young people. Few adolescents—or adults—are immune to the effects of social neglect or rejection, often judging their worth to a considerable extent in terms of the way others react to them.

Unfortunately, unpopular adolescents are likely to be caught in a vicious circle. If they are already emotionally troubled and lacking in confidence, they are likely to meet with rejection or indifference from peers—which in turn further undermines self-confidence and increases the sense of social isolation. Other things being equal, social acceptance by the adolescent's peers is desirable—particularly if it is based on mutual helpfulness and shared interests. However, too great an emphasis by parents and adolescents on the pursuit of popularity—on "fitting in" in an organization-minded society, rather than pursuing private, "inner-directed" adolescent dreams and goals—simply invites the real pain of "not belonging" when some setback occurs.

Boys and girls together

During pre-adolescence, boys tend to associate largely with boys and girls with girls. There is a wariness towards the opposite sex that is at least partly self-protective and defensive, precluding, for example, premature heterosexual relationships.

As a young person enters adolescence, wariness of the opposite sex—or outright scorn—diminishes and heterosexual interests increase. Nevertheless, boy–girl relationships in early adolescence still reflect many pre-adolescent characteristics. Self-preoccupation and concern remain, strong, deep emotional involvement is rare and there is usually a superficial, gamelike quality to heterosexual interactions. At this stage, heterosexual group activities are common and provide the security of having familiar members of the same sex present.

Gradually, a young person becomes more familiar with members of the opposite sex and more confident of his or her ability to relate to them. At the same time, increased personal maturity—less narcissism and greater concern for others—is likely to lead to deeper and more meaningful relationships. At their best, such relationships include sexual attraction and social enjoyment, as well as feelings of mutual trust and confidence, a genuine sharing of interests and a serious involvement in the wellbeing of the other partner.

When allowed to develop at a pace that is natural and unforced, such relationships can play an important part in the growth towards maturity. Unfortunately, in a number of Western countries there are often artificial pressures, from parents, peers and the media, to speed up this process and to encourage "going steady" at ever younger ages.

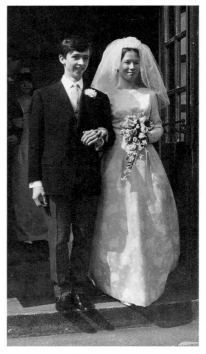

Does a boy or girl who marries a high-school sweetheart have a happier marriage than peers who do not? Adolescent marriages, often complicated by unwanted pregnancies, suffer higher casualties than marriages for other age groups—the divorce rate of both men and women married under the age of 20 is more than twice that of those married later. However, a significant number of such marriages do succeed but the road is seldom easy.

Psychological problems

Every young person will encounter problems in the course of growing up. No life can be, or should be, totally free of anxiety, frustration or conflict. Like joy or love, these experiences are part of being human. An adolescent may have emotional ups and downs, periods of discouragement and worries about being accepted by peers. He or she may experience anxiety before an examination, occasional outbursts of anger and rebellion, involvement with others in a minor delinquent act, sadness at the loss of a boyfriend or girlfriend. But this does not mean that the young person is psychologically disturbed or needs help beyond normal parental understanding and support. It is only when such reactions are exaggerated or look like becoming chronic that it makes sense to talk of a serious problem and to seek professional help.

The common problems

Some psychological problems are relatively easily understood. An adolescent girl who is constantly rejected by her peers may become anxious and withdrawn. A boy who has been subjected to harsh and inconsistent parental discipline may grow into an angry and destructive adolescent. Other kinds of problem, however, are less easily analysed. A suicide attempt may seem, on the surface, to have resulted from a relatively minor disappointment; acute anxiety or panic may have no identifiable source.

Such problems may be reflections of feelings which the adolescents have not identified or acknowledged or, even if they have, cannot articulate to others—fear of loss of love, of angry, hostile feelings, of sexual impulses or of personal inadequacy.

Anxiety reactions

These reactions are not restricted to specific situations or objects. The person may become agitated and restless, easily startled and complain of physical problems such as dizziness or headaches. Concentration and attention may be impaired, and sleep disturbances are common.

People experiencing such anxiety may be puzzled or alarmed about its apparently mysterious source. They may think they have some serious illness, or attribute the anxiety to a variety of external circumstances and incidents. On more careful enquiry, however, it usually becomes apparent that more extensive factors are involved—disturbed parent–child relationships, concerns about the demands of growing up, pervasive fears and guilt regarding sexuality or aggressive impulses—although the adolescent may not be aware of their role in the disturbance. It is easy to see how such factors might produce an apparently all-pervading anxiety which does not seem to be tied to a particular set of circumstances.

It is obviously important to bring in therapeutic intervention as soon as the anxiety reaction has been identified and before the beginning of a patterned response to it, such as psychological withdrawal, impairment of schoolwork, continuing physical problems such as pains, diarrhoea, shortness of breath, fatigue and the like. But how does the concerned parent go about allaying the fears of adolescents or improving their relationship with the youngster?

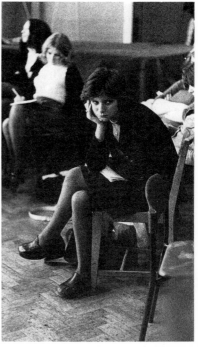

Adolescence is a demanding time—it is not surprising that psychological problems are common.

Body problems

With the adolescent growth spurt and awareness of developing sexual maturity, a teenager's anxieties become focused on his appearance and on the functioning of his body. Rates of growth vary considerably, and at any time someone may be feeling too short or too tall, that his or her shoulders are too narrow or breasts too large. In Western society boys are typically most concerned with muscular development—while girls try to combine their more rounded, maturing shape with fashionable slimness. Fitness and athleticism may be considered desirable for both sexes. But, when it comes to weight control, excessive dieting may lead to anorexia, while overeating provides some compensation for unmet emotional or sexual needs. The main pressure is to fit in with the peer group as far as possible in appearance and style. Sadly, minor problems or differences may result in teasing and insults, which add to the burden of coming to terms with a growing body.

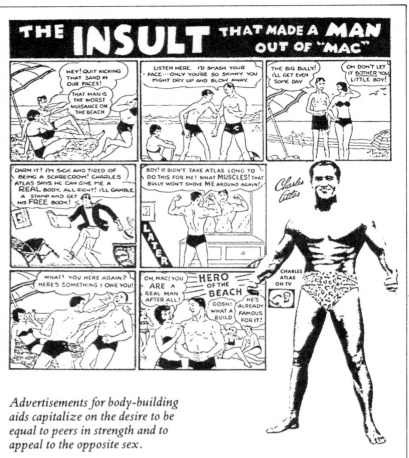

Advertisements for body-building aids capitalize on the desire to be equal to peers in strength and to appeal to the opposite sex.

Descriptive items

		% concern Boys	Girls
1	Pimples, blackheads and acne	51	82
2	Uneven teeth	39	42
3	Greasy skin	27	52
4	Large or misshapen nose	<10	38
5	Having to wear glasses	23	31
6	Skin blemishes, moles, birthmarks	13	30
7	Receding chin	<10	13
8	Heavy eyebrows	<10	11
9	Forehead too high or too low	0	13
10	Homely, unexciting appearance	0	42
11	Dry, scaly or flaky skin	0	43
12	Narrow lips	0	.13
13	Freckles	0	24
14	Face pudgy or too rounded	0	21
15	Face narrow or too thin	15	0
16	Large or sticking out ears	<10	0
17	Gaps between front teeth	26	0
18	Heavy growth of facial hair	13	0
19	Heavy lips or jaw, lack of beard	<10	0

Teenage facial concern

Teenagers are acutely aware of the physical changes taking place in their bodies and they often become highly critical of their appearance. The diagrams show common areas of worry caused by the face alone as experienced by both sexes.

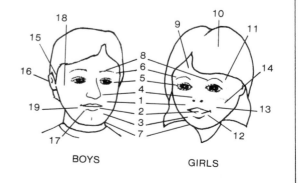

Depression

Saying that a person is depressed tells us little. The word is used when someone is sad over a loss or disappointment, and when the mood is so low the person is almost immobile and expressing feelings of worthlessness and severe guilt.

For most adolescents, low mood is transient, a part of the emotional ups and downs that are so frequent at this time. For some, however, depression may become the dominant mood; it is at this point that professional help may be required. If ignored, such depression may become chronic or even result in suicide.

Depressed adolescents may be unwilling to talk about their feelings and they may show "depressive equivalents" such as boredom and restlessness, which may confuse anyone trying to clarify the problem. A strong dislike of being alone, or a constant search for new activities, drugs, sexual promiscuity, delinquency, risk-taking (including reckless driving) may all be indications of depression, although obviously they may be the result of other factors.

In general, adolescent depression is most likely to take one of two forms. In the first, a young person may complain of a lack of feeling and a sense of emptiness. It is not so much that these adolescents have no feelings as that they are sadly unable to deal with or express those they have.

A second type of depression is usually more difficult to resolve. It has its basis in long-standing, repeated experiences of defeat or failure. A large number of adolescent suicidal attempts are not in fact the result of a momentary impulse, but of a long series of unsuccessful attempts to find alternative solutions to problems. The last straw is often the loss of a desired relationship, whether with a parent, friend or loved one.

Eating problems

Early adolescence is a period of rapid physical and physiological change, and it is not surprising that after the onset of puberty many adolescents go through a brief period of weight fluctuations.

Our society, in contrast with some others, places a great emphasis on being slim. Many adolescents, particularly those with a naturally large body structure, may eat less than good health requires in an effort to look like some currently admired model of attractiveness such as a film or television star. The result, though hardly desirable, gives no real cause for parental anxiety.

Some adolescents, mostly girls, undereat for so long that they become severely malnourished and their very survival may be threatened. The label given to this behaviour is *anorexia nervosa*. A girl often begins with what appears a sensible diet to get rid of a few extra pounds, but once she reaches an ideal weight or even slightly less, she does not stop dieting. She is fearful that anything she eats will result in an unsightly weight gain.

While this kind of behaviour is still relatively rare, it is becoming more common. Parents are often surprised by it, because their child has always seemed so "normal"—in fact, almost too good: quiet, obedient, always dependable, eager to please. Most have been good students.

When one looks closely, however, the picture is not so bright. Although they may not be able to articulate it, many of these girls feel they have been exploited and prevented from leading their own lives, and that they have not been able to form a strong identity of their own. They may have struggled to be "perfect" in the eyes of (often demanding) others. Perhaps in reaction they are likely to display a strong desire to be in control of every aspect of life, including their own bodies. Indeed, they may discover with pleasure that their weight is one area where they are now in control, however tenuously.

Studies of parents of these girls show that the parents had frequently exerted such firm control and regulation during childhood that the girl herself had had great problems in establishing independence, psychologically and physically. These parents are also likely to have encouraged their children to become perfectionists and over-achievers.

Because of the physical effects of prolonged undernourishment, carefully planned hospital treatment may first be necessary. But if long-term progress is to be made, psychological intervention, not only with the adolescent but also with the parents, is essential.

On the other hand, some adolescents may eat too much. Most obese adolescents become so through overeating. A few owe their large size to genetic or constitutional factors, and others may develop a physical predisposition to overweight as a result of overfeeding by parents early in life. Infants are born with a certain number of fat cells, and overfeeding during infancy can result in a permanent increase in the number and size of these cells, making normal weight difficult to achieve.

The psychological reasons for overeating to obesity are many and varied—feelings of emptiness or loneliness, anxiety about being taken care of, feelings of inadequacy. Overweight may be seen as a way of avoiding social or sexual relationships, or even of just getting out of physical exertion. In our weight-conscious society, obesity can be as good as a chastity belt. Obese adolescents—and adults—often seem bad at labelling their bodily feelings, including hunger. The average adolescent will eat when hungry and avoid eating when full, as will the slim adult. This is not typically true of the obese, who tend to eat if food is present or in response to cues other than hunger.

Helping an adolescent lose weight needs parental support and understanding as well as a sensible diet. It will not do to nag and deride. Where significant psychological problems seem to play a part in obesity—for example, anxiety over social relationships—an attempt must be made, if necessary with professional help, to clarify this and deal with it as with weight.

Delinquency

More than 2000 years ago, an Egyptian priest carved on a stone, "Our earth is degenerate. Children no longer obey their parents." Delinquency is no new problem. Today it includes not only the more serious offences such as burglary, assault and robbery, but also minor offences such as truancy, running away, sexual activity or "being beyond parental control", which would not constitute criminal offences if committed by an adult.

Nevertheless, current rates of delinquency are cause for serious concern in many Western countries, particularly the sharp rise in the rate of serious offences and for delinquency among girls.

Delinquency is both a psychological and social problem. The

Clues to suicidal risk

1 A persistently depressed or despairing mood.
2 Eating and sleeping disturbances.
3 Declining school performance.
4 Gradual social withdrawal.
5 Breakdown in communication with parents or other important people in the young person's life.
6 A history of previous suicide attempts or involvement in accidents.
7 Seemingly reckless, self-destructive, and uncharacteristic behaviour, such as drug or alcohol use, or reckless driving.
8 Statements such as "I wish I were dead" or "What is there to live for?"
9 Enquiries about the lethal properties of drugs, poisons, or weapons.
10 Unusually stressful events in a young person's life, such as school failure, break-up of a love affair, or loss of a loved one.

Teenage suicide
The suicide rate in teenagers and young adults (15- to 24-year-olds) is lower than in any older age group, but there is great variation between rates for different countries (right). Whereas the rate in the UK and the Netherlands is relatively low, young people in the USA and Switzerland, in particular, are more prone. Also, Japanese women exhibit a high suicide rate compared to men, but in the USA, the trend is reversed. The trigger for suicide is not always obvious—it is often high achievers rather than problem students in college who succumb.

incidence is higher in socially disorganized, economically deprived areas such as the urban ghettoes of large cities, although this does not mean that all young people raised in these areas are delinquents, or that children raised in affluent backgrounds are not.

What distinguishes the delinquent? Research studies indicate that delinquents tend to be more angry and defiant, suspicious of authority, resentful, impulsive and lacking in self-control. They also appear to have lower self-esteem and more feelings of personal inadequacy and emotional and social rejection.

Although influences such as peer-group pressure and a generally adverse social environment obviously play a part in delinquency, the role of parents appears to be crucial.

Fathers of delinquents are likely to be rated by independent observers as cruel, neglecting and inclined to ridicule their children (sons in particular). Mothers of delinquents are more likely to be rated as careless or inadequate in child supervision, and as hostile and indifferent rather than loving and responsive.

What can parents do? In the first place, keep the problem in perspective. Delinquent behaviour should never be ignored, but many people who become involved in minor delinquent acts go on to become perfectly responsible adults. Sneaking into a movie without paying, "borrowing" a peer's property, playing truant from school, even minor shoplifting are not crimes comparable with mugging and burglary.

Serious and honest discussions between parent and child, conducted in a calm but realistic atmosphere, can often be helpful, especially if the basic relationship between them is one of mutual trust, warmth and respect. When such communication is impossible or when it appears that emotional disturbance is playing a part in delinquent behaviour, professionl help should be sort. As we have seen, parents who encourage the development of independence and self-reliance are less likely to have a delinquent son or daughter.

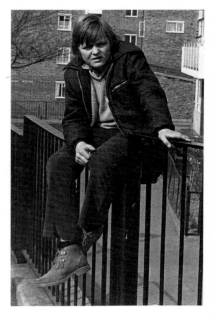

Adolescent depression may be manifested as boredom or restlessness.

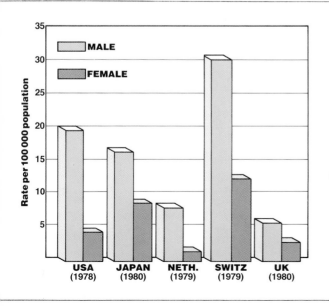

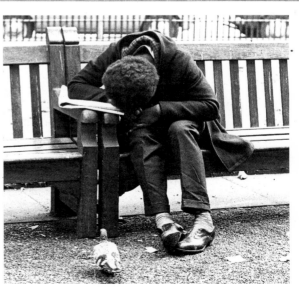

Ready for adulthood

Many of the challenges that young people will eventually have to meet and the adaptations they will have to make are impossible to predict: one need only look at last year's "expert" estimates of what today's world would be like to see the truth of this.

However, emotionally mature young people—those who are able to achieve a workable integration of their own needs and desires, their conscience and ideals and the demands of the real world—will be far better prepared to cope with the inevitable "slings and arrows of outrageous fortune" than the immature, the rigid and inflexible, the rootless and self-indulgent or the neurotic.

Being "mentally healthy" does not mean being able to go through life without conflict. No one can avoid conflicts between his or her needs, goals and desires, and the demands of reality—in any case, a reasonable amount of conflict often serves as an impetus to further growth and development. All we can hope is that, as they approach adulthood, adolescents should have been helped to tolerate a reasonable amount of conflict and frustration and to deal with it effectively.

Sigmund Freud was once asked what he meant by emotional maturity. "*Lieben und arbeiten*", he replied—the capacity to love and to work. By genuinely loving their children (which certainly does not preclude moments of acute frustration and irritation), by valuing them as people, by being worthy of their trust, parents can help them to become capable, in their turn, of loving and trusting others.

With emotional maturity comes the confidence and flexibility to cope with the great variety of situations presented by life.

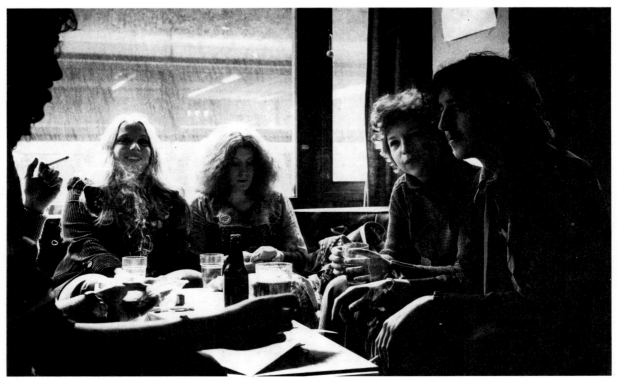

By encouraging sons and daughters to become independent, competent and responsible, parents can help them prepare to meet the challenge of changing vocational demands and responsible citizenship. As we have seen, this is best accomplished by authoritative or democratic parenting, not by *laissez-faire*, overly permissive or autocratic child-rearing—and certainly not by neglect or indifference.

Parents alone, in a modern society, should not be expected to do the whole job. Children need adequate nutrition and health care, they need to grow up in decent surroundings, they need to be around peers and adults who can provide models of socially responsible behaviour. And they need a good education, which can challenge and develop their talents and prepare them for rewarding careers and responsible citizenship. Finally, to be fulfilled, they need to find jobs and to be accepted as fully-fledged members of society.

Do we really care?
For all too many of our young people, these needs are not being met. Unless Western society begins to demonstrate a greater sense of responsibility to its young people—not just the socially, economically or ethnically favoured, but *all* its children—we will continue to see rising rates of personal failure and tragedy, of delinquency, suicide, psychological problems and alienation.

The importance of education
The situation is worst for those growing up in urban or rural slums. Here overburdened, discouraged teachers with inadequate resources and community support often have difficulty in maintaining even a semblance of order and discipline in the classroom, let alone providing an education relevant to the needs of their students. And even middle-class schools often provide little cause for wholehearted enthusiasm. Charles Silberman, in a nationwide survey of secondary education in the United States, found a tendency for many middle-class schools to concentrate on what he calls "education for docility". This means an over-emphasis on order, discipline and conformity at the expense of self-expression, intellectual curiosity, creativity and the development of humane, sensitive human beings.

Other countries will vary in their conformity to these findings according to such factors as social class, the split between private and state-provided education, emphasis on public achievement and so on. But there is no doubt that in general in the Western world, education is designed to shape rather than to encourage growth. This situation is likely to be most pronounced at the junior high-school levels. Adolescents are harder to "control" than younger children, and secondary schools are thus likely to be even more authoritarian and repressive than elementary schools.

Obviously, not all schools fit these dismal patterns. Even in some urban ghettoes, there are schools that are spectacularly successful. One such school is in a run-down section of New York City, where adolescent girls, who had previously been rejected as incapable or unmanageable by other city schools, proved able not only to stay in school, but to develop a sense of pride in themselves and their school, and to improve their education skills greatly.

How was this "miracle" achieved? Researchers studying this and other successful educational efforts found several essential ingredients.

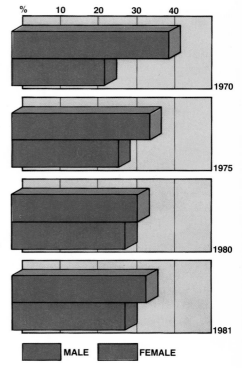

MALE　FEMALE

College enrollment
There has been a significant change in the pattern of enrollment in the USA over the period 1970 to 1981. Although the percentage of high school graduates enrolling has remained fairly stable, rising only slightly over the decade, the proportion of men has dropped from nearly 50 per cent and the proportion of women has risen from around 25 per cent—in 1981 about 30 per cent of both men and women were enrolling.

The atmosphere is much warmer and more supportive than in most schools. Disruptive behaviour is handled more positively, and there is the conviction that "disadvantaged" children can learn. Principals and teachers in these schools hold themselves accountable if their students fail (in contrast to the widespread labelling of such children as "learning disabled", which occurs in many conventional schools) and innovative, imaginative, pupil-centred approaches to the development of academic skills are flexibly employed. Far more such schools—and teachers—are badly needed.

From school to work

There are those who find the transition from school to work relatively painless, but for many school leavers the transition to work is neither easy nor welcomed. For some, this may be because they failed to get the kind of job they wanted. Two separate studies have found that one half of school leavers who had seriously set their sights on a particular kind of work failed to achieve it, even when their choices were realistic and consistent with their school performance. In times of economic recession, this figure would be considerably higher.

Others may find it difficult to come to terms with the contrast between school and work. The pace of work may be faster and may demand more energy than classroom activities. The new worker may have difficulty in grasping where everyone fits in the hierarchy.

Smoothing the transition from school to work

One important reason why the transition from school to work may be difficult is a lack of knowledge about the world of work in general or about particular jobs. There is a good deal of evidence that the process of job selection among school leavers, particularly those who have been low achievers at school, is very haphazard.

Many young people will take any job which comes their way, because they genuinely don't mind what kind of work they do, providing the pay and conditions are reasonable. Others, lacking any clear idea of what they would like to do or how they would like their career to develop, may find themselves in jobs which, had they known more about them from the start, they would have realized would be uncongenial to them.

A number of schemes now exist which try to introduce young people to the world of work, but in general far too little is being done. All too often, school leavers are not even given the kind of information which would help them make a more informed career choice and so approach their first job with the confidence that they have at least some idea of what to expect.

Schemes which do exist range from one- or two-day conferences, sometimes organized by trade unions, covering topics such as finding a job, attending interviews, and coping with the world of work, to day or block release schemes whereby young people gain experience of various working environments, either by extended visits or by actually working for short periods while they are still at school.

These schemes are valuable, but need to be backed by a school syllabus which, in its later stages, is much more work-oriented than at present. Although there is little direct impact an interested parent can make in this respect, it is always valuable for them to contribute as much as possible in parent–teacher meetings.

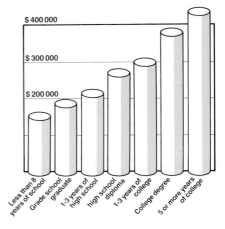

Education and income

The value of further education may not always be appreciated. A study by the US Census Bureau in the early 1970s equated lifetime income for a 22-year-old male with levels of education. Apart from obvious changes in figures due to inflation, higher incomes are now more widely enjoyed in the population due to the fact that more women and minorities are embarking on further education.

Health problems in adolescence

Adolescence is a time of great physical and psychological changes. The majority of health problems are due to the activity of sex hormones, e.g. acne and menorrhagia. Other problems are related to diet—many cases of anaemia are attributable simply to bad eating habits. Anxiety about their developing bodies may lead adolescents to seek reassurance that they are not suffering from serious illnesses. But generally this is a time of high energy and relatively few diseases are characteristic of this stage.

PROBLEM	SYMPTOMS	TREATMENT/ACTION
Anorexia nervosa	Obsessive dieting in girls, extreme thinness, cessation of periods, low resistance to infection.	There may be reluctance to admit a problem but advice is needed. A period in hospital may be advised when food intake can be monitored. These problems are usually part of problems within family relationships and may be difficult to treat in isolation.
Bulimia nervosa	Binge eating followed by self-induced bouts of heavy vomiting.	
Menstrual problems Pre-menstrual tension	Period pain, swelling of body due to fluid retention, painful breasts, backache, depression and irritability.	Consult a doctor. Hormone preparations, such as progesterone, are sometimes effective. A diuretic relieves fluid retention.
Menorrhagia (heavy periods)	Heavy bleeding during periods, often accompanied by pain; blood loss can cause anaemia.	Heavy periods may cease later when the menstrual cycle settles into a regular pattern. Bleeding between periods should be reported to a doctor. Hormone treatment may be effective.
Dysmenorrhea (painful periods)	Severe period pain and cramps, nausea, dizziness.	Self-help remedies include relaxation and physical exercise. Aspirin temporarily helps the pain. Seek medical advice for drugs to control pains and cramps.
Migraine	Headaches lasting up to several hours, nausea, dizziness, sensitivity to light.	The cause of migraine has not been identified. Some sufferers get relief from anti-histamine drugs; diet may be a factor. Seek medical advice.
Allergies	Sneezing, skin rashes, difficulty with breathing.	For severe allergies an allergy test is necessary to identify the cause, when suitable treatment can be prescribed.
Acne	Regular crops of surface pimples, some abscessing to affect deeper layers of skin and cause scarring.	Many proprietary brands of acne creams and gels are available. If the infection is deeply rooted it may respond to antibiotics given under medical supervision. For most people acne disappears at the end of adolescence when glandular activity settles.
Sexually transmitted diseases (STDs) Gonorrhea	In males, yellow discharge from the penis and pain when urinating. In women, unusual vaginal discharge.	Self help is not effective for STDs. Abstain from sex and seek immediate treatment. Since many people show no symptoms, it is important to consult a doctor if there is fear of infection.
Herpes II	Itching, small blisters on genitals.	

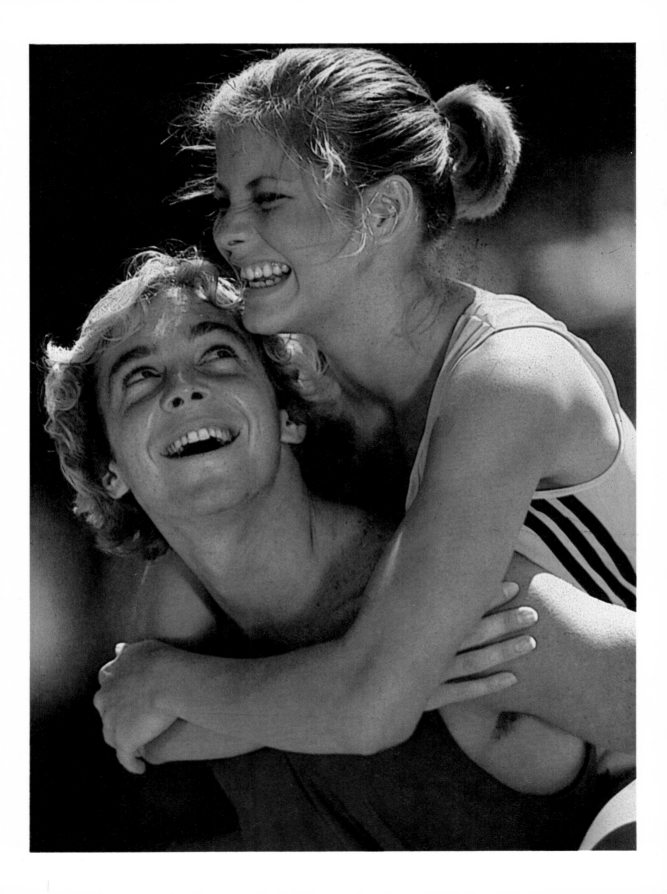

Young Adulthood

What matters is the kind of life which people lead and the satisfaction they find in it. And here, I suspect, most of us think too much of problems and too little of persons.

R.H. Tawney (from *The Observer* 1953)

The stage of young adulthood falls roughly into two parts: the transition phase, when the individual moves into work and into long-term relationships, and the establishment phase, marked by career development and the raising of a family. For some, the transition phase occurs while they are still adolescents, for others not until much later.

It is perhaps more accurate to think of these phases in terms of roles enacted and major preoccupations. The transition phase is the age of role rehearsals, in contrast with the more tentative explorations of adolescence. The two principal preoccupations of young adults in the transition phase seem to be the search for an intimate relationship or commitment and identification with social institutions. During the establishment years, most people's main preoccupation is with major life investments—work, family, friends and community activities.

A generation or two ago, most people's paths through these two phases would have been highly predictable, given a particular social class or educational level. However, the last few decades have seen remarkable changes in the pathways, or at least in their timing. Both men and women are much more willing to delay the establishment phase: for many, this phase is now marked by the disruption (often welcome) of divorce, setting up a new family, of career switches, of embarking on a new career for the first time.

In this section we will explore the problems, challenges and rewards facing young people as they attempt to find and consolidate their roles in adult society.

Left: Establishing ourselves, and with it the fulfilment of adulthood

Employment, study or neither

Once out of school, young people face several possibilities: going directly into work, travelling abroad, going into further education, living in "anti-institution" groups and adopting an alternative life style, or being faced with unemployment and thus starting adult life without an occupation—while work provides the prime role identity of adulthood in our society, particularly for men.

Students: time out of life

Full-time students comprise a substantial minority of young adults all over the industrialized world. In Britain, about 20 per cent of those aged 18 to 21 are students, and in the United States the figure is higher still. Even in countries where students are less numerous, they are likely to be an extremely important sector of the population. Students in institutions of higher education are in a position to develop a wide range of interests. They have time, opportunities and external encouragement to develop resourcefulness. This is true not only of their academic work, but of all their time and activities.

Developing skills in argument, finding evidence to support a point of view, getting to know many different kinds of people and life styles, taking part in sport and drama, are not only relevant to a future occupation, but to making one's way in life according to the prevailing ideas of a liberal education. Peter Marris wrote, in his study of British higher education in the 1960s:

> Most people who have faith in a university believe that [it] can give [a liberal] education and that this is its particular justification. The idea implies . . . both the development of a generalized rational understanding both from the courses themselves and, equally, the social environment in which the student learns. For him, the university is not so much an institution as three or four years of his life when living away from home making friends, falling in love or realizing his religious convictions may be as important as studying for his degree.

However, this ideal is not as widespread as it might be. At many universities and places of further education, getting a degree or qualification is of overriding importance; at others, students do not live in halls of residence but continue to live at home, in part under their parents' control. Nor is the ideal even as generally desired as it once was.

Where the research is focused

Of all young adults, most is known about university students. A good deal of the research tends to focus on things such as aptitude testing, teaching methods, student "wastage" and performance (which are useful to those responsible for financing further education), and not on how the students actually grow and develop as people.

Peter Marris's study, *The Experience of Higher Education*, is a wide-ranging analysis of what it means in the lives of young people to spend three or four years at an institution of higher education. Although carried out in the early 1960s, this study gives us some insights which are probably valid still.

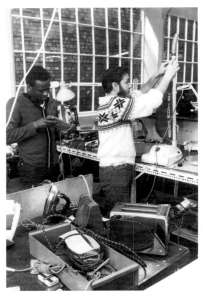

Schemes, such as the Job Corps of the US Job Training Partnership Act (JTPA), undertake the training and job placement of young people between the ages of 16 and 19. An equivalent project in Britain is "Brass Tacks", which trains and employs young people who would otherwise be unemployed.

Education and employment

The US Bureau of Statistics'
figures (below) confirm that
further education is an advantage
in terms of occupational status. In
general, the more education people
have, the more likely it is that
they will have a white collar job.
Educational qualifications increase
the chances of getting any kind of
job: the percentage of employed
with less than 4 years of high
school education dropped by
around 50 per cent between 1970
and 1981; for those with more
education the percentage
increased. The percentage of
women employed in any category
is lower than men, but women
with high qualifications in high
status jobs seem to be particularly
disadvantaged.

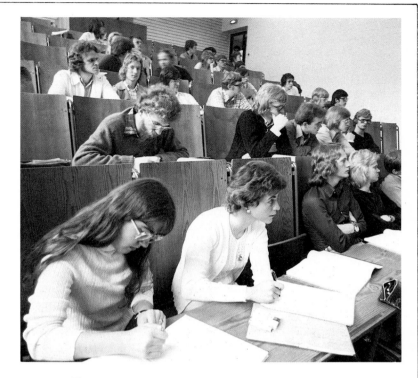

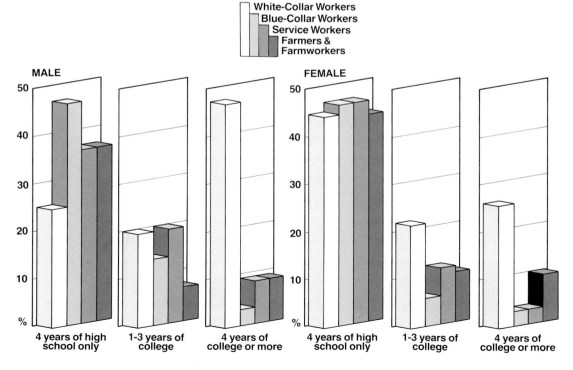

White-Collar Workers
Blue-Collar Workers
Service Workers
Farmers &
Farmworkers

MALE

FEMALE

4 years of high
school only

1-3 years of
college

4 years of
college or more

4 years of high
school only

1-3 years of
college

4 years of
college or more

Most students in British universities had accepted the logic that it followed from their success at school that they should proceed to higher education. They did an honours degree at university if they were judged to have the ability; they went to what is considered a "lesser institution" if they did not. They rarely went to an alternative institution because they liked what it had to offer.

The present recession has not diminished the numbers seeking higher education in Britain. On the contrary, they continue to rise. In 1981, the number of applications to universities rose by 4.2 per cent, but the number of places available fell by 3 per cent. What has changed, however, is the pattern of applications to different subject areas. Demand for places is growing on vocation-based courses such as computer science and business studies, and falling in once popular areas such as sociology and politics, where jobs for such graduates are now harder to come by. The pattern in the USA is the same: in 1979 nearly 40 per cent of eighteen- to twenty-four-year-olds were enrolled for higher education courses. Overall enrollment figures have risen steadily, increasing by 15.5 per cent between 1974 and 1979, and increases for women, ethnic minorities and mature and part-time students were much greater. The same shifts in subject choice have also occurred, with students opting for business studies in particular.

Because of the pressure to get good examination grades at school and the assumption that university is the goal, many students arrive at college and "seem at first to wait passively for some inarticulate but great fulfilment". Many become disenchanted—academically and socially—when their romantic dreams of "gaiety, freedom, intellectual excitement and graceful surroundings" crumble. Further, they are so conditioned by the spoon-fed way they learned at school that they do not know how to learn on their own and rely on their own initiative. By the time they have mastered self-directed learning, their final exams may be almost upon them.

College: a social necessity or social advancement?
The majority study the subjects they were best at in school. A sizeable proportion of students switch from pure to applied sciences, adopting a more calculating attitude about the usefulness of their studies, especially middle-class students. Marris compares the middle-class student who "sees his university career primarily as a means of qualifying for an occupation similar in status to his father's and . . . feels his parents to have been a more important influence than his school", with the working-class student who "sees the university more as the final prize in the competition for education, whose vocational usefulness he takes for granted. . . . Neither student has the social or intellectual opportunities of the university uppermost in his mind."

A broad education?
Most students did not feel their higher education had contributed much to the development of their general interests: "Altogether, a quarter of the scientists had not opened a book at all during the term, apart from their studies, and another quarter had read only light fiction or motor racing manuals, while 15 per cent of arts students had read nothing and eight per cent merely light entertainment."

Unemployment

In the USA, in 1981, 14.7 per cent of high school graduates between the ages of 16 and 21 were without a job — a total of 937000. The rate for school dropouts was much higher — 31.1 per cent. It is thought that youth employment schemes have not had much impact on these figures — a drop in the ocean compared to the effects of world economic recession. However, figures for the 16 to 25 age group for 1982 and 1983 do suggest that the rate of unemployment is showing a decrease, albeit a small one (just over one per cent). These are the findings of the US Bureau of Labor Statistics. In their comparative study of international unemployment rates, Britain had a higher unemployment rate by 1982 than Sweden, West Germany, France, Canada, the USA and Japan.

Unemployment in developed countries has affected all levels of society, but school leavers (whether they have completed their education or not) are perhaps the hardest hit. Members of ethnic minorities and those without experience, work references and with few qualifications are not finding work for months, and sometimes years. In the UK, one-third of men and one-quarter of women in the 20 to 24-year-old age group had been on the register for over a year, in statistics compiled in April 1982.

There were 25343 registered bankruptcies in the United States in 1982—the highest annual figure since the depression year of 1932. Hardest hit is heavy industry, and Chicago is a case in point, with 160000 unemployed over the past 10 years. By 1982 the rate had accelerated to 12.8 per cent of the working population.

The sight everywhere is of severe economic depression—the steel mills on the shores of Lake Michigan have idling outputs and at one point the huge industrial and agricultural automotive giant "International Harvester" teetered on the brink of bankruptcy. The Wisconsin steel plant has closed, with the loss of many jobs. Ironically, among all the chaos, Chicago is already deeply involved in planning for the 1992 World Fair. This picture of contraction is repeated to a greater or lesser degree all over Western Europe.

Above: When the "Mayor Jane Byrne" firm recently offered 3800 temporary jobs, 20000 people applied and stood in a line all night.

Below: Between 1973 and 1983 unemployment rose sharply in most industrialized countries. In the US, the rate dropped in the late 1970s, only to rise again

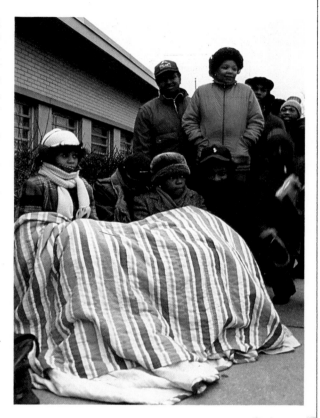

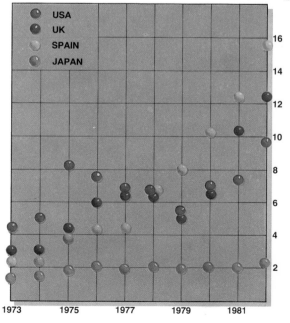

USA
UK
SPAIN
JAPAN

Occupational Group	Adjusted Ratio
Professional & Technical Workers	70.2
Managers, Officials & Proprietors	59.8
Clerical Workers	63.9
Salesworkers	50.7
Skilled & Kindred Workers	63.6
Operatives	64.3
Service Workers, excluding private household	68.3
Total	**67.2**

Left: Women's wages

In spite of legislation in the US, women still fall behind men in the wages stakes. Even after taking into account women's shorter working hours and other factors, there is still a significant difference between the sexes. In 1978, the ratio of female to male earnings in full-time, year-round employment was as shown. Furthermore, these differences are mirrored for specific occupations.

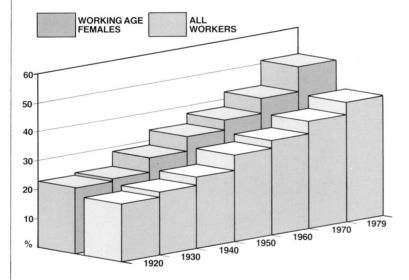

Left: Percentage of women in employment

The percentage of women in the workforce, in the US, has shown a large increase over the last few decades. Women in 1979 made up 42 per cent of the workforce.

Right: The role of women in the workforce

This chart shows some of the countries in which women form an important proportion in the various categories, eg wage earners, for different years. The patterns are unexpected—in only two categories do major Western powers come within the top four—USA and Germany—for women as wage earners. In all other categories, the USSR and other eastern bloc countries, and economically unstable countries rely much more heavily on women. It is impossible to disentangle the reasons for these trends whether through women's choice, male dominance or simple economic dependence.

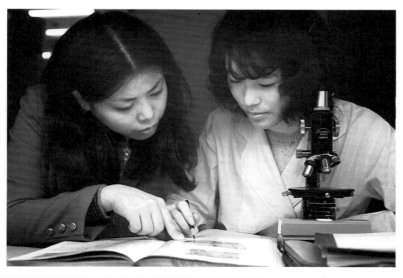

Left: Young scientists. However, more girls than boys still tend to specialize in arts and social science subjects, though the pattern is beginning to change.

Women as a proportion of all those economically active	
USSR	50.45 (1970)
TANZANIA	47.79 (1967)
BULGARIA	46.81 (1975)
E. GERMANY	46.27 (1971)
USA	39.75 (1976)
UK	36.52 (1971)

Women as a proportion of all employers and those working on their own account	
ROMANIA	57.87 (1966)
POLAND	55.29 (1974)
GHANA	53.04 (1970)
TANZANIA	52.88 (1967)
USA	22.45 (1976)
UK	20.13 (1971)

Women as a proportion of all wage earners	
W. GERMANY	85.29 (1975)
JAPAN	79.96 (1976)
NORWAY	79.71 (1976)
USA	79.25 (1976)
BELGIUM	77.21 (1976)
NETH.	75.40 (1971)

Women as a proportion of all salaried workers	
USSR	49.18 (1970)
FINLAND	46.67 (1976)
BULGARIA	46.08 (1975)
CZECH.	43.81 (1970)
USA	40.73 (1976)
UK	38.05 (1971)

Women as a proportion of all administrative and managerial grades	
USSR	63.57 (1970)
POLAND	47.28 (1974)
BRAZIL	46.75 (1974)
ARGENTINE	46.63 (1974)
USA	33.65 (1976)
UK	30.88 (1971)

Source: Social Trends 1983

Studies in the United States have shown similar overall patterns. Available research on drop-outs from college indicates that the largest proportion typically attributed dropping out to "lack of interest". Those with vocation motives are more likely *not* to drop out, but there is no simple relationship between personal growth and staying or leaving.

Youth unemployment

Unemployment in general will be considered later, but for young people there are special problems. The percentage of 1980 high school graduates in the USA still unemployed in October of that year was 18.9 per cent, and in Britain less than one in three school leavers can expect to find work six months after leaving. Adult unemployment rates are much higher among the unskilled and unqualified, so school leavers lacking training or work references are particularly hard hit in times of recession. The unemployment rate for high school dropouts in the USA is over 30 per cent.

The graduate pool

University graduates also face unemployment, and there is a feeling that the community has made an investment in their education that should not be wasted. Of the batchelor's degree recipients in the USA in 1977, 5.9 per cent were unemployed in 1978 and 16 per cent were employed in jobs for which they were overqualified. In Britain, over 11 per cent of graduates are unemployed, despite the efforts of placement services, and there is a similar problem concerning overqualification.

Work in the establishment phase

The establishment phase is often seen as a time of career development and consolidation. For many, however, it is a time of resignation to a job which offers little personal satisfaction, or a time of frequent job changes in an effort to find congenial employment.

Why work? The cynical answer to this question is because it enables us to earn money. That may be the case, but there is, in Western societies, a very strong work ethic. We work partly because it is expected of us, at least until retirement age, particularly men.

However, we also work for more positive reasons. Work broadens our horizons and introduces us to a much wider range of people than would be possible if we remained at home. Work may give us power and prestige. It can provide friends and a social life. It gives a sense of achievement.

What makes for satisfaction at work?

The idea that personal satisfaction with work is important is a relatively recent one. The idea grew alongside an increasing concern with psychological factors in general (a change already mentioned in "Childhood"). This preoccupation partly arose from the fact that many of the physical hardships imposed on workers by the Industrial Revolution had been alleviated. Employers were also interested in the job satisfaction of their employees, sometimes for altruistic reasons, but also because it was assumed that improving satisfaction would improve performance and productivity. It has, however, proved surprisingly difficult to demonstrate any relationship, or at least a simple relationship, between satisfaction and performance at work.

Partners for life?

The vast majority of adults in Western society marry, at least once. They also tend to contract their first marriages during the early part of young adulthood. The rising divorce rate has led some observers to conclude that marriage is becoming an outmoded institution, but this view is not supported by the data. If anything, a slightly higher proportion of the population now marries than 50 years ago; in addition, a substantial number of the divorced and widowed (especially divorced men) remarry, showing that, at least as far as marriage is concerned, once bitten is not twice shy.

What is changing is the form of relationships into which people enter before marriage. (It is interesting to note the extent to which the phrase "trial marriage" has virtually disappeared from the language, thus elevating living together to the status of a separate relationship in its own right.) More people are also marrying more often, sometimes in the process creating families so complicated that even their members have difficulty in describing the relationships within them.

We have noted that a major preoccupation of early adulthood is the search for a "mate"; the figures for the number of marriages which take place would seem to indicate that most people are, at least initially, successful in their search.

The social geography of marriage

In contrast with studies of opposite-sex attraction, where the couples studied may or may not eventually marry, studies of social factors in mate selection have concentrated on married couples, partly because the kind of information in which researchers were interested is often obtainable from public records of marriage.

The research which does exist is, however, meagre but the results are surprisingly consistent. In three different countries (France, Britain and the United States) the crucial factor of "residential propinquity" (as living near each other is grandly described) has been highlighted. This factor is particularly important in lower social classes. In the American study, for example, it was found that the median distance (the distance above and below which there were equal numbers of people) travelled by an unskilled worker to find his eventual spouse was five blocks.

Bernard Ineichen of the University of Bristol in Britain has recently carried out a detailed study of mate selection in that city. He found that, before marriage, over 30 per cent of the 232 couples studied came from the same or an adjoining district as one another. Similar studies in the USA have shown that the tendency for people to marry partners who come from the same socio-economic background is increasing, and that partners from all social classes tend to have lived within three miles of each other before marriage. This may be connected with people's increasing freedom to choose their own spouses without parental pressures.

Why him, why her?

Forming a partnership involves three processes. The first is the initial attraction between the pair, the second the decision to take the relationship beyond the first meeting or two, and the third the decision to marry or live together for an indefinite period.

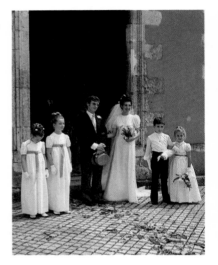

In spite of opinions to the contrary, marriage is still very popular: one-half of all men who marry do so by age 24, and women on average marry two years earlier. Nearly all Americans eventually marry, the current figure being 94 per cent of men and 96 per cent of women. At the moment there is a trend to delay marriage. The median age has increased by over two years and is now the same as it was in 1940. Such fluctuations can be attributed to a variety of social and economic factors, such as the increase in pre-marital sex, rising numbers of female college graduates, unemployment etc.

What determines whether people will find each other attractive? Social psychologists have identified two extremely powerful factors, which are, in order, physical appearance and similarity of attitudes. The ideas that we are attracted to people by their personalities, or that opposites attract, have found very little support. People are generally reluctant to admit that they are attracted to people because they look good, perhaps because this seems such a superficial and unfair way to judge others. It is also possible that we are unaware of the powerful effect of physical attractiveness and rationalize our liking for others in terms of their personalities. However, there is now overwhelming evidence that people's appearance is one of the prime determinants of whether we find them attractive (in the psychological sense)—not only that, but physically attractive adults (and children) are judged, *a priori*, to have more attractive personalities, even if the judgements are made from photographs.

In one large-scale experiment, Elaine Walster and her colleagues invited students at the University of Minnesota to fill in questionnaires describing their backgrounds, attitudes, interests and so on. They were told that the answers would be fed into a computer which would match them with a partner of the opposite sex, to whom they would be introduced at a "computer dance". The students were, in fact, matched randomly. As they entered the dance, they gave their names and were rated by two observers for physical attractiveness. A few weeks later, the students were contacted again and asked how much they liked their dance partners, whether they wanted to see them again and whether the relationships had actually continued. It was found that the most powerful factor in determining whether

Adjustment to a mate

The ease of adjustment to a partner in a long-term relationship depends to a great extent on the expectations of each person. Where the reality falls short of the "ideal" and one partner feels that his/her needs are not being fulfilled, adjustment becomes more difficult. Similarity of outlook, background, values and interests makes adjustment easier. Both partners will have to make considerable changes to their patterns of living to accommodate the other, and this is a potential cause of friction, particularly when each has a definite, conflicting, concept of the roles of husband and wife. Considerable emotional adjustments are also being made at this time, and these affect the stability of the relationship. In general, the further the mate is from the individual's ideals, the harder the adjustment is.

Difficulties in adjustment

Inevitably, difficulties are experienced when first adjusting to a mate; but certain factors can prolong and exacerbate the problems. An overly romantic concept of marriage and unrealistic expectations can lead to disappointment and emotional difficulties. When one partner feels that he/she is seen from outside as merely the spouse of the other, the loss of identity is resented. Sexual adjustment is generally easier than in the past because of the availability of information. But few couples have advance experience of child-rearing, coping with in-laws or even many of the routine domestic tasks. Early marriage and parenthood can lead to a feeling of having 'missed out' on life; and socially and racially mixed marriages usually need extra adjustments. Finally, changes in society's attitudes to marital roles of men and women can make adjustment more difficult than when roles were rigidly prescribed.

Stability of marriage

A number of factors affect the stability of a marriage. Generally speaking, divorce is more common among partners who come from different cultural, racial, religious or social and economic backgrounds. Those who married because the wife was pregnant have a higher than average divorce rate, as do couples who married in their teens. The shorter the interval between marriage and the first child, the higher the divorce rate. There are more divorces between childless couples and couples with one or two children than among those who have large families— mainly because the former have less to cope with after divorce. The couples who maintain their separate identities instead of one becoming submerged by the other are far more likely to have a lasting marriage.

partners liked each other and whether they continued to see each other was physical attractiveness.

The second important determinant of attraction is attitude similarity. Presumably this is partly because we find it reinforcing to have our view of the world validated. Not all attitudes are equally important, of course. It is those dealing with social, moral and political issues which seem to influence people most.

There are, however, certain circumstances under which we will find people who share our attitudes less attractive than people who do not. In one experiment, subjects were introduced to someone who apparently shared their attitudes to important issues. They were told, however, that this person had once received psychiatric care and still felt bad from time to time. Under these conditions, the subjects declared themselves to be more attracted to someone who, they were led to believe, did not share their attitudes but who, on the other hand,

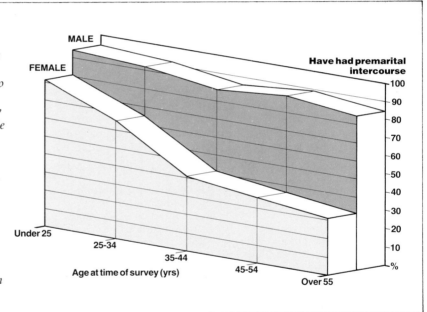

Pre-marital sex
Recent surveys have shown that pre-marital sex is increasingly common, and the trend is towards earlier experience. A large proportion of the statistics refers to couples having sex before marriage. But some surveys show that it is becoming more acceptable for young people to have sex whether or not they intend to marry each other. Thus, as the graph on the right shows, there is a marked increase in the percentage of people, especially women, who engage in pre-marital sex — in 1974, 81 per cent of women under 25 had engaged in pre-marital sex as compared to 31 per cent of women over 55.

MALE

FEMALE

Have had premarital intercourse

Under 25
25-34
35-44
45-54
Over 55
Age at time of survey (yrs)

had no history of mental illness. Nevertheless, in everyday social interaction the rule holds: we are attracted to those who are similar to us in important ways.

From dating to mating
Unless our attitudes are extremely deviant, most of us will have few problems finding others who share them. Though most of us are neither extremely beautiful nor handsome, yet the majority form lasting partnerships. Invoking clichés such as "Love is blind" or "They see each other through rose-tinted spectacles" does not really help in understanding why these particular partnerships are formed.

The common belief in Western society is that people marry because they are in love. This belief tends to go with a positive attitude towards marriage. In one cross-cultural study, it was found that a strong tradition of arranged marriages and a relatively low level of economic development went with a low motivation to marry, while a high level of economic development and a "romantic" rather than a contractual tradition of marriage went with a strong motivation to marry eventually.

The belief in romantic love as the basis of marriage is tied to the idea of "true" love as altruistic, selfless and caring. Agreeable as these sentiments may be, they are not supported by research. There is, in fact, an increasing amount of evidence to indicate that people form partnerships (or begin to think about forming them) with a particular person when they believe that what they have to contribute to the partnership is matched by what they will receive from the other person—physical attractiveness, personal attributes, material possessions, homemaking skills and so on.

Put beside notions of selfless love, such a view of relationships seems crude and superficial. If we examine some of the common ways

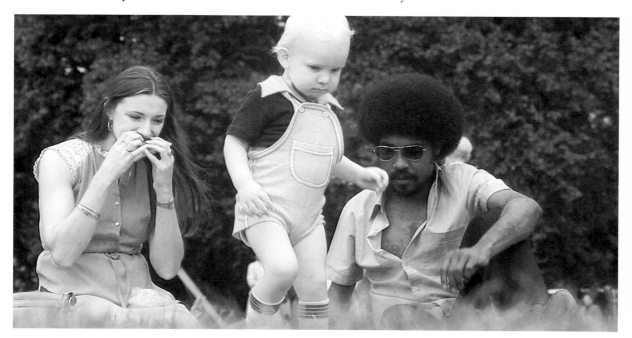

in which people talk about relationships, however, it is clear that we *expect* them to proceed along these lines. Phrases such as "She could have done better for herself", "He's marrying beneath him", "They're well-matched", "I'm not getting anything out of our relationship", "You're not giving me what I need"—all imply that a good relationship is one in which there is a balance of exchange. Further evidence that we assume this to be the case comes from a study where observers were asked to make judgements about a (pre-arranged) couple where the woman was much more physically attractive than the man. The observers assumed, without any evidence, that the man possessed other desirable characteristics.

We may expect people to choose partners on the basis of matched attributes, but does this actually happen? One area where it certainly happens is in physical appearance. In a naturalistic study, couples in a bar were discreetly photographed. Judges, who had not seen the

When partners come from different racial backgrounds (so-called 'mixed' marriages), adjustments to in-laws and parenthood may prove more difficult.

couples together, were then asked to rate each photograph for physical attractiveness. When the couples were reassembled, it was found that the majority had received highly similar ratings of attractiveness from the judges. We only have to look around to see that this matching principle operates in the majority of couples.

In another set of studies, subjects were shown all possible pairings of a set of pictures of the opposite sex, and asked, for each pairing, to say which they would most like to date. On a separate occasion, they rated each photo for physical attractiveness and for the likelihood that the person would accept them as a date. It was found that subjects based their decision about the desirability of the photographed people not only on their physical attractiveness, but also on the likelihood that they would be accepted by them. In other words, whom we choose as "desirable" depends on whether we think they will like us.

The meeting of equals
A number of scales have been developed which attempt to measure the extent to which couples see their relationships as balanced in terms of exchange, or matching of rewards (including personal attributes). As expected, it has been shown that "Individuals who are matched with equally desirable partners are happier, more satisfied with the relationship and more confident that it will last . . . than respondents who are mismatched". (Mismatched in this case means that one partner has more to offer than the other.)

Ted Huston, a social psychologist from Pennsylvania State University, has described the development of intimate relationships within this "exchange" framework. Most first encounters, whether planned or not, are superficial. The majority do not proceed beyond this stage, Huston suggests, because either the rewards exchanged are easily available from other sources ("everyone I go out with tells me I've got nice eyes") and/or the encounter is not sufficiently rewarding to motivate the partners to step up their involvement ("she didn't laugh at my jokes"). Only when partners find such superficial interactions unusually rewarding, or when they suspect that the rewards they can offer each other are not readily available from other people, will their relationship intensify. As it does so, the partners will be constantly monitoring and reviewing the balance of exchange and the probability of getting the same rewards elsewhere.

When relationships go wrong
We have seen that satisfaction in relationships is associated with maintenance of a balanced exchange of rewards. There are two main ways in which this exchange can go wrong and result in unhappiness. Firstly, couples may reward each other much less than they did in the past—the wife may complain that her husband does not try to please her any more, the husband that his wife is "letting herself go". Signs of appreciation and affection may become much rarer than they were during courtship. In these cases, couples are likely to describe their dissatisfaction as boredom, or being in a rut with the relationship.

The second way in which this exchange can go wrong is when the exchange of rewards becomes unbalanced—one partner continuing to reward at a high rate while the other partner reduces his or her rate of reward. When this happens, the "over-benefited" partner, who is getting more than he or she is giving, or whose partner is more

Divorce
Marriage rates are dropping and divorce rates are rising, as the graphs for the US (bottom right) and the UK (bottom left) show. In 1980 there was about one divorce for every two marriages in the US and one in three in the UK. The frequency of divorce is not evenly distributed; for example, it is lower for Roman Catholics and much higher for those who marry young or who come from lower socio-economic groups.

These figures are not as gloomy as they first appear. Remarriage is common, and three out of four women who divorce before the age of thirty do so. However, the rate of remarriage is levelling off while divorce continues to rise. Another factor which makes the figures hard to interpret is the increase in non-traditional family structures.

Source: Social Trends 1983

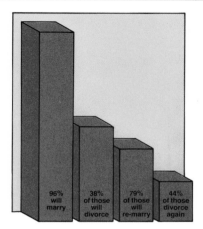

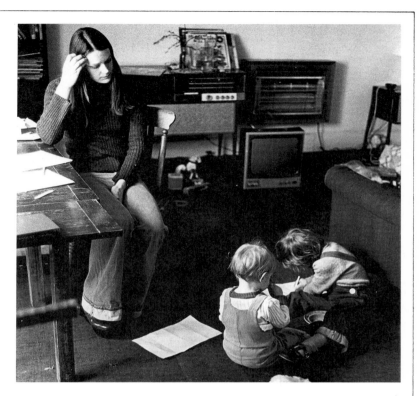

The marriage odds

In the USA in 1978, more than 38 per cent of first marriages ended in divorce. 79 per cent of the divorcees remarried and, of these, 44 per cent were divorced for a second time.

96% will marry

38% of those will divorce

79% of those will re-marry

44% of those divorce again

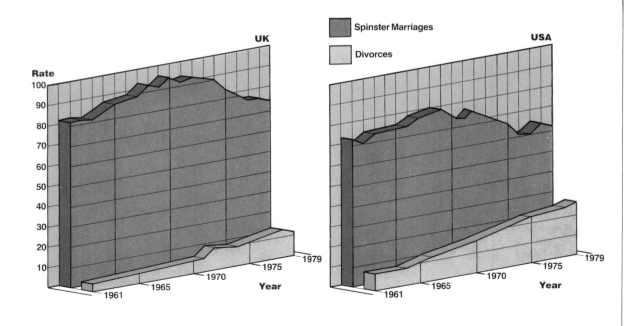

Spinster Marriages

Divorces

UK

USA

Rate

desirable, is likely to report feeling guilt or shame, or being insecure or fearful of losing the partner. The "deprived" partner, on the other hand, who is giving more than he or she is getting, will probably describe the distress felt in terms of anger, or resentment, stemming from feelings of not getting fair rewards from the relationship.

Restoring the balance

Under these conditions, we would predict that both partners would be motivated to try and restore a balance of exchange to the relationship. Social psychologist Elaine Hatfield of the University of Wisconsin has described a number of ways in which couples might do this. For example, in the area of physical appearance, the deprived partners might become more careless about dress and appearance. They might become more reluctant to make any effort to please their partners sexually. They might feel entitled to stop making sacrifices for the benefit of their partners. More constructively, the over-benefited partners might try to make themselves more desirable, perhaps by improving their appearance, becoming more stimulating as persons and in general putting more into the relationship.

The importance of good communication

Marital therapists (and divorce lawyers) have long realized that dissatisfied couples do not communicate with each other very effectively. At extremes of dissatisfaction, communication is used to score points or exchange insults rather than to gather information and to exchange views.

The importance of communication is highlighted when we consider that inequity may result from, or be maintained by, poor communication. A woman, for example, may not tell her husband how she likes to be stimulated sexually, either because of shyness or the mistaken belief that he should somehow "know". A husband may not tell his wife that he preferred her when she was slimmer. Couples in an imbalanced relationship will almost certainly try to restore equity through verbal communication. Constructive and positive attempts would include the woman asking her husband to touch her in certain ways and rewarding him (by her response) when he does. The husband might tell his wife how attractive she was when she was slim, try to find out why she is no longer controlling her weight and ask if there is anything he can do to help. Unconstructive and negative attempts would include the woman complaining that she is not interested in sex or "punishing" her husband when he does not stimulate her in the way she wants. The husband might tell his wife how ugly she looks, shout at her if she overeats and often remark on the attractiveness of other, slimmer, women.

Marital therapy

Richard Stuart, of the University of Utah, has developed a comprehensive and very successful scheme of marital therapy, based on the exchange theory. It is now used by a large number of clinical psychologists. Briefly, the scheme consists of three parts. The first is aimed at increasing the rate at which rewards are exchanged by couples. The second aims to restore reciprocity, or balance, to the relationship by ensuring that rewards are only given by one partner if they are returned by the other. Thirdly, couples are taught to change their pattern of communication so that it comes to resemble the positive patterns shown by the couples who report high levels of satisfaction with their relationship.

This procedure may sound simple, but when applied to individual cases it becomes extremely complex, not least because couples generally do not think of their marital problems in these terms. Instead they use phrases such as "She doesn't care about me any more" or "He takes me for granted", and it can take a considerable amount of skill on the part of the therapist to translate these unhelpful descriptions into specific behaviours.

Does dissatisfaction equal breakdown?

We noted that people take the decision to marry when they feel that the rewards from marriage will outweigh those from remaining single. It follows that couples may tolerate an extremely high level of dissatisfaction in their relationship as long as they do not feel that any better alternative exists. Indeed, some couples may marry only because the alternatives are so bleak—loneliness, remaining with disliked parents, even social rejection. Until relatively recently, our society operated on the assumption, to paraphrase St Paul, that "it is better to marry than to do almost anything else".

Alternatively, some couples may break up when dissatisfaction is relatively low, but when an extremely attractive alternative presents itself to one of the partners. In this case, the deserted partner is likely to use phrases such as "I don't understand why she left me" or "She always seemed quite happy".

Is marital break-up inevitable?

In order for there to be no divorce (apart, of course, from legally banning it), individuals would have to remain perfectly matched throughout their married lives. This would mean that neither of them changed at all, or that each change in one was matched by an equivalent change in the other. Secondly, the married state would have to remain the most attractive option throughout the lives of both partners. Some couples manage to achieve this state of affairs, though often more through luck than judgement.

There is a great deal we could do to try and ensure that fewer marriages end in divorce. We could try to make sure that young people know something of the reality of marriage, so that their choice of it as an alternative is based less on fantasy and more on reality. It is ironic that in order to reduce the number of marriages breaking down we must reinforce the idea that marriage is, by no means, the perfect institution we first thought. Not only that, but actively discouraging people from marrying when young may also prevent disaster—as we age we are less likely to change, although it becomes more difficult to adapt to a new partner. We could encourage young people to experiment with alternative styles of living so that the choice of marriage as an option is an informed one. Last, but not least, we could take marriage off its pedestal and regard it as only one of a number of rewarding ways of living. Even if all this were achieved, however, it is difficult to see how a certain rate of marital breakdown could be avoided. People are constantly growing, changing, and meeting new experiences. We regard this as desirable, but it must inevitably affect the ways in which people relate to each other.

Marriage around the world

There is no society which does not recognize the marriage relationship. Sometimes it is a contract between individuals and families and sometimes it has religious significance. But in all cases it is accompanied by ritual and rites which last anything from an hour to several days. In Western society marriage is monogamous and is solemnized by a religious or civil ceremony—or, in France for example, by both. Polygamous marriages survive in a few countries: in patrilineal societies marriage often means polygyny (one man having several wives) where the elders, in particular, accumulate wealth from their wives' and children's labour and use it to gain and maintain power; in matrilineal societies, which are now rare, polyandry is practised (one woman and several men). In some societies marriages are made when the parties concerned are children; in others men do not marry until aged 35. In some societies even death cannot break the bond. One thing is certain—it seems that marriage is not decreasing in popularity worldwide, although there may be regional fluctuations.

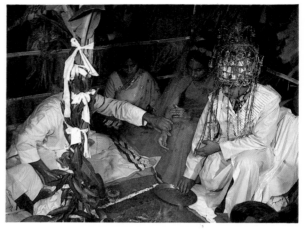

Above: An Indian wedding. The bride is dressed in an elaborate costume and adorned with ceremonial jewels. The couple rarely see each other before the ceremony.

Below: A Greek Orthodox wedding. After the ceremony well-wishers pin money to the bride's and groom's clothes.

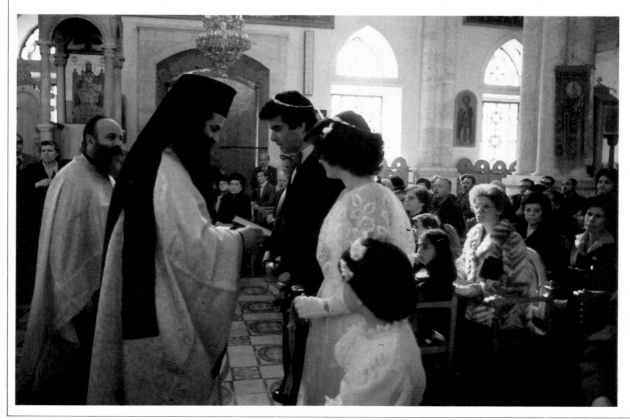

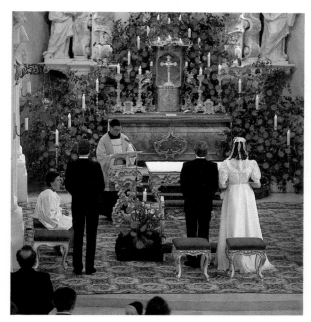

*Above: Formal European Christian marriage ceremony.
The basic requirements are a qualified priest and two
witnesses. In the Roman Catholic church, marriage is one
of the seven sacraments and the ceremony of instruction
and exhortation by the priest, followed by the answering
of questions and giving consent by the couple, is crowned
by a Nuptial Mass. The wedding ring is worn as a
symbol of fidelity.*

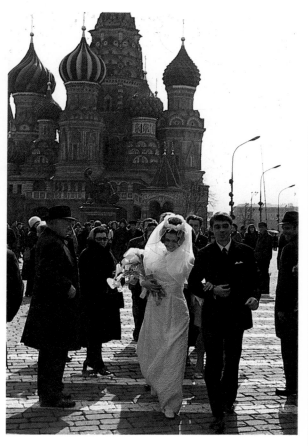

In all countries of the world, marriage is still the most
significant domestic festival in both the secular and the
religious realms.

*Above: A Russian wedding. The couple are walking
through Moscow's Red Square. In Orthodox weddings
crowns are placed on the heads of the bride and groom, a
ceremony known as the 'matrimonial coronation'.*

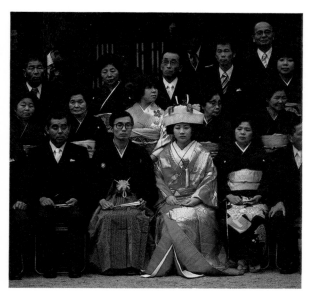

*Left: A Japanese wedding group, formally posed.
Traditional ceremonial robes, as shown here, are often
worn. About fifty per cent of Japanese marriages are
arranged.*

Sexual reactions and problems

Before the pioneering work of American sexologists William Masters and Virginia Johnson in the 1960s, our information on the sexual responses of men and women was very limited indeed. Men, of course, knew that when they were sexually aroused they experienced an erection and, eventually, ejaculation. What happened to women was anybody's guess. In Victorian times and later, it was suggested that women did not experience sexual arousal or, if they should be so remiss, it certainly could not be compared to that of men. Freud, on the other hand, recognized the existence of female sexual response but, again speaking from a platform of ignorance, made his now famous statements about vaginal and clitoral orgasms.

Masters' and Johnson's important contribution was not only to chart the course of sexual response in men and women, but to show that this course was virtually the same regardless of the type of stimulation being responded to. Over almost a decade, they studied 10 000 orgasms experienced by almost 700 volunteers of both sexes, aged 18–89, who were not having any sexual problems.

The way in which the response cycle is divided up is somewhat arbitrary, and different researchers have divided it in slightly different ways. Ultimately, the best system will probably be that which is most useful in helping us understand sexual problems. The point to note,

The control of the testes
The chief male sex hormone is testosterone (the chief female sex hormone being oestrogen) which is secreted by the sex glands or male gonads—the testicles. The hormones are produced in response to stimulation from other hormones (gonadotrophins) released by the pituitary gland. Testosterone stimulates and maintains sexual arousal and desire, and induces the production of sperm in the testes. It also affects the body by increasing muscle mass and body hair.

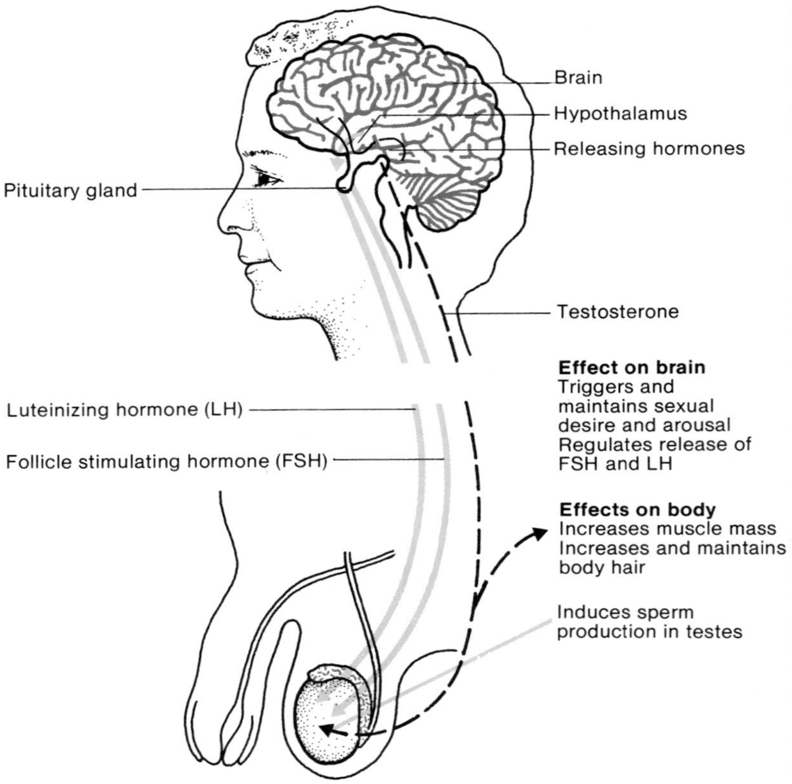

Brain
Hypothalamus
Releasing hormones
Pituitary gland
Testosterone
Luteinizing hormone (LH)
Follicle stimulating hormone (FSH)

Effect on brain
Triggers and maintains sexual desire and arousal Regulates release of FSH and LH

Effects on body
Increases muscle mass Increases and maintains body hair

Induces sperm production in testes

however, is that people who have no sexual problems experience roughly the same cycle on each occasion, but that there will be wide variations, both within and between individuals, in the duration and intensity of each part of that cycle. A large number of people, particularly men, are unaware of this and think that there is something wrong with them if their response is not the same each time. This misconception partly arises from the still prevalent belief that sexual behaviour and sexual arousal are instinctive. The capacity to experience sexual arousal and to respond sexually to others is certainly inborn, but the responses and behaviour of individuals are profoundly influenced by their learning experiences—a phenomenon well established in both human and non-human animals.

The male response cycle

Erection phase. Within a short time of receiving sexual stimulation, men respond with a swelling and stiffening of the penis, caused by congestion of its spongy tissue, which in turn results from blood flowing in one direction into the sexual organs. Early in the response cycle, the erection may be quite easily lost if there are extraneous distractions; this is less likely to happen later in the cycle. During this phase, the skin round the scrotal sac thickens and the testicles gradually rise within it, so that this area becomes "tighter". Later, a clear fluid may flow from the penis. This can serve a lubricating function, but it may also contain a considerable number of sperm cells. More general changes in this phase include raising of the heart rate and blood pressure, skin flushes and increased muscle tension.

Ejaculation phase. Ejaculation is preceded by a heightening of all the responses of the erection phase. This second phase has two parts. In the first, the prostate gland, seminal vesicles, vas deferens and testes undergo contractions which result in semen being deposited at the entrance to the urethra. In this stage, the man will feel that ejaculation is inevitable, as indeed it is. In the second part of the phase, semen is expelled from the urethra by a series of contractions involving the urethra and the muscles at the base of the penis. Afterwards, a man is physically incapable of attaining another erection or of ejaculating for variable periods of time which, because they are so variable, cannot be specified.

Resolution phase. As its name implies, it is during this phase that things "resolve" or return to normal. Like the previous phase, it has two parts. Men usually lose a good deal of their erection within a short time of ejaculation, but this will vary depending on how long the erection had been maintained before ejaculation occurred. In the next half-hour or so (again there are variations) the remainder of the erection will subside and the scrotal sac regain its usual slackness. The general bodily changes which accompany sexual arousal and which reach a peak at ejaculation will also return to normal.

The female response cycle

Lubrication phase. Like men, women respond to sexual stimulation with congestion of the sex organs. Lubrication of the vagina quickly follows, and the inner two-thirds of the vagina lengthen and expand. The increased blood flow to the vulva causes a colour change in the labia minora, which become bright red, or a deeper red if the woman has had children. The clitoris does not become engorged until late in

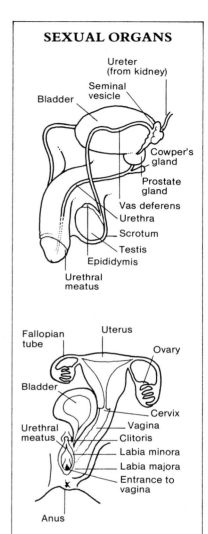

SEXUAL ORGANS

Top: the male sexual organs. These are situated both outside and inside the pelvic region. Outside the body are the testes which produce the sperm and the penis.
Bottom: the female sexual organs. The external organs are known collectively as the vulva (the mons pubis, the labia majora, labia minora and the clitoris). The vagina leads to the cervix, the neck of the womb.

THE STAGES OF SEXUAL RESPONSE

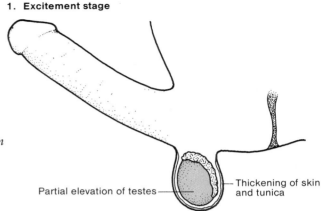

1. Excitement stage

Men

1 *When the sex centre in the brain responds to a stimulus (usually touch or vision) blood rushes to the penis. The heart beats faster, the breathing rate increases, blood pressure rises and body muscles (both voluntary and involuntary) tighten. The testes rise.* 2 *Muscles in the inner pelvis massage seminal fluid from the prostatic area along the urethra. The ejaculation centre (in the lower spine) passes messages to the muscles surrounding the shaft of the penis which contracts, releasing sperm.* 3 *The penis begins to retract and the testes descend.*

Partial elevation of testes—

Thickening of skin and tunica

Women

1 *The body's reaction to sexual stimuli causes blood to engorge the clitoris and to swell the entrance to the vagina. The vagina itself becomes moist and lengthens and expands to accommodate the penis. The cervix and uterus balloon upwards. Breathing rate and heart beat increase, the nipples become erect, body muscles tighten and there may be a rash on the skin.* 2 *The muscle tension is released in orgasm when the vagina and uterus contract rhythmically.* 3 *After orgasm the uterus drops and the vagina begins slowly to return to normal.*

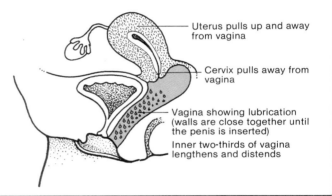

Uterus pulls up and away from vagina

Cervix pulls away from vagina

Vagina showing lubrication (walls are close together until the penis is inserted)

Inner two-thirds of vagina lengthens and distends

this phase, and just prior to orgasm it retracts under the clitoral hood. The woman also undergoes general physiological changes in muscle tension, heart rate and blood pressure. Some women develop what Masters and Johnson called a "sex flush"—a rash which starts in the chest area and spreads to other parts of the body.

Orgasm phase. The physiological mechanism which triggers orgasm in women is still unknown. The orgasm is made up of a series of rhythmic contractions which involve the womb, the pelvic muscles and the vaginal entrance. For most women, orgasms are triggered by clitoral stimulation; even if they are not, they still involve identical changes in the clitoris. Thus, while an orgasm may result from different kinds of stimulation, there are not two "kinds" of orgasm.

Unlike men, women do not have a refractory period when they are incapable of being aroused. Women are capable of having several orgasms in succession if they continue to receive stimulation.

Resolution phase. Within a few seconds of orgasm, the clitoris returns to its usual position, and the labia minora resume their normal colour. Other changes occur over a longer period—about 15 minutes. The vagina contracts to its usual size, and the womb, which has risen in the pelvis, returns to its usual position. The general bodily changes also decline slowly.

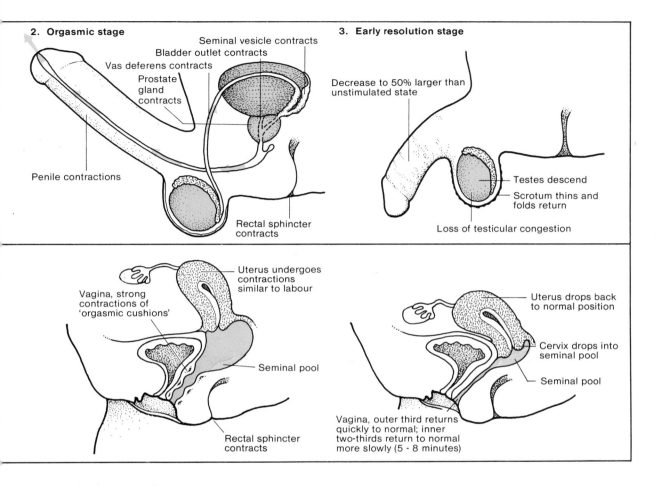

2. Orgasmic stage

Seminal vesicle contracts

Bladder outlet contracts

Vas deferens contracts

Prostate gland contracts

Penile contractions

Rectal sphincter contracts

3. Early resolution stage

Decrease to 50% larger than unstimulated state

Testes descend

Scrotum thins and folds return

Loss of testicular congestion

Vagina, strong contractions of 'orgasmic cushions'

Uterus undergoes contractions similar to labour

Seminal pool

Rectal sphincter contracts

Uterus drops back to normal position

Cervix drops into seminal pool

Seminal pool

Vagina, outer third returns quickly to normal; inner two-thirds return to normal more slowly (5 - 8 minutes)

For both men and women, this response cycle remains essentially the same from puberty to old age. What does change with age is the intensity and duration of each phase.

New findings

For some years after their publication, Masters' and Johnson's findings were regarded almost as the last word on the subject. Certainly, their contribution has been immensely valuable and the broad outline of their discoveries remains.

Increasingly sophisticated measurement over the last few years, however, has added some new findings. It was assumed, for example, that women did not "ejaculate" during orgasm. There is now, however, some very limited evidence that some women may discharge prostatic fluid through the urethra during orgasm. This may go unnoticed if there is a good deal of vaginal lubrication, or may not occur at all.

It was also assumed that only women were capable of multiple orgasms. Researchers have now gathered some mainly anecdotal evidence that men may be able to exercise control over their responses so that they are able to experience several "orgasms" within one session of lovemaking, before ejaculating, after which, of course, they will have a refractory period. This evidence was gathered from only a tiny number of men, and mainly through interviews, so that we cannot yet be certain that what the men are reporting would constitute an "orgasm" in the physiological sense. Certainly, men who only experience one orgasm per lovemaking session should not feel inferior! Nor, indeed, should women. In spite of women's undoubted capacity for multiple orgasm, most do not experience them regularly, and those who experience them do so mainly through masturbation.

Responses to stimulation

Masters' and Johnson's research told us a great deal about what happens to men and women when they receive effective sexual stimulation. What it did not tell us—nor did it set out to—was what constitutes effective sexual stimulation for men and women. Most people believe (because they have been taught that it is the case) that men respond to visual stimuli (hence their liking for pornography), while women respond to tactile stimuli or to "romantic" visual stimuli, and that the male response is swifter and stronger.

Right: graph showing sexual response in women. Again, tension builds rapidly in the excitement stage. The plateau phase, however, can differ greatly. There may be a single orgasm with a fairly quick resolution; or a longer plateau phase followed by several orgasms; or a prolonged plateau phase without orgasm followed by a very slow resolution. There is no resistant stage in women.

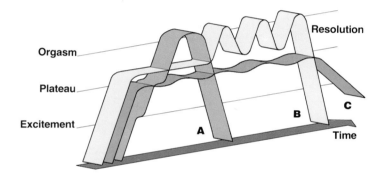

Sexual response in women
A Short plateau single orgasm
B Longer plateau multiple orgasms
C Plateau but no orgasm, slow resolution (this may also occur in men from time to time)

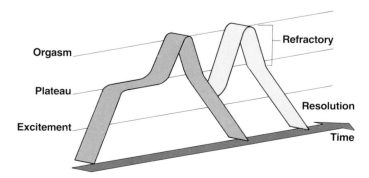

Sexual response in men
Only men have a refractory stage, which may last minutes or hours

Left: graph showing sexual response in men. Sexual tension builds rapidly during the excitement stage and intensifies in the "plateau" phase. At this stage the tension may be dissipated by outside factors. If not, the orgasm or ejaculation phase follows and the cycle ends in the resolution phase. Men then experience a resistant period when they are unresponsive to additional stimulation.

It is only since 1974 that it has been possible to monitor female vaginal arousal, with apparatus that measures pressure pulse and blood volume change (such equipment for measuring male penile arousal as been available for some time). Using such instruments, Julia Heiman, of New York's Stony Brook University, investigated the responses of male and female students to verbal descriptions of sexual material. She used four kinds of tape—explicit erotic, romantic erotic, romantic only and non-romantic, non-erotic. The erotic tapes were further divided into those where the woman "took charge" and those where sex was initiated by the man. Contrary to popular opinions, *both* males and females showed the strongest response to the explicit erotic tapes, with romantic erotic, romantic only and non-romantic, non-erotic following. In addition, both men and women responded more strongly to the erotic tape in which sex was initiated by the woman.

Where the men and women did differ was in the "accuracy" of their self-reports of arousal. Heiman examined the women's responses

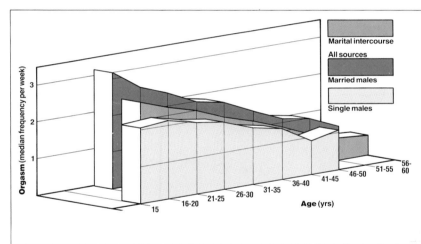

Decline in the male sex drive
A measure of the male sex drive is the frequency of sexual outlet, or orgasm. This graph is based on a study by Kinsey, Martin and Pomeroy, and shows that there is a marked decline in sex drive as age increases. As men get older, they tend to become more alike as regards the frequency of their behaviour. There is no equivalent decline in the sexual capacity of women. Of course, sexual activity depends not only on physiological changes but also on the partner.

to the first tape they heard, regardless of its content. She found that, of those women showing the *largest* change in vaginal blood volume, i.e. those who were most aroused, 42 per cent said they felt *no* physical response, 54 per cent said they had not experienced any vaginal sensations and 63 per cent said they felt no signs of lubrication. Needless to say, none of the men made similar mistakes—an erection is much more difficult to ignore. These results have been repeated using visual as well as verbal material.

There can be no doubt that women are as responsive as men to sexually explicit material—with or without romance—but that the women may not recognize or will deny that they are aroused.

Sexual problems

Before we consider those problems which are commonly reported by men and women, some general points need to be made. Firstly, we have to be very careful about labelling someone as having a sexual problem. Humans are immensely varied in their sexual behaviour— sexologists are only beginning to realize just how varied. This is a particularly important point because self-proclaimed experts, whether professional, religious or publishers of pornography, are much given to making pronouncements about sexual behaviour which may bear no relationship to reality. This would matter less if people freely discussed their sex lives, because they would soon discover the truth!

Secondly, the new insights we have gained from research, such as Heiman's, may help us understand why men and women tend to report their problems in different ways. Men usually use mechanical terms, while women tend to talk in terms of not becoming aroused.

Thirdly, researchers are gathering an increasing amount of information about the neurological pathways involved in sexual responses, and this may have implications for our understanding of sexual dysfunction. Touch, for example, can evoke the mechanical aspects of arousal independently of the brain. The erection centre is in the lowest portion of the spinal cord. A man who has an injury which has separated this part of the cord from the brain can still have an erection if the genital area is stroked.

It also seems that the physiological processes of initial arousal and vasocongestion and the process of orgasm are controlled by different parts of the nervous system. Thus, full arousal can occur without orgasm, and orgasm without vasocongestion—it is quite possible for a man to ejaculate while his penis is flaccid. This distinction between arousal and ejaculation is important, because it used to be assumed, at

The courtship ritual—the process between meeting and mating. In contrast with the past, the choice of a partner is determined by the individual, rather than the parents or some other elder of the community. In the absence of a chaperone, couples are free to have sexual intercourse relatively unhindered.

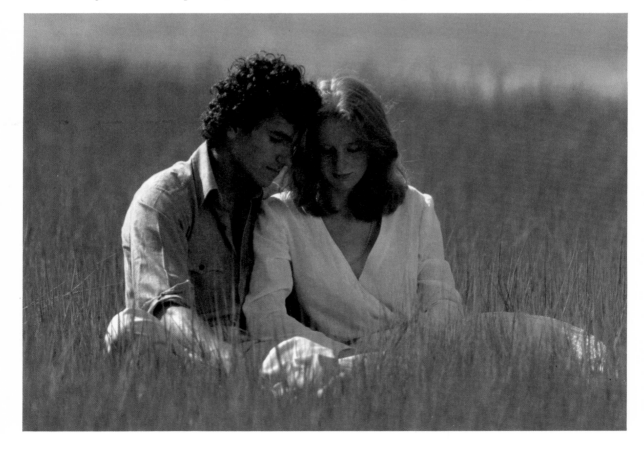

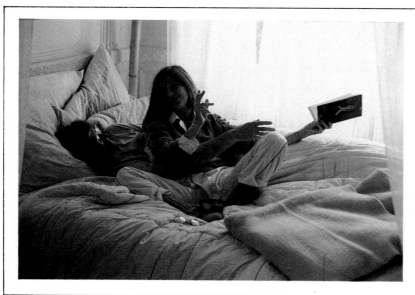

Communication
Communication about sexual matters is as essential for the successful continuation of an intimate relationship, as communication about more mundane and practical matters. Sexual reactions and responses differ from person to person and in each person may differ from day to day. Fear of rejection, inability to come to terms with sexual fantasies or needs, or the persistence of a sexual hang-up can all inhibit communication and lead to problems within long-term relationships.

least in the case of women, that a lack of orgasm meant lack of arousal. It seems to be very difficult for writers on the subject to assume an equivalent lack of interest in men. Even if they cannot have an erection, ejaculation or both, they are still assumed to be interested! This, of course, reflects the prevailing beliefs about patterns of sexual response which were discussed earlier.

Men's sexual problems

Erectile dysfunction. This term has now replaced the earlier, more derogatory label "impotence". Every man experiences difficulty in getting or maintaining an erection at some time in his sexual career. It is only if this happens over a long period of time or in a variety of situations that it is likely to be reported as a problem.

The men who would be included under this heading are a very heterogeneous group, which means that the label itself conveys very little information about the person. The group will include men who have never had an erection at all (extremely rare), men who have erections only, say, on waking or during masturbation but have never had intercourse with a partner, men who have had intercourse in the past but now cannot, men who can have intercourse with some partners but not others, even though they are attracted to them, men who get an erection and then lose it if they try to have intercourse, men who lose their erections during intercourse and men who have erections of varying quality.

Premature ejaculation. Initially, Masters and Johnson defined this problem in terms of the man's inability to satisfy his partner on at least 50 per cent of their sexual encounters. Obviously, this definition cannot be used, as it assumes an unvarying response not only from all women but from each woman on every occasion. Definitions based on time between the start of intercourse and ejaculation are equally problematic as (fortunately) there are no rules about how long intercourse *should* last. It is better, in describing this problem, to

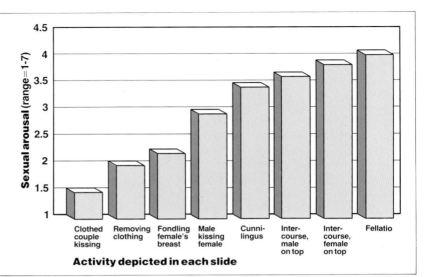

Arousal to erotic photos

Right: graph showing arousal in men and women in response to erotic photographs. A study in 1971 by Byrne and Lamberth showed that individuals became sexually aroused when observing the sexual activities of others. It did not appear to make any difference if the event was real, on film (there was also no distinction between colour and black and white films), or still photographs. What did make a difference, however, was the content of the scene.

concentrate on the man's feeling that he cannot control his ejaculatory processes even when he tries to do so. Again, most men will experience this problem at some time, and with new partners it is almost commonplace. It is only when control is not established over a reasonable period with the same partner that a problem could be said to exist. Premature ejaculation is almost never a problem during masturbation.

Retarded ejaculation. When Masters and Johnson carried out their initial research into sexual problems, they encountered only 17 men (or 3.8 per cent of their sample) with this problem. These men were unable to ejaculate during intercourse even though they were fully aroused, or they were able to ejaculate, but only after a much longer period of time than they and most people would judge to be reasonable.

Many men experience retarded ejaculation when they are tired or have had sex a short time before. For some men who experience this problem regularly, it may still be limited to certain partners or certain situations, but even if it is more general, the man will still usually ejaculate during masturbation or have nocturnal emissions.

There is some evidence that Masters' and Johnson's figures may have underestimated the scope of this problem. Out of 486 men who reported sexual problems at one clinic, 72 (15 per cent) said that they had never ejaculated during either masturbation or intercourse. The figure for men who experience this problem to a lesser degree is probably much higher.

Women's sexual problems

Disorders of arousal. We have seen that women are often unaware of (or fail to report) that they are sexually aroused. If a woman complains of this as a general problem, it is therefore important to find out whether she is actually experiencing physiological arousal (vasocongestion and lubrication) and is mislabelling it, or if she is not experiencing any physiological changes at all. Strictly speaking, we can only speak of a

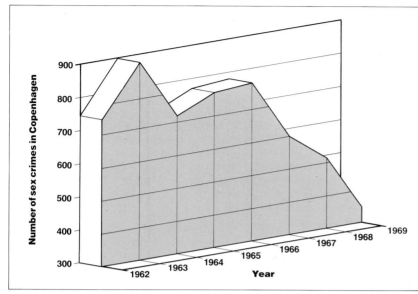

Pornography
Left: graph showing the rate of reported sex crimes in Copenhagen from 1962 to 1969. In 1965 pornographic material became freely available to the general public throughout Denmark, through shops, the post and vending machines. This 1971 analysis of police statistics shows there was a sharp decline in the number of reported sex crimes following the legalization of pornographic material.

problem of arousal if the physiological changes that go with it are absent.

As in the male equivalent of erectile dysfunction, this group is very heterogeneous. A woman may be unaroused only with one particular partner or with a number of men (or women). She may be unresponsive to a wide variety of erotic stimuli or become very aroused during masturbation, but not with partners.

Vaginismus. This can be seen as a problem of arousal and more besides. We have seen that the usual female response to sexual stimulation is a lengthening and widening of the upper part of the vagina. Some women, however, respond to attempts at intercourse with a massive tightening of the muscle walls of the lower third of the vagina, so that penetration is impossible. It is usual to find that these women respond in a similar way to medical attempts at internal examinations (general anaesthetics are sometimes resorted to if the examination is essential) and that they have never used tampons during their periods. The label "married virgins" is often applied to these women. Some never seek help and their marriages remain unconsummated or break up; some seek help because they very much want to have children.

Orgasmic dysfunction. Most women who do not become aroused with sexual stimulation also fail to experience orgasm. A large number of women, however, do initially become aroused, but do not have orgasms. Again, this problem may be a global one, with the woman never having experienced orgasm even during masturbation—if she has ever masturbated; it may, however, be confined to particular partners, or to partners in general, or occur only in specific situations—as, for example, when there is a possibility of lovemaking being interrupted by the children. A woman also may experience orgasms in response to manual or oral stimulation, but not during intercourse (the reverse is unusual).

Both men and women sometimes report that intercourse is painful. For women, it is important to rule out vaginismus, as many women will, not unnaturally, report this problem as "intercourse being painful". Painful intercourse, however, may itself cause vaginismus. It is important for both men and women to define not only the type of pain experienced—sharp, throbbing, aching and so on—but also its location (groin, testicles, penile head, vaginal entrance, deep in the vagina) and its timing (when intercourse is attempted, during intercourse, when thrusting and so on).

What causes sexual problems?

We have to be very careful indeed about suggesting any particular factor as a cause of sexual (or, indeed, any) problems. In order for us to be able to say that x is the cause of some problem, we would have to demonstrate that we could reliably bring about the problem in someone who previously did not have it by exposing them to x. Readers will quickly realise that for sexual—and almost all—problems, this has never been done. Furthermore, it almost certainly never will be done because of the ethical issues involved.

On what, then, are theories about the causes of sexual dysfunction based? In most cases, the answer is, on the information received from people who seek help for sexual problems.

People who seek help for their problems, including sexual problems, are a highly selected group. We have no way of knowing, except through large-scale surveys, how many people in the general population have had similar experiences to those reported by a clinic population, but who have not developed any sexual problems. Equally, we have no information on those who have developed a sexual problem but who have not sought help, either because the problem resolved itself or for some other reason. This is an important point, because people may not seek help for sexual problems until they have had them for a long time.

Anxiety as a major factor

One of the most important maintaining factors in sexual problems is anxiety about the problem itself. Masters and Johnson spoke of people adopting a "spectator" role in which they constantly monitored their responses to check that they were functioning "correctly". It is easier to imagine the effect this monitoring has on sexual responses if we recall occasions when we have tried to get to sleep. The more we try, the less we succeed, and it is only when we stop trying that we finally drop off. Performance anxiety, of course, may also be a precipitating factor. This is particularly likely to be the case in those who are sexually inexperienced or who are concerned about how they will function with a particular partner.

A second, related, maintaining factor is the response of the partner. People sometimes assume that it is only if the partner is hostile, unsympathetic or even amused that the problem will worsen. Reports from people who seek help for sexual problems reveal a more complex picture. Some people are put off by too much sympathy and understanding, which can make them feel even more "inferior", while others find the common "it doesn't matter" response equally off-putting. But there are no rules which can be offered about how partners should respond. The best course is for them to find out from their partner what they could do (or refrain from doing) that would be most helpful or least harmful.

Common sexual problems

For any problem, there will be a variety of causes, some of which are no longer operating (precipitating factors), and some that operate after the problem has established itself (maintaining factors). Anxiety in particular is an important factor—the more anxious we become about our performance, the worse the problem becomes.

Organic factors

A variety of drugs induce erectile problems, and some are implicated in retarded ejaculation. The contraceptive pill may impair arousal in women.

Psychological factors

A very restrictive upbringing may be associated with problems, especially vaginismus in women. Lack of attraction to a partner is a second important factor—whether due to marital circumstances of the couple, or simply boredom. Anxiety can also cause problems, which are compounded by resulting performance anxiety.

Premature ejaculation has its own set of factors—possible causes are previous sexual experiences a man is used to, or anxiety.

Coping with problems

1. Communicate with your partner.
2. Seek information about sexual functioning.
3. Do not assume that sexual attraction will withstand time—make an effort.
4. Seek professional help if you are still having problems. Not only does the therapist provide reassurance, and re-educate where necessary, but instructs on various techniques that have proved a success.

Pregnancy and motherhood

Social attitudes towards women and motherhood are confused, to say the least. A woman is bombarded by contrary advice and opinion from every side. The influence of psychiatrists such as John Bowlby and Renée Spitz has emphasized the vital and irreplaceable role of the mother in the first months and years of a baby's life. Some sections of the women's movement, however, appear to be saying that motherhood is a denigration and denial of human potential. They may state that "women are denied personhood". However, such statements are not meant to denigrate motherhood as such, but are made in reaction to widely held assumptions about the mother's role.

The accepted standard
In Western society, people still tend to assume that most women will remain at home when they have children and spend most of their time looking after them (which often includes the care of a husband as well). At the same time, full-time mothers are given a low social status (for example, on official forms) and little help with vital issues such as child-care facilities. The assumption is that motherhood is the most important role in a woman's life—it must therefore be fulfilling and rewarding in itself. So, women who strive to free themselves from this role, or who choose not to take it up at all, are somehow seen as deviant.

At the same time, the media present a distorted, but powerful, image of pregnancy and motherhood. (Fatherhood rarely appears until the child is much older, and usually only then if it is male.) Photographs in women's magazines are a novel extension of the glamour photographer's work. Pregnant women are shown as elegantly slim—apart from that interesting bulge—and radiantly at peace with themselves and their state. You will rarely see a photograph of a pregnant woman doing the housework, going shopping or changing nappies on an older child. One might imagine that pregnant women are rarely indoors, but live entirely in beautiful parks and gardens. Similarly, early motherhood is depicted as a time of joy and tranquillity, with babies who are either laughing or sleeping.

Conflicting attitudes towards motherhood
These contradictory attitudes, and the conflict between media images and reality, are all the more confusing for today's woman because, for the first time in history, she can choose marriage or other committed relationships without motherhood as an almost inevitable result. In spite of the existence of this choice, however, the social pressures towards motherhood are enormous—not only motherhood, but motherhood within a family unit. The old idea of marriage, ordained by the Church as being primarily for the begetting of children, is still very much with us. Illegitimate children are still, as they have been throughout history, seen as a challenge to the economic stability of the family and society. The strenuous (and not conspicuously successful) efforts of some psychologists and psychiatrists to "prove" that children brought up outside the traditional family unit—apart from those in institutions—suffer in consequence can in part be seen as stemming from this view.

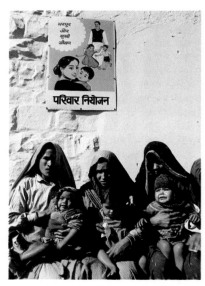

The role we conform to as adults and parents is deeply rooted in our culture, whether Eastern or Western. Only by consistent and persuasive application of pressure by the media will the pattern of parenthood change, for instance this attempt to promote contraception in New Delhi.

The signs of pregnancy

The first sign of pregnancy is nearly always the "missed period". Pregnancy, however, is only one of a number of possible causes of amenorrhea, so that, in a woman who has irregular menstrual periods, this is not a very reliable early sign.

Breast tissue is very sensitive to hormonal changes and many healthy women experience a feeling of fullness and even some tenderness in their breasts just before menstruation. These changes are related to the female sex hormones, oestrogen and progesterone. In early pregnancy, the high levels of these hormones may be a cause of breast tenderness. At the same time there is an increase in blood supply to the breasts, development of the milk ducts and enlargement of breast tissue. The nipples become larger and the circular patch around them, the areola, darkens and may swell slightly.

So-called "morning sickness" is another common early sign of pregnancy, but it certainly does not occur only in the morning. The cause of the nausea, which is usually mild, is unknown, but it may be related to the large increase in circulating sex hormones that occurs early in pregnancy. There may also be psychological elements involved and these will be discussed in more detail later.

The pregnant woman may find that in the early weeks she urinates more frequently than usual. The kidneys work overtime early in pregnancy, probably again as a result of the increase in sex hormones, so that the bladder fills more quickly than usual.

The later stages

Pregnancy becomes obvious as the foetus and the uterus grow in size. At about 20 weeks of pregnancy, the top of the uterus has reached the level of the mother's navel. This is regarded as roughly the mid-point of pregnancy. Until 20 weeks, the top of the uterus rises the breadth of two fingers above the front of the pelvic bone every two weeks of pregnancy, having appeared above this bone at about 10 weeks.

After 20 weeks, the top of the uterus rises the breadth of two fingers every four weeks until it has reached the front centre of the rib-cage at 36 weeks. Towards the end of pregnancy, the foetal head is pressed downwards and engages in the birth canal entrance of the pelvis. This means that the top of the uterus is lowered and at 40 weeks (term) it will be where it was at about 30–32 weeks.

Around the 18th to 20th week in first pregnancies and the 16th to 18th week in later pregnancies, the first foetal movements may be felt. They are initially very slight and feel like a tremor. The movements become much stronger as pregnancy proceeds. The developing foetal limbs push against the uterine wall and can be seen and felt through the abdominal wall.

Activity in the womb

Foetuses have quiet periods (perhaps actual sleep periods) and these vary in length and degree of activity. These phases are often not synchronized with maternal rest or sleep periods and this, while normal, can be disturbing to the mother. The pregnant woman can become anxious when the foetus is quiet for a day or more after being notably active. However, this prolonged rest is quite common and does not signify that anything is amiss unless it lasts longer than a couple of days, in which case medical advice should be sought.

AGE AND PREGNANCY

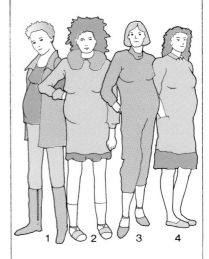

Dividing women into four age groups, variations in several aspects of pregnancy are evident, especially for the first baby. Not only are medical factors important in pregnancy and health but also financial, social and psychological factors.

1 *The youngest group (under twenty) usually have easier labours. But there is a higher risk of congenital abnormality in the baby and of anaemia and toxaemia in pregnancy.*
2 *Young women aged twenty to thirty are less likely to have still-born babies and the figures for perinatal mortality are also lower.*
3 *Women aged thirty to forty have longer labours, with more complications in birth and pregnancy. Their babies tend to be heavier and they are more likely to have twins.*
4 *Older mothers (aged over forty) run a higher risk of giving birth to mongoloid children. Though labour is sometimes very short, there is a high risk of complications.*

Obstetricians listen to the foetal heart sounds, their rate and regularity, for many reasons. These sounds not only confirm that the foetus is living, but are also a good monitor of its health, especially as labour nears. Foetal sounds can usually be heard from the 12th week, and are almost always detectable after the 16th week.

Antenatal care

A pregnant woman may be looked after by her family doctor, who knows the background and her medical history. In Britain and the rest of Europe, the mother-to-be may also be attended by a midwife, with whom she builds a continuous relationship up to, during and immediately after the birth.

On the other hand, it may be more desirable to attend a regular antenatal clinic (which has all the expertise, tests and so on) for regular examinations. Here the "doctor" may, in fact, be a team.

It is vital that a pregnant woman has regular medical examinations. If trouble is spotted early, there is more chance of its being dealt with successfully.

The best time to start antenatal care is when the second missed menstrual period would have happened. At the first visit, a medical history will be taken, and a complete examination will determine the woman's present state of health. Important base-lines will be deter-

DEVELOPMENT FROM CONCEPTION TO BIRTH

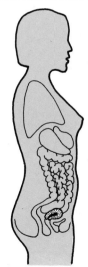 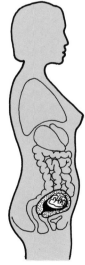 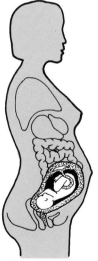 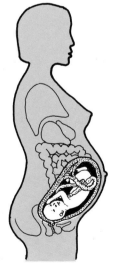

Weeks 1–13 The illustration shows week 4 of the pregnancy: the fertilized egg has implanted itself in the uterus and the embryo has started to form. But the uterus has not begun to grow in size, so there is no visible swelling of the abdomen.

Weeks 14–26 As the foetus and uterus grow in size, the mother's abdomen starts to swell. Week 16 is shown here; at about 20 weeks—the mid-point of the pregnancy—the top of the uterus is level with the mother's navel. At week 26 the foetus is about 33 cm (13 in) long.

Weeks 27–39 The baby's size and weight increase rapidly and the uterus continues to grow (week 28 is shown here) until about week 36, when the baby's head is engaged in the pelvic cavity. During this stage the mother's posture alters to adapt to the load.

Week 40 The baby's head is shown here engaged in the birth canal entrance to the pelvis, ready to be expelled by the contractions of the uterus. (The contractions first open the cervix.) The top of the uterus has retreated to its position of about weeks 30–32.

Pregnancy exercises

There is plenty that the expectant mother can do to help herself keep in good physical shape throughout the pregnancy. This will favour her health and well-being both during the pregnancy and birth and after the baby is born, when she will want to recover her health and strength as quickly as possible.

The abdominal and pelvic muscles and the back all work particularly hard during pregnancy and should not be subjected to unnecessary strain. Outlined below are ways for the expectant mother to move about that will help avoid this. There are also simple exercises to keep the hard-worked muscles in the best condition possible while they are performing their important task.

Rest is also essential for the expectant mother. Deliberate relaxation rests the body and also trains the mother to relax at will, which is invaluable during the pregnancy, during the birth itself (between contractions) and after the birth.

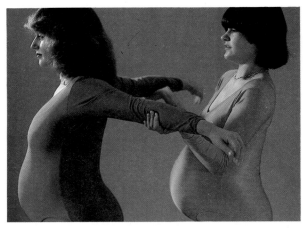

Exercise during pregnancy is important both for the general health of the mother and to ensure that she is in good physical condition for labour.

Posture

There is a tendency for the pregnant woman to adopt the stance shown by figure A, leaning back slightly and with a hollow back. This may be unavoidable late in the pregnancy, but earlier on the stance shown by figure B is the correct one, with the spine as straight as possible. This stance gives the best support to the abdomen and chest.

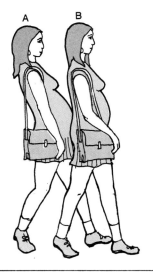

Daily activities

To prevent unnecessary strain being put on the back, which is already burdened by the extra load being carried, the expectant mother should avoid bending the spine. She should try to adjust her movements so that she is doing as much as possible with the back straight. When reaching for the floor, for example, she should bend the knees so that the legs take the strain, rather than stooping down with a bent back. Where possible, working surfaces, etc., should be raised to avoid further unnecessary bending.

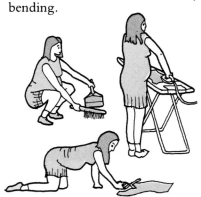

Lifting

Care should be taken when lifting during pregnancy, so that there is no unnecessary strain, and lifting heavy objects should be avoided. Again, the general rule is, as far as possible, to keep the back straight. When picking up a child, for example, bend at the knees with the back straight and then rise slowly with the child close to the body. Objects can be lifted from the floor by putting one foot in front of the other and bending at the knees with the back straight. Bags should be held high in the arms.

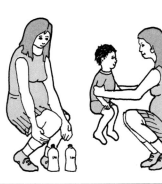

Relaxation

The expectant mother should be sure to make time for some physical relaxation during each day. One good position is to sit well back in a chair, with the legs up (the feet supported) and a cushion supporting the lower back. Another is to lie out-stretched on a sofa or bed with both the head and feet supported by cushions or pillows.

General exercises

Here are a couple of simple exercises to help keep the muscles well-toned and improve circulation. Firstly, lie on your back on the floor with the knees bent and the feet flat on the ground. Stretch out each leg in turn, and then pull it slowly back in again. Secondly, lie in the same position, pull the buttock muscles tight, hold, and then release.

Sport

It is a good idea to continue with sports in a non-competitive way during pregnancy; especially swimming, long walks, bicycling and even some athletics. All forms of exercise during pregnancy should be directed towards maintaining good posture, muscle control, control of breathing and relaxation. One word of warning though—it is important not to overdo it and become exhausted.

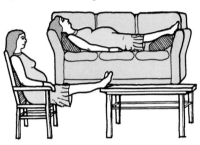

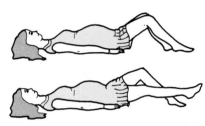

Regular swimming provides many of the most useful features of pre-natal exercise. It strengthens muscles, improves circulation and respiration and it adapts to increasing weight and change of balance.

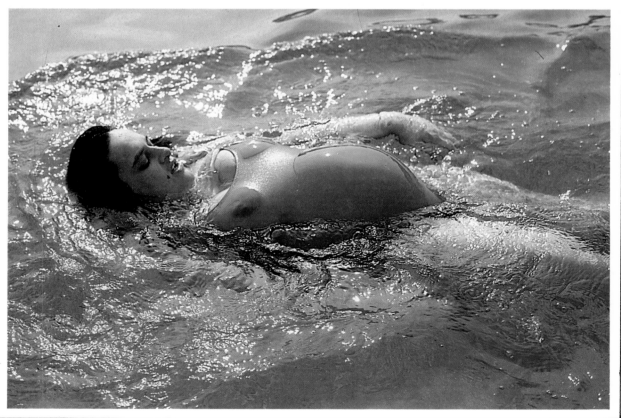

mined, including body weight, abdominal size, blood pressure and breast size. At subsequent visits, the physician or midwife will see if things are progressing normally and whether changes from these baselines are acceptable. Ideally, visits should be every four weeks up to 28 weeks of pregnancy, then every two weeks until 36 weeks and, finally, weekly.

Exercise in pregnancy

The uterus is a muscular thick-walled container that gets bigger and bigger in pregnancy. It is supported within the abdominal cavity by two strong ligaments on either side—like guy ropes. The mother's abdominal wall, which is quite thick, regardless of the amount of fat present, covers the abdominal cavity.

The uterus contains the amniotic fluid or "waters" within two tough membranes or "envelopes". Inside this fluid compartment the foetus floats, grows and develops. In this way, protection is provided. A pregnant woman's fall need not mean damage to the foetus. On the other hand, it would not do to imagine that the foetus is immune from all damage.

When labour comes, it is ideal for the woman to be in good physical shape. During the pregnancy, she should continue to practise her usual exercise or sport as far as she can without strain. There is no need for the busy housewife, who may not usually exercise or play a sport, suddenly to go overboard and start. But if swimming is usual and enjoyed—continue swimming; similarly riding, gardening, walking. There is no need to avoid travel during pregnancy, although some airlines may need a certificate of "good" health for a woman who is more than 30 weeks pregnant.

Weight gain and diet

Different female frames react differently to pregnancy. At one extreme, some healthy women can carry their normal-sized foetus, remaining virtually sylph-like and able to wear their usual clothes almost to the end. At the other extreme, some healthy women look and feel very large from quite early on.

Generally, pregnancy does not permanently ruin the appearance. However, if a woman puts on excessive weight and lacks exercise, it may seriously affect her figure afterwards.

Obviously, all pregnancies result in weight gain. Some of this is accounted for by the growing foetus, the placenta and the amniotic fluid. The enlarging uterus and breasts also increase in weight. But there are also less obvious factors. The hormones which increase during pregnancy cause both the retention of water and the storage of fat, probably as an energy source. Also, the volume of blood circulating increases.

The *average* normal gain of weight over the duration of a pregnancy is about 28 lb (12.5 kg). This gain does not take place regularly and smoothly. Up to 20 weeks, it amounts to about 8 lb (3.5 kg). Then the foetus grows rapidly, fat is deposited and water starts to be retained. So the second 20 weeks produce an average weight gain of 20 lb (9 kg).

There are wide individual variations in this pattern. Women who are overweight before pregnancy are usually advised to watch their weight carefully; underweight women are encouraged to put it on.

Problems of pregnancy

About half of all women who become pregnant in Western countries suffer from a feeling of nausea or actual vomiting, especially during the first three months. This phenomenon is widely believed to be a normal part of pregnancy. Yet in other parts of the world it is virtually unknown.

On the basis of research by a French doctor, Léon Chertok, it seems that women who vomit in pregnancy tend to be ambivalent about the coming babies, although it would be an oversimplification to state that this is always the case.

Nausea apart, there are very few clear physical concomitants of pregnancy. There may be a very slight swelling of the ankles, or of the breasts.

Pre-eclampsia and eclampsia (toxaemia)

Another common complication which occurs in pregnancy and seems to be peculiar to Europe and the United States, is pre-eclampsia, characterized by raised blood pressure, oedema and protein in the urine.

In very rare cases, pre-eclampsia leads on to eclampsia, in which the symptoms are much more serious and the woman may also suffer from convulsions. The condition is probably caused by the interaction of physical and psychological factors. The body malfunction may be more likely in some women because of their constitution. But in some cases at least, it is triggered by a psychological event. It can occasionally be brought on in normal pregnancy by sudden very severe stress. Pre-eclampsia usually goes with very high levels of anxiety during pregnancy, perhaps with other psychological disturbances, especially depression.

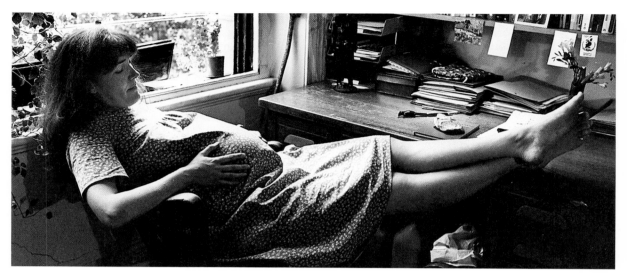

Normally, after pregnancy, the figure and weight will return to what they were before. But if a very large weight gain, say 33 lb (15 kg) was allowed, then it can be a real problem to lose that excess.

The diet itself

The pregnant woman must see that she eats sufficient nutrients and provides sufficient energy for the growth of her foetus and for her own needs. Clichés such as "eating for two" do not apply. A normal, healthy pregnant woman does not have to bother with a special diet. In general, provided it is within a usual and normal range, the diet has very little influence on the pregnancy or birth or on the size or survival of the newborn baby.

However, pregnant women may need an extra protein component and iron-containing foods in the diet. In some countries, health services provide mineral and vitamin pills, as precautionary supplements but this is by no means standard practice.

Day-to-day hygiene and care

Without spending extravagant sums on special maternity clothes, it is possible for a pregnant woman to dress well and feel attractive. But comfort is important: constricting clothes below the waist are to be avoided, as they restrict the blood flow and may cause varicose veins. The breasts are enlarging and need adequate support.

The antenatal team should advise on daily breast care. The nipples need to be gently drawn out and stroked for a short time daily. After about 30 weeks, the pregnant woman needs to be shown how to press the body of each breast towards the nipple. This is called "expressing" and can help the milk to flow when it first comes in.

Long, soothing, warm baths are perfectly safe, and so is ordinary swimming. During the last four weeks, however, in rare cases, the doctor may advise a woman to take showers and not lie in water that *could* enter the genital tract.

If the natural drinking water is low in fluoride, a doctor is likely to prescribe a daily fluoride tablet to help the baby's teeth develop strongly and so prevent decay in late foetal life and early infancy.

During pregnancy it is important to learn how to relax properly so that energy can be conserved during labour. Mental relaxation is also essential and women who are used to meditation or yoga will be well-equipped. The body must be completely supported so that no muscles are working.

There is no reason why a pregnant woman should not have any necessary immunizations or boosters during early pregnancy—except where the inoculation is with a live virus, as in smallpox or German measles (rubella) inoculations. In these cases the virus from the inoculation can reach the foetus and could cause malformation. Rubella is especially dangerous. Careful discussion with the doctor is therefore always necessary.

Emotions in pregnancy

It is commonly believed that the mood changes in pregnancy are caused by hormonal changes. Many of the books written for pregnant mothers give hormones as the cause of emotional disturbance. On the other hand, some people dismiss their role and say that it is "all in the mind".

Two main hormones play major roles in pregnancy: progesterone and oestrogen. The responsibility for mood changes has been laid at the door of both of these and also on the possibility that in some women the two become "out of balance". A third hormone, human chorionic gonadotrophin, which is manufactured by the embryo in its early stages, has caused particular interest, because it rises to a peak at about week 10 of pregnancy and then drops again. It would seem to be a good candidate for the villain of the piece, because its life corresponds so closely with the duration of sickness in the first three months.

However, not all women experience similar emotions during pregnancy. Something extra is needed to explain why some women suffer more (or feel better) in response to their bodily changes, and this appears to be the influence of psychological expectations. These are formulated by the culture in which the woman lives and adapted by her own personality and family experience. So although the hormonal changes during pregnancy are unlikely in themselves to produce changeable emotions, except perhaps in a few women where the changes are very large, they do make it more likely that a woman is going to react both to the changes in her own body and to the role to which society allocates her.

The role of anxiety

The medical profession tends to take it for granted that childbearing is a normal function for women. This being so, some doctors have tended to brush aside the feelings and anxieties of many pregnant women as irrational and irrelevant disturbances in what is a perfectly healthy process. Other doctors recognize the stress of pregnancy and are more inclined to react sympathetically to women's fears. But they still treat these fears as an unfortunate side-effect.

Our culture and our history are such that we do not make things easy for pregnant women and so a certain measure of distress is inevitable for most. Most women handle it quite adequately, with support from their husbands and families. Childbirth classes run by childbirth educators are also very helpful, especially because they are usually arranged to allow the mother-to-be to play an active role. Such classes may be more help to a woman experiencing some distress than the standard classes given in many hospitals and antenatal clinics, helpful though these are. The classes given by medical institutions tend to concentrate, understandably, on the biomedical aspects of

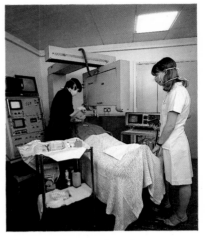

An increasing number of women undergo an amniocentesis test in early pregnancy, usually at between 14 and 16 weeks.

A pain-killing injection is given in the lower part of the abdomen and about 2 tablespoonsful of fluid drawn off through a needle inserted through the mother's abdominal wall and into the uterus. The fluid contains cast-off cells from the foetus which can be grown to form a culture and then analysed. It is possible to tell from this whether or not a child will be affected by a number of inherited disorders. Over 100 different possible abnormalities can be detected in this way, including Down's syndrome and haemophilia.

Testing is regularly carried out on women who already might be at risk. However, if the test is done too early or too late in pregnancy, there is a risk to the foetus.

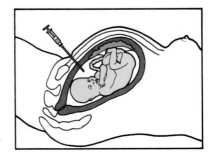

childbirth and are usually straightforward teaching sessions. Since pain in labour is associated with high levels of anxiety and good classes reduce pain, it appears that they are beneficial in helping women cope with the anxiety linked with pregnancy and giving birth.

Anxiety levels typically rise during the first three months and fall again during the middle months. The early anxiety can usually be attributed to the need to adapt to pregnancy, a task which is comfortably completed by most women by the end of the third or fourth month. Anxiety rises to a new peak as birth approaches, reflecting the large changes in the woman's body and the approach of the birth and the new baby.

Women who experience no anxiety at all during pregnancy are likely to be as badly off during and after birth as those who experience unusually high levels. It is women who experience moderate levels of anxiety who are likely to have the easiest time in labour and after the birth. The reason is that these women are doing what Irving Janis calls "psychological work". They are presented with a problem, a coming "crisis" and an encounter with the unknown—and they work at it. They learn about the things they may expect. They rehearse in their minds what they are likely to experience and they sort out which possibilities are more or less likely, which fears are reasonable and which are beyond any bounds of plausibility.

Much of this work does not take place consciously. But fantasies often emerge into consciousness and may themselves be frightening; often a woman does not know that she is capable of such nightmarish thoughts.

Sex in pregnancy

With few exceptions, there is no reason why a couple who want to make love during pregnancy should not do so. It is true that lovemaking can cause contractions in the womb. These may be a temporary exaggeration of the regular small contractions that the womb undergoes throughout life, or they may be caused by the hormones contained in semen. In any case, they are insignificant compared with the contractions of labour. Only where there is already a high risk of miscarriage should a woman abstain from intercourse or from orgasm. It is sometimes said that lovemaking when birth is very near can bring on labour, but at least one study has found no evidence of this.

However, many women simply do not want to make love during pregnancy. Although it is not common for interest in sex to be lost as soon as pregnancy begins, it does happen. There is wide variation in the amount of interest pregnant women feel in sex (as there is in non-pregnant women) and in how it changes during the course of pregnancy.

Some women, perhaps a quarter, feel an increased interest in sex which lasts until the seventh month. About a quarter feel less interest from the beginning, rising to three-quarters in the ninth month. Overall, however, there is a steady reduction in sex interest and activity throughout pregnancy. Masters and Johnson found a greater decrease in sex interest in women expecting their first child than in women who were already mothers; others have not found any difference. The change appears to be in the basic sex drive rather than in any physical problems over intercourse.

Husbands and pregnancy

The ability both to ask and to refuse is an important ingredient of sexual happiness, and never more so than during pregnancy and immediately afterwards. Many men will be pleasantly surprised at the responsiveness of their wives to their needs, if only they can find the right way of expressing themselves.

Other problems with sex may arise when men find that the girl they married is turning into a mother—a class of person with whom sexual relations are forbidden. The fact that many couples keep up love-making until late in pregnancy suggests that either this is not a problem for them, or it is one that they are able to cope with.

Many find that they are put off sex by the presence of the unborn child. Sometimes they have fantasies or ideas that they will damage the child, either by lying on top of it or by their thrusting. Some men feel as though they are being watched by the child. All these feelings are nonsense objectively, but they are perfectly understandable fantasies which form part of the process of adapting to change.

Few couples need to be advised to change from the traditional man-on-top position for lovemaking during pregnancy. The most favoured alternative is side by side.

Some fathers-to-be find their partners less attractive as soon as the bulge begins to appear; others not until it is a large and inescapable protuberance. Other men find their partner's new shape enticing. In the middle three months, many women go through the well-known "bloom" of pregnancy. Their skin takes on a radiant transparency, their eyes sparkle and their hair gleams.

Birth—a family event

How conditions have changed

A hundred years ago childbirth was a dangerous business for both mother and baby. Before 1914 statistics are unreliable, but in the nineteenth century the risk from infection, especially in hospital, was very high—one hospital in England recorded a maternal mortality rate of 33 per 1000 births. In the 1930s and 1940s the rate began to fall and has continued to decline dramatically: in 1940 the US rate was 3.76 per 1000 and by 1979 it was just 0.096. Most of these deaths either follow abortions or are caused by medical conditions such as heart disease, which have nothing to do with pregnancy.

Mortality risks aside, childbirth is still a big, mysterious event. Apart from freak achievements during emergencies, it is probably the hardest work performed by humans. It is not called labour for nothing. And yet, until recently, the exact nature of the work to be done, and how it was achieved, was concealed. It is not unknown for middle-aged women to report that they went into hospital to have their first child not even knowing by what means babies were born. The word "labour" was not used in polite society. A woman was "confined" or "brought to bed"—terms lacking any specific meaning, one carrying overtones of imprisonment, the other of illness.

The problem of pain

There is an unspoken rule among women that one does not tell a first-timer what to expect so as not to terrify her in advance. On the other hand, there is an opposite feeling that it is not fair to let a woman arrive at her first delivery in complete ignorance. The result, as one woman put it, is "you try to let them know without actually telling them". Medical staff may collude in this and some standard hospital and antenatal classes gloss over the subject. They do not ignore it, but they may deal with the question of pain by talking of technological prevention by gas or an injection. At the same time, old-fashioned nurses talk about the "pains", enquiring in labour, "How often are the pains coming?"

THE STAGES OF LABOUR

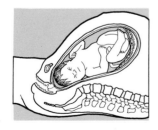 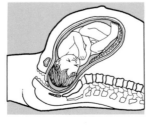 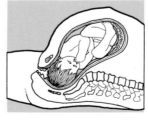 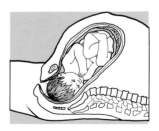

1 *When the mother comes to term, the baby is in position for the birth, usually upside-down with its head engaged in the mother's pelvis.*

2 *Contractions (of the muscular walls of the womb) start, stretching open the cervix as the baby pushes down against it.*

3 *The contractions continue, growing stronger, until the cervix is fully open. This first stage of labour lasts about nine hours.*

4 *At the end of the first stage, the amniotic sac breaks, releasing the amniotic fluid (the "breaking of the waters").*

The result is a confused state of half-knowledge. Many women who arrive in labour without the benefit of good childbirth classes are utterly unprepared for what happens to them.

Does childbirth have to be painful? In order to answer this question, we must first ask a more fundamental and perhaps more surprising question: is childbirth painful at all? Many women in the West would say, "Of course; it is the most intense pain known to humanity: you men can know nothing like it." But the British pioneer doctor Grantly Dick Read was alerted to the possibility of painless childbirth when he encountered a woman in labour in London who reported no pain at all.

Childbirth without pain?

In many societies, women apparently do not feel pain as such while giving birth. In some societies, where *couvade* is practised, the father is the one who retires to a darkened hut and groans in pain, taking several days to recover, while the woman goes back to work soon after the birth.

Grantly Dick Read first suggested the "triad" of pain in childbirth, in which the anticipation and fear of pain produces anxiety, which in turn produces pain. According to Read, if fear could be removed, then pain would disappear as well. Research on the nature of pain broadly supports this suggestion. If pain is anticipated, then anxiety levels rise and the experience of pain increases.

However, it is not the anticipation of pain which itself leads to pain; if it were, then the most effective way of avoiding pain would be to deny that it exists. In fact, denial beforehand actually increases pain, perhaps by producing a shock reaction to it. The real culprits are fear and ignorance.

Childbirth pain has an added dimension: it is likely to be more severe in women who are negative or ambivalent about their pregnancies. Studies in Sweden have shown that the women who have the most pain in birth are on the whole those who have had the most psychological disturbance during pregnancy. This includes those with most marital problems, those who are reluctant to tell their own mothers about the coming baby and women who are late in contacting the antenatal clinic.

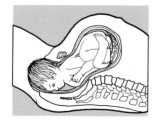

5 *In the second stage of labour the baby is forced out through the birth canal. The mother "pushes" to expel the baby.*

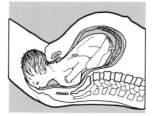

6 *The baby is born, facing the opposite way from the mother. The second stage of labour lasts half an hour to two hours.*

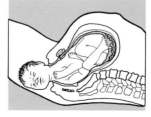

7 *Once the baby's head has passed out of the mother, the rest of the body follows easily.*

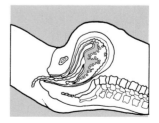

8 *The umbilical cord is cut and, as the final stage of labour, the placenta and remains of the umbilical cord are expelled.*

Training for childbirth

Childbirth classes have been found to be a help in that they teach women about pregnancy, birth and motherhood. A number of experiments have investigated the effect of the psychoprophylactic (meaning psychological preventative, and known as PPM) techniques in childbirth and other types of pain.

One of the most comprehensive studies of the effects of actively preparing for childbirth was carried out with 269 American women who were all married and living with their husbands. Half had taken a full course in psychoprophylaxis and half had had other kinds of preparation in varying degrees.

Level one contained those women who had had no training and those who said things such as "I don't want to know *anything*." At level two were those women who had read books about pregnancy and childbirth and who knew about the psychology involved but who had not attended classes and did not know about coping techniques. At level three were those women who had level two knowledge plus some knowledge of psychophysical techniques. This group included those who had attended classes based on Grantly Dick Read's philosophy. Level four was composed of those women who had had a full PPM training.

It was found that the more training a woman had had, the more aware and conscious she was likely to be at birth. Among level four women, 84 per cent were fully conscious and only 5 per cent unconscious. Even a small degree of preparation—such as that achieved by level two women—was enough to increase the proportion who were partly conscious or aware from 37 per cent to 69 per cent, although only 4 per cent of these women managed to remain conscious and aware throughout. It is only in the United States that such high rates of general anaesthesia apply. Elsewhere, it is used only for Caesarian sections and very difficult forceps deliveries, in 5 to 10 per cent of women at most. How much medication a woman receives in childbirth is strongly influenced by the policy of the unit where she is giving birth. Some will allow her complete freedom of choice, but many will wish to apply their own standards.

When a woman "fails"

Some women arrive at labour with all they have read or been taught about natural childbirth in their minds and determined to go through with it without an anaesthetic. Then, during the labour, they find the pain more than they can stand and accept an anaesthetic injection or a spinal block.

After the birth, many women who have changed their minds in this way feel remorseful and consider that they have failed. The tendency then is to comfort the woman and to reassure her by denying her feelings of having lost control. It is doubtful whether this is wise. Much the better course is to allow the woman to accept that she has failed the target she set herself, but also to examine whether it was a realistic target in the first place. No woman can predict in advance how much pain she is going to feel. But it is more helpful for her to come to terms with this than to pretend that she never really intended to do without anaesthetics. On the other hand, perhaps she never really did intend to do without them. Many women arrive at labour with all sorts of feelings of what they ought or ought not to feel or do,

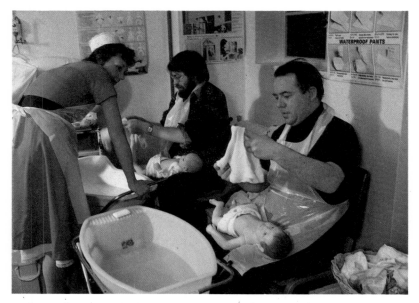

Help from fathers
For any woman, the time of her baby's birth and the following weeks can be a time of great emotional and physical strain. It is now appreciated just how important is the role of the father in fostering an atmosphere of warmth and security for both the baby and mother. Apart from providing moral support, men are encouraged to take a part in the day-to-day business of washing, changing and feeding the newborn—formerly the domain of the females in the family. Many pre-natal classes provide training for fathers in these matters.

and not always with the training to go with these ideas. If a woman's intention to do without drugs was really only lip-service to ideals she did not genuinely share, then it is going to be more useful to her to be allowed to re-examine these ideals than merely to be soothed down.

Fathers in pregnancy and birth

Some writers suggest that modern society has pushed the father out. However, men are excluded from births in societies of many different economic types throughout the world.

Whether they admit it or not, men are profoundly affected by their partner's pregnancies, especially the first. This impact is demonstrated by the number of men who become disturbed, to a greater or lesser degree. Women's symptoms could be put down to alterations in their hormones and other physical systems, but this could not explain changes in moods and behaviour in their partners. So the tendency was simply to ignore such changes, unless the disturbance was very serious.

In men, mood and behaviour may become disturbed, changeable, perhaps erratic. These are the reactions of a person called upon to make profound psychological changes without reliable guidance, because nobody recognizes that the crisis exists.

Recently, we have moved towards giving the father a much more central role in pregnancy and childbirth. Many fathers now attend classes with their wives, as well as attending the birth. This makes it easier for the father to adapt to his partner's pregnancy and to form a good relationship with the child from the moment it is born.

There are, in fact, good grounds for suggesting that the father is the linchpin that ensures the smooth turning of the whole cycle of a woman's transition through pregnancy to motherhood. Several studies of married couples have found that the husband's personality is at least as important as the wife's in determining the psychological outcome of her pregnancy. The more secure and emotionally supportive the husband, the more complete and successful the wife's

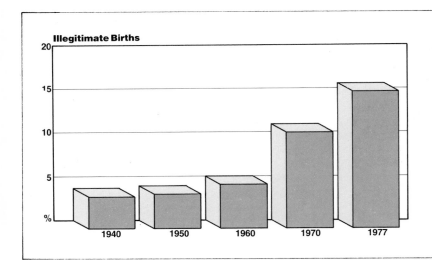

Illegitimate Births

20
15
10
5
%

1940   1950   1960   1970   1977

Illegitimacy
There has been a large increase in the rate of illegitimate births in the USA over the last few decades. One out of every seven children born in 1978 was born outside of marriage—three times the rate in the mid-1960s, although the number of total births has declined. Currently, over half of all black births and 8 per cent of white births are illegitimate. Also, the majority of such births are concentrated in the under-20 age group. Older women are more likely to use contraceptives.

adjustment to the changes that are required of her.

The extent of the support the husband is called upon to give naturally depends on the wife. Some women are so well prepared for pregnancy that their husbands need provide little support. At the other extreme, some women are so unready for the transition to motherhood and so unable to cope with the burden of pregnancy itself, that the husbands are crucial to the whole outcome. It is also easier for a woman to form a good relationship with her unborn baby when her husband takes a clear interest in her pregnancy and the development of the child, and gives her emotional support throughout.

Fathers at the birth
The nervous father waiting in helpless ignorance in a hospital in the middle of the night has long been a standard subject for cartoonists. Today, however, such men are becoming figures of the past. The time when it was suggested that there was actually something wrong with a man who wanted to attend the birth of his child has gone.

Men are discovering, with their wives, that the birth of their child can be one of the most joyous experiences that life has to offer. One study has compared the experiences of two groups of fathers. One group had attended "natural childbirth" classes with their wives and stayed with their wives throughout labour and delivery. The other group (standard fathers) had not attended classes and retired to the waiting room, usually at the end of the first stage of labour.

Richard Gayton found that the groups had very different experiences. He tracked how their anxiety levels changed throughout the birth process. Standard fathers were more anxious throughout until they received the news that mother and child were well, when their feelings of anxiety dipped below those of the other fathers. At the beginning of labour, the anxiety level of the standard fathers was substantially higher. When the wives were in hard labour, towards the end of the first stage, the anxiety of the "natural childbirth" fathers reached its highest point. Thereafter they became calmer, while the standard fathers, removed from the scene, continued to become more anxious, reaching a peak when told that birth was imminent.

Husbands and doctors

One of the reasons that is sometimes offered for resistance by medical staff to the presence of husbands in the delivery room is that the layman might not understand all that the doctor does and might "get the wrong idea". Richard Gayton's study shows that, on the whole, doctors have little to fear and much to gain in parental attitudes from the presence of fathers.

To a large extent, how a father feels about the medical staff during his wife's delivery depends on how they treat him. If they make him welcome and permit him to play a useful and active part in labour and delivery, he reacts favourably. If they tend to exclude him, he may react at least as negatively as those fathers left outside in the waiting room in a completely passive role.

What fathers can do

One aspect of the father's role during labour and delivery has been likened to that of a sportsman's coach. He brings his wife drinks, wipes away sweat, massages her, monitors her contractions and keeps track of her breathing and relaxation. But apart from such caretaking activity, the very presence of the father is profoundly calming and reassuring in the hospital environment, which many women find unfamiliar and hostile. Many women find that it is easier to respond to a voice that they know and love than to instructions from a stranger, particularly when a change of staff may occur with a new shift in the middle of labour.

One study in West Germany, in which husbands were introduced for the first time into a hospital, noted that as well as helping their wives and the medical staff, their presence "produced an atmosphere of calmness and dignity in the delivery room".

No doubt because of this calming effect, the presence of her husband often has the effect of lowering the woman's experience of pain. There is another side to this too. Pain is an intensely private experience, and the cues by which others estimate it are subtle and easily misinterpreted. It is not surprising, then, that husbands are often very much better at judging how much pain a woman is feeling than midwives, doctors or even childbirth educators.

After the birth

As many as four-fifths of mothers experience a brief period of tearfulness at some time during the first few days after the birth. Sometimes the mood creeps on slowly; more often, however, the onset is sudden and many women are quite unprepared for it when it happens. A woman may be astonished to find herself bursting into tears without any apparent provocation at the moment when she "should" be happy, such as when her husband arrives for a visit. Then, after perhaps as little time as an hour, the mood is gone.

A much smaller proportion of new mothers find themselves with a depression that may last a few weeks or months or, occasionally, even longer.

In the first few days after giving birth, some women find themselves confused and disoriented, feeling not quite sure where or who they are, or what age. Except in a very tiny number of cases, these feelings pass after two or three weeks at the most, leaving only the depression.

Avoiding depression

Richard and Katherine Gordon have studied ways to help to avoid or alleviate postnatal depression. They instituted a scheme in which mothers-to-be were instructed and advised on the following points:

1 The responsibilities of motherhood are learned: hence, get informed.
2 Get help from husbands, friends and relatives.
3 Make friends with other couples who are experiencing child-rearing.
4 Don't overload yourself with unimportant tasks.
5 Don't move house soon after the baby arrives.
6 Don't be over-concerned with keeping up appearances.
7 Get plenty of rest and sleep.
8 Don't be a nurse to relatives or others at this time.
9 Confer and consult with husband, family and experienced friends and discuss your plans and your worries.
10 Don't give up outside interests, but cut down on responsibilities and rearrange schedules.
11 Arrange for baby-sitters early.
12 Get a family doctor or see the one you have early.

Women who followed such instructions before they gave birth were much less likely to become depressed or to be disoriented after birth. Their babies were also less likely to be irritable and to have sleeping problems six months later. If their husbands received the same instructions, the results were even better. Women who had not been given the instructions and who had become depressed were helped by receiving the course after they had given birth.

The birth

Regular contractions of the uterus signal the onset of labour which can last anything from four to 24 hours or more. Women's experiences of labour differ widely: some describe the baby as having 'slid out', others see the whole process as 'a battle'.

The newborn is covered with vernix, a thick greasy white substance which assists the passage through the birth canal. He or she may be spattered with the mother's blood and covered with a dark body hair (lanugo) which disappears by four months at the latest. Stores of fat, sugar and fluid, which sustain the baby until the mother's milk is ready, may make him or her look fat.

Directly after the birth, mucus is cleared from the air passages and the baby begins to breathe.

Difficult births are not common but may occur if the baby is born feet or buttocks first (the breech position) or if the mother's pelvis is too small or the baby is in danger of suffocation. Forceps may be used to help the baby or an incision (an episiotomy) made in the perineum to ease the passage of the baby's head. A complicated birth may necessitate a delivery by Caesarian. For potentially difficult babies, women are advised to deliver in hospital.

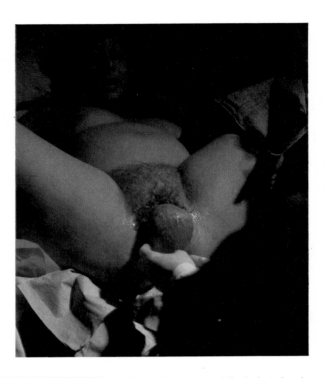

Above: Crowning. The baby's head is forced into the vagina and can be seen. (In the majority of births, the baby's head is born first.) Once it passes the bones surrounding the birth canal the mother is told to bear down to push the baby outwards.

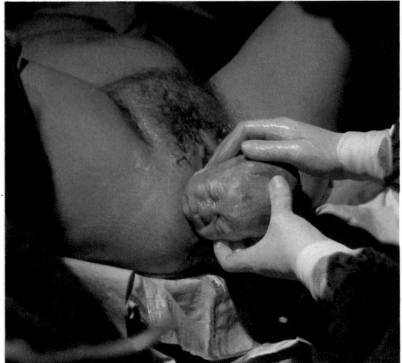

Left: As the baby's head leaves the birth canal the mother's backbone is forced down to let it pass and the head and neck are bent backwards (extension). Once outside the mother's body they untwist so that the baby faces the mother's right thigh.

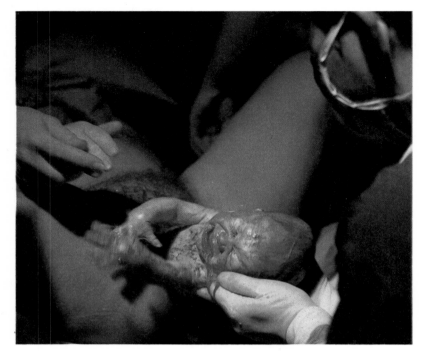

Left: One shoulder, then the other follow, and the rest of the body is born almost immediately. The whole process described here takes an average of 1¾ hours. The placenta is pushed out after the birth of the baby.

Below: The newborn infant and mother resting. The baby may suckle soon after birth. The milk will not come for several days but the baby will receive colostrum, a clear, slightly sticky fluid which contains valuable proteins and can provide immunity to infections.

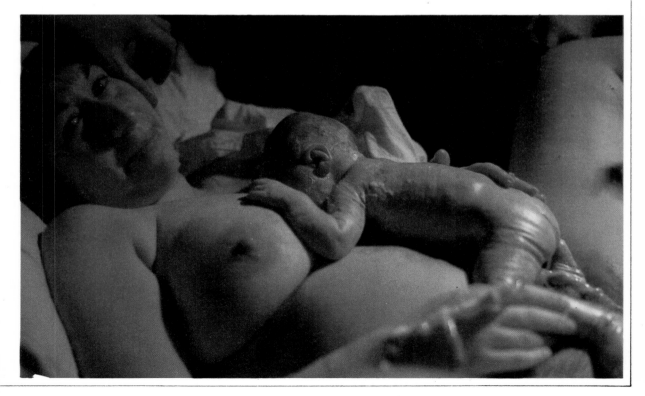

Life with infants and children

For many people, the realization of how different life with children can be from the life of the childless (or childfree) comes slowly two or three months after their child is born. During labour, delivery and the period immediately after the birth, the baby and parents are likely to get a lot of attention and there is a novelty about all that happens. However, a few weeks later, feelings can change. The novelty has worn off, and days seem completely filled with feeding and changing the baby. Nights are disturbed by crying. Constant child care seems to stretch ahead into an unlimited future, unrelieved by any of the activities that were important to the parents before the baby was born. The parents may feel that things will never be the same again and are panicky about what they have let themselves in for. The baby is, of course, sweet and adorable—at least, that is what it is easiest to say in public—but privately the parents may bitterly resent the constant demands for attention, and wonder how they could have been misled by all the glossy pictures of smiling, well-scrubbed babies dressed in immaculate clothes.

Reactions, of course, vary as do capacities to cope and what needs to be coped with. However, our culture does tend to idealize parenthood, and many parents find themselves let down with a bump when they discover that reality does not square up with this ideal.

The "average" modern family

What are the key features of middle- and lower-middle-class families in Western societies today? We tend to marry fairly young, in our early twenties, and have an average of two children fairly soon after marriage. Our households are small, usually containing only parents and children. Links with a wider network of relatives are not particularly strong and, on the whole, the family is fairly isolated. Social life usually centres on the family, and couples spend the bulk of their leisure time together with their children. Work and home life are very separate.

The roles of husband and wife are separate, but less so than, say, for a Victorian middle-class family. Because of the smaller number of children and the longer lifespan, a much briefer proportion of a woman's life is spent in child care than has been true in the past. In recent decades, there have been some shifts in the distribution of work within the home, but it is still only a small minority of men who share the responsibility for their children and take an equal part in their care.

Life after Freud and Spock

Our society is often described as child-centred. Certainly, we pay a lot of attention to the needs of our children. But perhaps the main thing that sets us apart from earlier times is that we have a very strong belief that what we do with children matters for their future development. There is not a great deal of agreement about what kinds of early experience lead to particular aspects of later development. Our approach to child care is less punitive than that of some of our forebears, and distraction and rewards are now seen to be important techniques in teaching discipline.

It seems likely that at every period in history some parents have

---

ADJUSTMENT TO PARENTHOOD

The advent of parenthood is a major development in a couple's lives, involving not only altered practical circumstances, but also changed roles and a more complex network of relationships in the home. A number of factors can be identified which affect the ease with which an adult will adapt to parenthood.
1 The woman's attitude is initially coloured by her experience (physical and emotional) during pregnancy, though the adverse effects of an unhappy experience of pregnancy will normally lessen with time.
2 Parents with a child (or children) of the sex(es) they want will adapt better. Their attitudes to parenthood will also be better if they have the number of children they want.
3 Younger parents tend to adapt quickly, adjusting their life style to the baby without compromising their own interests too much.
4 Parents who wanted a child because of social pressures will tend to adapt less well.
5 Anxiety about the best way to bring up children will have an unfavourable effect. Also, parents with a preconceived ideal of what a child should be like will tend to react badly when they are disappointed. However, a child who is happy and easy to manage will have a favourable effect on the parents' view of parenthood.

been concerned with the emotional happiness and wellbeing of their children. Perhaps such concerns are more widespread today; it is hard to know. But there is now an interest in long-term consequences. A satisfying emotional life is thought to be important for a child, because it has beneficial effects for adulthood. Such a belief causes much anxiety for parents, because they are seen as the people who have the responsibility of ensuring that children grow up in the "right" emotional atmosphere. Their task is made harder because there is no agreement about what the right climate is or, indeed, about the degree of importance which should be attached to early experience. So whatever they do there is the possibility that a child will not develop satisfactorily, and they are the people who are likely to be blamed.

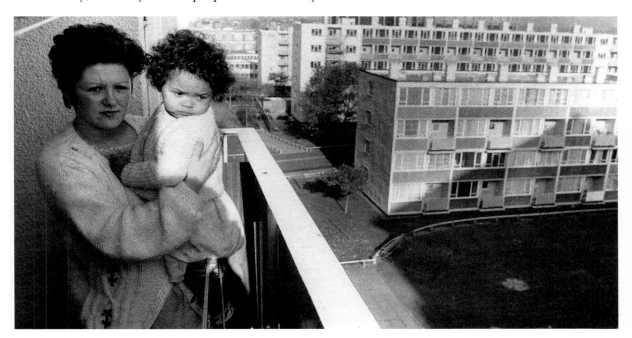

The isolation of the new mother

Some of the common problems that parents face in living with infants stem from the isolation that many women experience when they are at home with a small baby. This isolation not only arises from the structure of the small nuclear family, but also because of the common expectation of mutual dependence of the couple. Before their children arrive, much of their social life consists of activities undertaken not necessarily involving any other friends or family members. For many women, the social contacts at work form an important part of their social world. This and much of what a woman did with her husband disappears once she has children and is left at home all day. Before she had children, she may not have spent much time in the neighbourhood of the home, so may not have many friends in the range that can easily be covered with a small baby and without a car.

The table overleaf shows who mothers tend to call on for help in the period immediately after their babies are born. It demonstrates how only the close family are significantly involved (and only female relatives) and how friends and neighbours become more important as

The responsibility for a new life can be frightening and many parents do not realize how much their lives will change with the arrival of a child. Many women alone at home with a baby feel isolated and it is important at this time to establish links with people in similar circumstances who can be supportive.

more children are born. This is presumably because, having lived in a neighbourhood longer, they make more local friends.

What stems from this isolation? One of the commonest results is depression. Several surveys have shown that up to 40 per cent of women with children under five years old 'suffer from depression serious enough to warrant professional attention. The link with social isolation is demonstrated by the fact that rates are much lower for married women of the same age group who do not have children, and for women with children who go out to work. Pointing in the same direction is the finding that women who have a close, confiding relationship with their husband, a relative or friend are less likely to suffer from depression. Children of depressed mothers can also suffer, and it often causes problems in the marriage relationship. This is one reason why 9 to 12 months after a child is born is a very common time for marriages to break up.

Sources of mothers' help	Number of children			All mothers
	1 %	2 %	3 %	
Husband	89	90	87	89
Mother	50	52	45	49
Mother-in-law	27	25	25	25
Sister or sister-in-law	26	27	30	27
Other relatives	11	9	13	12
Friends or neighbours	25	38	48	35
Paid help	—	2	2	2
Other	5	5	3	5
No one	3	2	2	2

The mother–infant relationship

A consequence of the frequent isolation of women at home with children is that the relationship between mother and child becomes all-important and dominates all the others that the child may have. This emphasis on the mother–infant relationship is probably a relatively new phenomenon in the history of the family. Some psychologists have taken it for granted and see it as the necessary and sufficient basis for the development of children.

Current evidence, however, supports the view that children are most likely to develop satisfactorily if they grow up with *several* strong and close relationships. The idea that mothers should have sole charge of their young children certainly contributes to the problems of depression and isolation. Few adults find the exclusive company of infants satisfactory, but fear of "damaging" infants by leaving them with other people can deter mothers from seeking adult company.

However, parents need their own social life away from the demands of young children. We need to balance our concern about creating long-term psychological problems for our children with providing a satisfactory life for all members of the family in the present. The persisting belief that men are unwilling or unable to care for young children needs to be constantly challenged. Erroneous beliefs about infants—especially the supposed need for a mother to be

NAMING YOUR CHILD
A person's Christian name is such an integral part of his or her identity that the name you choose for your child can have important psychological consequences. Certain categories of name that could possibly adversely affect the psychological wellbeing of an individual can be identified. Bear in mind, too, that a perfectly normal Christian name may not combine well with a particular surname.
1 Very common names.
2 Very unusual names.
3 Names that are difficult to pronounce or spell.
4 Names identified with an ethnic or religious group subject to prejudice.
5 Names that can be given to either sex.
6 Names identified with unattractive characters in literature, history, on television programmes.
7 Names that may give rise to embarrassing nicknames.
8 Old-fashioned names.

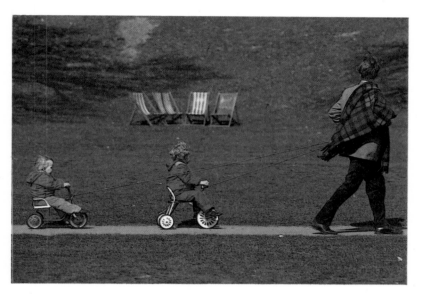

Fathers actively involved in the child-rearing experience are founding the basis for good lines of communication in the future.

a constant and exclusive caretaker—have often prevented the evolution of family life in desirable directions. It is interesting to contrast this belief with our society's strong opposition to single parents, based on the equally strong belief belief that children "need" both parents, although the point at which the child suddenly comes to need two parents, after being exclusively attached to his or her mother, has never been made clear.

Sibling rivalry

We have tended to talk, so far, as if all babies were alone with their parents. But, of course, many have older brothers and sisters. Siblings, particularly if they are well into the toddler stage or older, are usually very interested in the changes in their mother through pregnancy and in the new baby. Their first reaction to newborns, much like that of adults, is to want to touch and hold them. However, these reactions may often be followed by signs of resentment and anger. A toddler may revert to bed-wetting or demand a bottle.

The strength of these reactions seems to depend on the kinds of relationship that existed with the parents and others before the new baby's birth, and the extent to which old-established patterns are disturbed. If an older child is used to spending most of his time with his mother, he will be deposed by the new baby and is likely to resent it. Toddlers' resources for coping with such developments are more limited, and they will need more help and support to make an easy adjustment. In the working-out of new routines, space needs to be found for older siblings, so that they get some periods at least when they can still feel that they are the centre of things. This, of course, adds to the pressures on parents in the first few months, but in the long run awareness of the siblings' needs at this stage can do much to prevent a little rivalry becoming a deeper resentment.

Coping with violent feelings

Parents who injure their children are sometimes depicted as monsters whose feelings are quite outside the normal range. This is usually not the case. They are simply parents who are under more stress than most and who do not control their angry feelings about their children, expressing them in a violent form.

Studies of child abuse by Diana Russell of the University of California show that it occurs in as many as one in six families. It is more common in socially isolated families and where the child's behaviour is especially difficult and frustrating. Victims are often handicapped children. It is more likely to occur when parents get on badly, do not have a close, confiding relationship and do not cooperate over sharing child care. When parents themselves have been treated in a violent or abusive way as children, they are more likely to treat their own children in the same way. This is probably because the kinds of deprivation that create stresses for parents and lead to an increased chance of violence towards children tend to be passed on to the next generation. Another reason is that children who receive violence from their own parents are less likely to develop the controls over their own · behaviour which are needed to prevent violence.

Often, however, if parents find that they are becoming irritated with their children, it is because there is some other problem in their lives which is worrying them. Especially when a parent is alone with a baby for long periods of time, it is not surprising that the baby becomes the butt of his or her frustrations.

Keeping healthy

Young adulthood is a time when increasing responsibilities in the home and at work may mean less leisure time for sports and other active pursuits. At the same time, changes in life style (involving catering for children, for example, or more entertaining at home, or business lunches) may bring alterations in diet that are not altogether healthy. Obesity and a general lack of fitness are dangers. They can be guarded against by keeping a sensible (not fanatical) watch on your weight (cutting down on calorie intake if necessary) and making sure that you take some form of regular exercise. This latter need may be answered by a simple, regular exercise routine done at home, every day or even 20 minutes twice a week.

Body weight (kg) (1 kg = 2.2 lb)		Calories
MEN 18 - 35	55 - 69	2400 - 2650
	70 - 84	2700 - 3000
	85 - 95	3050 - 3400
WOMEN 18 - 35	40 - 49	1550 - 1750
	50 - 64	1800 - 2100
	65 - 75	2200 - 2400

Various factors affect the daily calorie requirement of an individual. The figures shown above take account of a major factor—body weight.

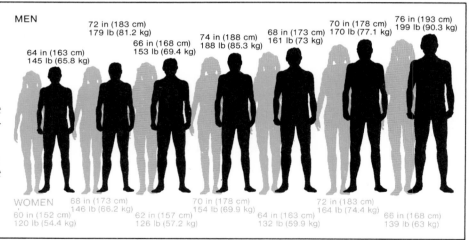

Weight and height
This chart shows the average weight (in indoor clothing) for men at different heights. The heights are for a person of medium frame and aged 30–39 years. (Ideal weight changes with age, with 30–39 years being the time of least change for men, apart from old age, while women increase slightly throughout life.)

MEN

64 in (163 cm)
145 lb (65.8 kg)

72 in (183 cm)
179 lb (81.2 kg)

66 in (168 cm)
153 lb (69.4 kg)

74 in (188 cm)
188 lb (85.3 kg)

68 in (173 cm)
161 lb (73 kg)

70 in (178 cm)
170 lb (77.1 kg)

76 in (193 cm)
199 lb (90.3 kg)

WOMEN
60 in (152 cm)
120 lb (54.4 kg)

68 in (173 cm)
146 lb (66.2 kg)

62 in (157 cm)
126 lb (57.2 kg)

70 in (178 cm)
154 lb (69.9 kg)

64 in (163 cm)
132 lb (59.9 kg)

72 in (183 cm)
164 lb (74.4 kg)

66 in (168 cm)
139 lb (63 kg)

STAYING FIT
Exercise
Combined with healthy eating, you should take some form of exercise; as little as 40 minutes a week is all that is required, though, of course, the more you have time for, the better.

The average single man in Western Europe spends a quarter of his leisure time in physical recreation—particularly in swimming, football, table tennis, athletics and jogging. Single women favour dancing, swimming, tennis, table tennis, horse riding and skating. This picture of activity usually changes after marriage and children. The family unit is consolidated and both partners spend more (if not all) of their free time on home-based pursuits. Fortunately, exercising has recently become both popular and fashionable (and a profitable industry) so there are now many sources of information to encourage you to exercise in the home—books, tapes, records and video-recordings.

Basic exercises
If you cannot or do not want to exercise outside the home, or from a recording, you can still keep fit and healthy on a minimum of 40 minutes a week, in two or three sessions.

A typical routine will involve exercises for warming up, for developing strength and for building up stamina. Each movement is repeated several times and as you progress you will be able to increase the number of repetitions week by week. Before beginning any programme of exercise you must be sure that you are physically able to cope with it. If you have any doubts, consult your doctor. If you are extremely overweight, you must lose weight before you start exercising.

The warming-up exercises are designed to loosen up the muscles—never start with anything too energetic: it could be dangerous. Wear loose, comfortable clothes and find a place that will allow you enough room to lie flat on the floor and swing your arms and legs around. Warming-up exercises include bending and stretching. For example, stand with your feet wide apart and legs straight. Bend over each leg alternately, reaching to your foot with your arms and bending your head towards your knee. Or stand with your feet slightly apart, with your arms above your head and stretch up as far as you can, first with the right hand and then with the left.

Exercises for developing strength condition and tone the muscles. They include push-ups on the floor or to a chair, which strengthen arm muscles, and sit-ups (sitting up from a lying position without using the arms and keeping the legs straight on the floor) to strengthen the stomach.

Stamina-building exercises involve repeating movements at speed (for example, running on the spot) to increase the pulse rate.

Do not leave more than four days between each exercise session, and do not attempt to do too much too soon. It takes about three months on average to get fit and you should continue exercising in order to stay fit.

Physical illness

Infectious diseases have declined in recent years and the most common cause of death in men between 20 and 30 is an accident, principally a car accident. The death rate for women in this age group is less than half that for men and the accident rate is considerably lower. Over 30, the female death rate rises more rapidly than the male.

Cancer: this is the major medical killer for young adults, attacking the lung, brain or testes in men, the brain in younger women and the breast, ovary and cervix in women over 30. Treatments include surgery and chemotherapy. If detected early, it can be eliminated.

Heart disease: stress and obesity are major factors. It is increasingly found in younger men.

Multiple sclerosis: two-thirds of those suffering from multiple sclerosis contract it between the ages of 20 and 40. It is a disease which causes degeneration in the nerve sheaths in brain, spinal cord and optic nerves, resulting in muscular weakness.

Diet

For most people at this time of life, the necessity to eat properly may not become apparent until physical bodily changes are experienced. But more than ever, when we are encountering major changes in lifestyle, it is wise to pay attention to the kind of food we eat, and when we eat it. Faced with a barrage of information on food and diet, it is difficult to know just what is healthy.

* Try to eat a balanced diet, that contains fats, proteins, carbohydrates, fibre, vitamins and minerals. By avoiding processed food, it is possible to obtain all of these nutrients without resorting to vitamin or mineral supplements.

* Try substituting brown sugar and wholemeal flour for the bleached varieties, and steer clear of too much animal fat, alcohol or added salt.

* Eat at regular intervals. Of course, the individual will vary in his or her requirements, but there is evidence from studies of premenstrual women that regular meals can allay their symptoms. Breakfast is particularly important after a night's sleep.

* Avoid eating between meals and do not overeat at mealtimes. It's much easier to resist large helpings that it is to shift those extra pounds.

* As much of your food as possible should be fresh—aim to eat more vegetables and less meat, particularly fatty cuts.

AVOIDING ILLNESS
Mental health

Depression is a major problem, particularly for women, during this time. It is estimated that one-third of women in lower socio-economic groups at home full-time with children under six are seriously depressed. Some house-bound women develop phobias about going out or become obsessed with cleanliness in the home, and need expert help to overcome their problems.

Sexual problems

Impotence: most men experience this from time to time and it should cause no concern unless it becomes a permanent condition. It can be caused by physiological factors, such as certain illnesses or drugs used to treat them, or by psychological factors, such as guilt or anxiety.

Infertility: in about 40 per cent of cases this is due to male sterility. In women the cause may be a hormone deficiency or a physical obstruction which can be cleared by surgery.

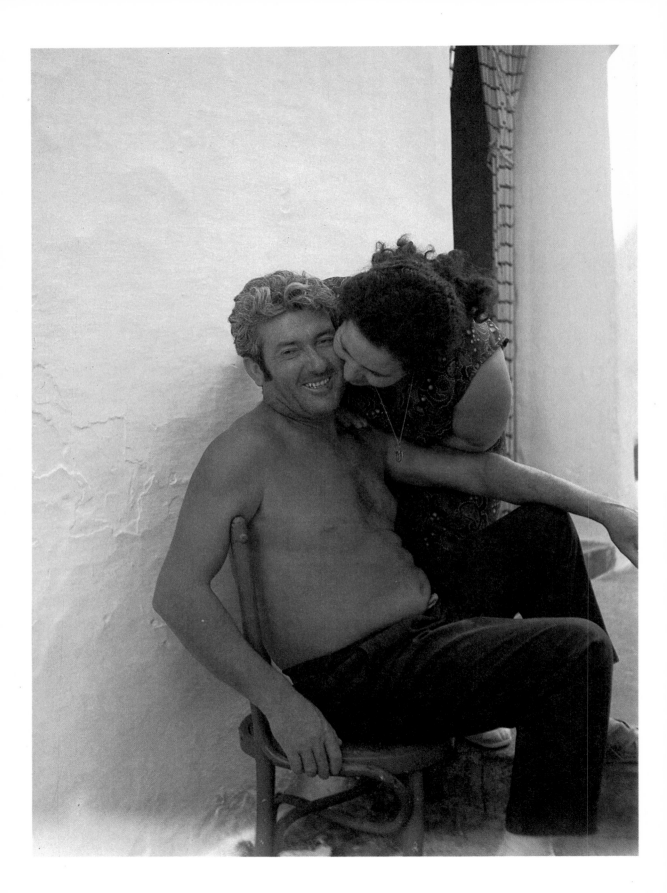

Middle Age

*The mutual conquest of difficulties is the cement of
friendship as it is the only lasting cement of marriage.*
Apsley Cherry-Garrard *The Worst Journey in the World*

Until recently there was à yawning gap in the human lifespan that
was largely ignored by social and behavioural scientists. Freud's
message (only slightly exaggerated) was that once the Oedipal
period ended at the age of seven or eight, the individual's
problems, conflicts and adaptability were more or less set for the
duration of life. However, one consistent research finding which
is emerging (which tends to disprove Freud) is that people do
change in the later phases of life and that, in nearly all the
important spheres of living, change for the better is almost as
frequent as change for the worse.

These findings have led to a heightened sense of the
flexibility and growth potential of the middle-aged. They have
also raised questions about some of our earlier assumptions, such
as the continuing influence on the capacity for change, in later
life, of various kinds of deprivations in infancy and early
childhood. For example, how long can you go on blaming early
circumstances, and those who peopled them, for your current
problems? If middle age can now confidently be viewed as
growth-oriented, then some adult changes may altogether offset
the negative consequences of early life events.

However, the process is by no means automatic. Studies
exploring the effects of early life experience on adaptation in
middle and later life will help us to understand the circumstances
under which unfortunate early experiences may be kept where
they belong—firmly in the past. The negative emotions which
accompanied them may not be forgotten—rather, they become
accepted and integrated parts of oneself.

Left: The prime of life? Many of life's deepest satisfactions come to the middle-aged

The changing family

The direct study of parenthood is one of the neglected areas of middle age. It is often mentioned as part of more general research where the emphasis has been on the parents as individuals rather than on their relationship with their children. Even then, there is a common assumption that the parenting role is ending in middle age as grown-up children leave home. We can, of course, question whether parenting ever actually ends, even when the children have created families of their own. But if we concede conventionally that the middle years span roughly the ages 40 to 55 or so, it is clear that many of the middle-aged will be parents of adolescents and still some way from the pleasures and problems of the empty nest. Given that both adolescence and middle age are times of considerable physical and, we suspect, psychological change, then this phase of parenting should be a particularly interesting area of study.

The middle-aged as parents
In one of the few research projects which has been carried out, Alice Rossi of the University of Massachusetts collected information from 68 women in mid-life, whose children had not yet left home.

One of her most striking findings was that the family emerged as a very significant source of pleasure for these women—more so amongst those in late than in early middle age. By contrast, when asked to name "the worst thing about being your present age", few women mentioned their children—most talked of themselves or other aspects of their marriage. Having already put one child through adolescence seems to make things easier the second time round and this may be one reason why the older mothers derived more pleasure from the experience. However, they may also be subjected to more criticism over such things as being old-fashioned or too strict.

It is not only age which makes a difference. The more education a woman had, the easier she found it to bring up adolescent children. Interestingly enough, the opposite held for younger children: they were rated as more difficult to raise by better-educated as opposed to less-well-educated women.

The effects of ageing
Those women who experienced ageing symptoms such as deteriorating eyesight or hearing, or a reduced energy level, tended also to report less emotional closeness with their children. Ageing symptoms were also associated with stress in the marital relationship, and with a desire on the mother's part to be much younger. It is impossible here to tease out cause and effect, but it is certainly possible that a poor relationship with her husband and children, for whatever reasons, might affect a woman's perception of the physical changes of middle age.

We cannot be sure that these findings would be replicated in a few years' time with a new sample of middle-aged women. Not-yet-middle-aged mothers are having smaller families, successful careers and, probably, do not see their families as their only source of fulfilment, which will affect their relationship with their children. It may be that signs of ageing do not appear until later in life.

CHILDREN'S SPOUSES

For many of the middle-aged, one of the major adjustments that has to be made is to their children's spouses. Not only is there a new relationship to be developed—with the son- or daughter-in-law—but the parents' relationships with their own child can also be expected to alter. Parents who expect no change in their relations with their child, or who expect to relate to the son- or daughter-in-law in exactly the same way as they do to their own children, may have difficulty in adapting.

Equally, problems can be caused by a son or a daughter who fails to adapt to the changed pattern of relationships—a married child who remains psychologically dependent on his or her parents may make his or her spouse resent them.

There may also be extra difficulties in adjustment for the middle-aged parents where:
1 the younger couple have to live with them
2 they do not like their child's spouse, or there is a difference in social, racial or religious background
3 they would like grand-children, but none are born
4 the younger couple live nearby, giving the parents more opportunity for interference.

The empty nest

Until recently, the term "involutional melancholia" was used to describe middle-aged women who became depressed. While the menopause was seen as an important contribution to this "condition", so too was the exit of children from the home. The assumption was that most women would find this event traumatic, especially as it tended to coincide with the menopause. These assumptions are now being challenged, or at least recognized as over-simplifications of the facts. One problem was that many of the theories about how women felt about children leaving home were based on reports from women who had sought help for problems such as depression. Obviously, the theories ignored the vast numbers of women (and men) who did not experience these sorts of problems in middle age.

Looking ahead

The exit of children obviously means different things to different people; it is also, apparently, differently viewed in anticipation than in reality. In her study of transitions, Marjorie Fiske of the University of California at San Francisco found that middle-aged men facing the departure of their youngest child made very little reference to the event, but were more preoccupied with their own retirement. Women, on the other hand, while not directly admitting it, seemed to view the future with some trepidation as unpredictable and unplanable. But this is by no means a general finding for all women. Fiske's results, and those of other researchers, show that it is those women who have assumed the traditional female role, who are housewives, who remain married and who are not overtly aggressive, who are most likely to respond to the "empty nest" with depression.

On a more hopeful note, Marjorie Fiske found that, five years on,

The family situation of the middle-aged can vary from parents with children of their own still at home, through those whose children are "flying the nest", to those with grandchildren to enjoy.

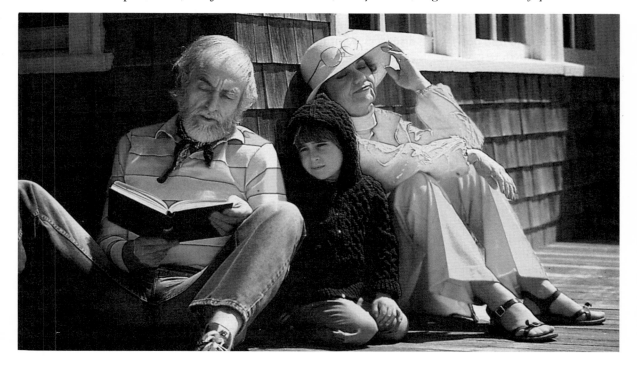

many of the women who had anticipated the empty nest with dread had in reality adapted well. They had made important changes in their lives, ranging from divorce or beginning a career to redecorating their homes. They were, in their own terms, well satisfied, often happy. Had they been born 10 years earlier, it is unlikely that as many would have had the courage to assume control over their lives. Perhaps those born 10 or 20 years later will not wait until middle age to take such initiatives.

The critical problem of ageing parents

Middle-aged parents may find themselves caught between two generations—their children and their own parents. It is the woman, however, who is likely to feel a heightened sense of responsibility for ageing parents. This anxiety is experienced by those who do not yet have dependent parents or parents-in-law, as well as by those already taking care of one parent or more; and it often emphasizes their own anxieties about becoming dependent on their own children. They know that the actual assumption of such responsibilities, often on a daily basis, can be a severe emotional, physical and economic drain, and a strain on marriages as well.

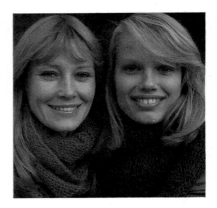

Children grow up and eventually leave home, but the family does not necessarily become less important for the parents. It can still be a major source of pleasure—and an adolescent child and a middle-aged parent can be a very happy combination.

In her study of middle-aged people at various transition points in their lives, Marjorie Fiske spoke to many women who had cared for ageing parents who had since died. In retrospect, they had come to consider it by far the most difficult period in their lives. The physical and emotional burden almost invariably fell most heavily on the wife's shoulders, whether the ageing parents were hers, his or both. The husband, who may run errands, provide money or visits, tends to have a greater capacity for emotional distancing and is therefore less likely to be pervaded by guilt feelings. This attitude is, of course, reinforced—or engendered—by society's assignment of the caring role to women.

With the rapid increase in the divorce and remarriage rates among the middle-aged and late middle-aged, there are now frequently double sets of parents and in-laws—as well as double sets of children—to feel responsible for. Marjorie Fiske's subjects were drawn from a strongly family-oriented segment of our society and were mainly white and lower-middle-class. But similar findings are being reported from a shorter-term study of a very large cross-section of the population being studied by Leonard Pearlin and Morton Lieberman at the University of Chicago. Their group also reports that young adults are at least as concerned about their parents as are the middle-aged, and that the men are just as anxious as women.

In the United States, where these studies were carried out, it is the middle-aged women who not only carry the day-to-day burden of ageing parents, but are most likely to be guilt-ridden about not doing enough. If they could perhaps find or develop small groups of others in like situations (as already exist in Britain for single women caring for their parents), they might jointly muster the courage to persuade their husbands to share the burdens or at least to be more supportive and understanding, rather than resentful, of the deflection of their wives' attention from themselves and their children to the older generation. The husbands should also be reminded that when they themselves get old, they will probably also turn to their daughters rather than to their sons for emotional and other forms of support.

Love and intimacy

There have been few rigorous studies of the significance of intimate relationships in adulthood, but most adults of sensibility are aware of their importance for growth and as a rich resource in the inevitable transitions and problems of the latter half of life. Marjorie Fiske defined certain aspects of the relationships which participants in her study had with their friends and spouses. These components include similarity, reciprocity and compatibility.

Their importance is shown in both verbal and non-verbal behaviour. On the verbal level, close relationships with others include sharing intellectual ideas, similar attitudes and exchanges of information, and also open and spontaneous emotional exchanges and self-disclosure. They may also include expressions of affection and love. Non-verbal expressions range from similarity of behaviour, perhaps in movement and dress, to closeness and frequency of looking and touching. Physical expressions of intimacy range from a casual handshake or touch on the shoulder, kiss on the cheek or a quick hug to the kind of "earth-moving" sexual encounters described by Hemingway in *For Whom the Bell Tolls* and by D. H. Lawrence in *Lady Chatterley's Lover* and other novels.

Desmond Morris delineates 12 stages which he believes a man and a woman move through in order to establish an intimate bond, which he considers necessary for survival. He believes sexual intercourse is the ultimate stage, which deepens and strengthens the other meanings of the relationship. This is not to say that sexual contact necessarily improves or deepens relationships. The few researchers studying these very personal matters agree that supportiveness, dependability, trust, empathy and mutual understanding are essential components of satisfying close relationships.

Friendship

Most studies of friendship focus on such questions as numbers of friends and amount of contact, rather than on the quality of relationships.

Marjorie Fiske asked her subjects to describe the nature of their relationships with their three closest friends and also what they thought an ideal relationship would be. There was enormous variation in what they considered to be the attributes of a close friendship. Many revealed little emotional depth; perhaps they experienced it, but reticence or lack of an appropriate vocabulary prevented them from talking about it. Many, especially among the middle-aged and late-middle-aged, expressed regret over the lack of closer and richer friendships and marriages. These regrets were expressed more by men than by women.

Women, on the whole, seem to find it easier to establish and maintain close friendships than do men. But it is doubtful that this results from any innate biological difference between the sexes. Women are traditionally responsible for establishing and maintaining the social networks of the family. Most men contribute to support this division of effort, but recently some have come to regret it as they become more interested in strengthening their bonds with others in middle or late middle age. Wives' control over the social sphere of

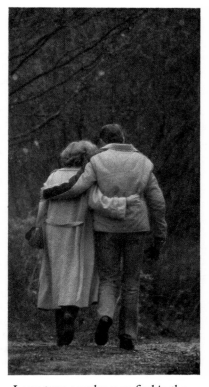

Long-term couples may find in the middle years that their intimacy is affected by outside factors such as unemployment or, conversely, a promotion and changed place of work for one of the partners, or by children leaving home. During the middle years many marriages break up, patterns of communication having been fatally disrupted by one or both partners who feel that time is running out and that their lives lack excitement. Equally, the stimulus of such changes may reinforce a couple's intimacy and the relationship may gain strength from it.

their lives may have shut out people who used to be the husband's friends. After widowhood or divorce, most women strengthen and extend their existing friendships with other women. The lack of closeness between men, by contrast, helps to explain the frequent hasty remarriages after the loss of a wife.

The course of marriage

Researchers who have studied marriage across the lifespan have produced results which suggest, rather depressingly, that the longer a marriage continues, the less satisfying it becomes. Younger and older women certainly talk of their marriages in different ways. Alice Rossi, for example, found that women in late middle age were more inclined to mention negative aspects, for example lack of communication, than were young women; when they spoke of activities such as travel, many of the older women did not mention their husbands at all. By contrast, younger women tended to see such activities as opportunities for enjoying time with their husbands, perhaps away from their children.

One consistent finding of mid-life studies, which may help to explain the older women's negative attitude to marriage, is that men and women seem to become aware of changing needs at this time. Men, who had previously shown a strong commitment to career development, become more interested in strengthening their relationships with others (including their wives). Women, on the other hand, are seeking to strengthen their competence and creativity or to satisfy their curiosity about the world outside. These changes can be seen as a genuine wish to balance their lives better, as first suggested by Jung and later documented by Bernice Neugarten and David Gutmann. But it is easy to see how such changing needs might lead to conflict or threaten a possibly neglected marriage.

Second honeymoon

Amongst her sample of middle-aged men whose children had recently left home, Marjorie Fiske found a good deal of optimism; some of it was almost certainly engendered by the expectation or realization of stronger bonds with their wives. However, five years later, the hoped-for second honeymoon seemed not to have come to pass. Poor physical health or the pressures of aged parents may be important here; some of the men, however, complained that their wives had changed—they were, for example, becoming bossier. Is this an accurate description or a male construction of any move to autonomy by a previously passive wife? What does seem likely is that the men's skills in establishing the intimacy which they wanted had atrophied from misuse. It is unfortunate that they should be trying to relearn these skills at a time when women are less receptive, partly because they are becoming aware of a different set of needs and partly because they have created intimacy elsewhere. For example, men in all life stages name their wives as confidantes far more often than women name their husbands as intimates. Women too are more likely to complain of poor communication with their spouse than are men. These findings raise the interesting but as yet unanswered question as to whether men and women have different ideas about what constitutes "intimacy" or "good communication", or whether these are more important to women than men, at least before middle age.

PHYSICAL AND SEXUAL CHANGES IN MIDDLE AGE

Both men and women experience changes in their sexual responsiveness in later middle age. For example, post-menopausal women take longer to arouse, produce a smaller quantity of vaginal lubrication, show lesser breast changes during arousal, have less enlargement of the vagina during arousal before intercourse and experience a shorter orgasm. Men, in much the same way, take longer to develop a firm erection, often find the firmness of the erection is reduced, take longer to develop another erection after ejaculation, have shorter orgasms, have a smaller volume of ejaculated semen and eject it with a diminished force.

For women, most of the changes, however, can be seen as part of a general slowing down. They certainly do not spell the beginning of the end of sexual activity. Those who have been sexually active before middle age, seem to experience less physical change.

In line with this, many women experience a post-menopausal resurgence of sexual interest. This, coming at a time when the male response may be slowing down, can create problems if the woman wrongly interprets this as rejection and the man becomes fearful of being unable to satisfy his partner. As "performance anxiety" increases, the man may find it increasingly difficult to get an erection, thus confirming his initial fears.

These problems can be avoided by acknowledging that sexual functioning probably will change and by altering sexual habits. Sex in the morning, for example, avoids late-evening fatigue as well as capitalizing on the erection many men awaken with.

Sexuality in mid-life

If mid-life in general has been neglected by researchers, then the sexuality of the middle-aged has been almost completely ignored. Whatever the reasons, much of the information we have about sexuality in mid-life has been gathered incidentally, as part of larger projects on lifespan development.

The middle-aged, it seems, may erroneously believe that their sexual interest should wane or disappear. It might well, but this is by no means the rule. Recent and more direct studies of sexual interest using, for example, reports of sexual dreams and fantasies, indicate that the vast majority of the middle-aged retain a strong interest in sex. Given the reticence which surrounds the reporting of this kind of material, the results are probably an underestimate of the true amount of interest. It seems, however, that for women an important factor in maintaining interest is prior experience of orgasm either through intercourse or masturbation. Obviously, this process could operate in a circular fashion where the absence of orgasm, for whatever reason, could reduce sexual interest, which in turn reduces sexual response, making orgasm seem even more remote and so on.

Finding a partner

Opportunity to engage in sexual behaviour may decline sharply in mid-life. One obvious reason would be the death of a partner, or divorce. It seems, however, that previously married women continue to form sexual relationships and do so more frequently than those who have never been married. This may be related to differences in opportunity; there is certainly no reason to suspect that it reflects greater interest on the part of the once-married woman. On the contrary, one study found that never-married women were less likely to report a decline in sexual interest after the menopause than were those women who remained married.

Even when partners are available, other factors may reduce opportunities for sexual activity. An aged parent who moves in with his or her son or daughter may have much the same—or a greater—inhibiting effect as children on a couple's sex life. Physical illness, especially cardiovascular and rheumatic disorders, may unnecessarily lead people to curtail or end their sex lives. What is needed here is adaptiveness and inventiveness in reorganizing sex around physical limitations. In fact, it is impossible to think of an illness which would eliminate all of the many components of sexual functioning.

Disability and sex

Sexuality, however, can and does survive any kind of illness or injury, albeit in an altered form. Technique books for paralysed individuals are now available; cardiologists are increasingly attuned to sexual counselling for heart-attack victims. The adverse side-effects of sexual performance of many high blood pressure medications, tranquillizers and anti-depressants are becoming better known and patients are—or should be—cautioned about these possibilities. But patients themselves must be willing to ask questions and seek information from their doctors rather than wait in the hope that the subject will be mentioned. This two-way communication will help to foster a view of sexual function as an important ingredient of life satisfaction at all stages of the lifespan.

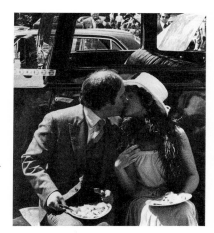

Just because a relationship is well established doesn't mean it's boring! A little romance can go a long way to relieving the monotony.

Health and fitness

The middle-aged can reap the benefits of fitness with a routine of moderate exercise done regularly two or three times a week. The exercises shown here are recommended by the Health Education Council. Start slowly, spending perhaps five or ten minutes on a session, and increase gradually until you are exercising for twenty or thirty minutes.

If you suffer from a physical disability, are receiving medical treatment, or experience pains or breathlessness when doing ordinary household tasks, consult your doctor before embarking on any exercise programme.

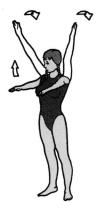

Arm swinging
Stand with the feet apart and the arms hanging by your sides. Lift both arms together, moving them forward, up, back and sideways, in a circular motion.

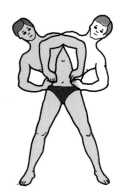

Side bends
Stand with the feet wide apart and the hands on the hips. Bend alternately to the left and right, keeping the head at right angles to the shoulders, reaching as far as possible.

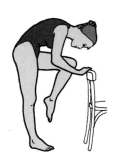

Trunk, knee and hip bends
Stand behind a chair, resting the hands lightly on the back of it. Lift the knee and bring the forehead slowly down . (Later, leave out the chair.)

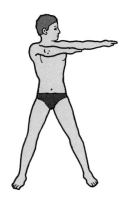

Trunk rotating
stand with the feet wide apart, the arms reaching forward. Rotate the head, arms and shoulder as far as you can alternately to left and right. Don't move hips or legs.

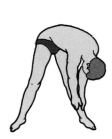

Alternate ankle reach
Stand with the feet wide apart. Bend slowly forward over the left and right leg alternately, sliding both hands down the front of the leg towards the foot.

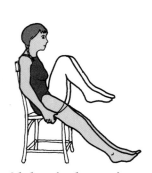

Abdominal exercise
Sit on the front part of a chair, legs straight out in front of you. Leaning back and gripping the chair for support, gently lift the thighs to the chest. Slowly lower and straighten them.

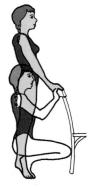

Leg exercise
Stand behind a chair, hands on its back. Lower into a squat, feet flat or (women) on tiptoes. Straighten the legs, rise on your toes and return to the squat position.

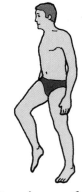

Running on the spot
Stand with the arms hanging loosely by the sides and gently run on the spot, gradually lifting the knees higher. Run for a little longer and a little faster each session.

Weight and height

If your weight falls within the shaded area, for your height, you are a suitable weight. Weights outside are not, and steps should be taken to alter them. Obesity in particular is a health hazard.

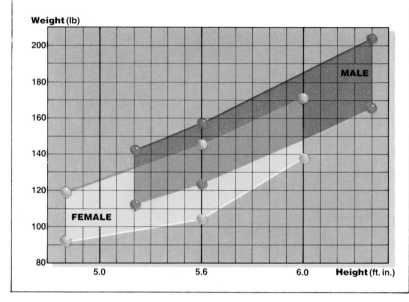

Self-help to fitness after sixty

A self-help approach will do much to maximize physical and psychological health for the over-sixties. Here are some guidelines.

1 Eat less (you need fewer calories now), but make sure you don't miss out vital nutrients.

2 Have a full medical examination once a year.

3 Drink more water (you need more liquid now).

4 Avoid alcohol, except at meals. If you must drink spirits, add plenty of water.

5 Take some gentle exercise every day. Don't nap for more than an hour in the middle of the day.

6 Avoid fruitless worry.

7 Keep busy, planning each day and avoiding a daily routine that never varies.

8 Stop smoking, or at least cut down to 30–40 cigarettes a week.

9 Make sure that you eat plenty of roughage.

Other ways of keeping fit

Sports are an obvious form of exercise. Bear in mind, though, that a non-competitive sport may be preferable for someone looking for a sport to take up in middle-age—you can move at your own pace, without the pressure of competition. Running, swimming, cycling and hill climbing are all good. Activities such as dancing are also beneficial, and there is now a great variety of classes available—dance, exercise, yoga and so on.

Finally, daily life contains many opportunities for exercise. Don't waste them. Walk rather than using the car or bus, and climb the stairs in preference to taking the lift. Such activities as digging and lawn-mowing are also good exercise.

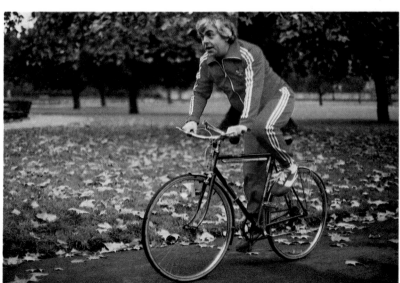

Keeping fit may provide other pleasures too—this cyclist is enjoying the fresh air and scenery, and providing himself with a relaxing 'breather' to break the day's routine.

A mid-life crisis?

The idea of mid-life as inevitably crisis-ridden is very speculative. It is possible that preconceptions about what *should* happen at middle age have somewhat biased researchers' interpretation of the material they have gathered from their subjects. It is also worth noting that these subjects have usually been well-educated and probably more given to introspection. So while some people may experience middle age as a sort of watershed, we should be very wary about generalizing from them to everyone in middle age.

Viewing ourselves

An alternative view of the adult years is that crises, rather than being an inherent part of them, are manifestations of asynchrony in the timing of life events. Thus, to become a widower at 30 or a mother at 50 may be stressful because cultural expectations of appropriate timing have been violated. It has been shown that many middle-aged women "feel" a different age to their chronological age—sometimes there is a considerable gap—and that their perceived age bears a strong relationship to their evaluation of their social and work roles, as well as to physiological changes.

However, our chronological age is a powerful determinant of society's response to us, and one of the fascinating questions about middle age is the extent to which any personal re-evaluation is a product of this obsession with age, rather than an integral part of growing older. In the following sections, we will be describing the experiences in middle age of people in industrialized societies, which have a strong tradition of age-grading. Because most of the results have been gathered recently, subjects also share roughly similar historical backgrounds. We can only speculate on how their experiences might differ from people in another place or at another time.

Stress

What is stress? This question can be approached from two directions. We can think in terms of events, such as loss of a job, which are assumed to be stressful. Or we can look at the individual's response to certain situations and define stress in terms of particular response patterns, regardless of the events preceding them.

The problem with the first approach is that people vary enormously as to the kinds of events and circumstances which they consider stressful: few of us could contemplate, say, a severe earthquake with equanimity. But in the grey areas of everyday life, it is very difficult to make prescriptive judgements about what constitutes a stressful event.

On the other hand, if we look at response patterns, we face the problem of deciding what kind of response to consider and in what system—physiological, cognitive (mental) or behavioural? Unfortunately, in any given situation, responses across these three systems do not always agree with each other. If we concentrate on one rather than another, we might get a very misleading impression of how the individual as a whole is responding. If, however, we decide that certain response patterns are manifestations of stress, do we assume that those who do not show these responses are not stressed?

A compromise

Some psychologists have suggested that we might think of stress as a discrepancy between the demands of a situation and the individual's ability to cope with it. Others, in a similar vein, have emphasized the importance of events which the individual cannot predict or control.

Bernice Neugarten suggests that stressful events are those which are "off-schedule" for an individual. The 55-year-old skilled worker whose company suddenly reduces its retirement age is obviously going to be more distressed, at least for a time, than if he or she had always anticipated retiring at 55. A 40-year-old woman with four young children is under greater strain when her husband is suddenly killed in a car accident than are much older widows whose husbands have died after a long illness. Events which are off-schedule, of course, are also those which are less predictable.

The effects of increased flexibility

An interesting observation made by social historians is that there was more variation in the timing of events, such as marriage, in the mid-nineteenth century than in the mid-twentieth century. In the latter part of this century, however, we are seeing a return to more fluid social norms where marriage, divorce, starting a family, beginning a career or gaining new qualifications are seen as appropriate goals at a variety of ages.

We might predict, from the timing of events model, that a loosening of social norms would reduce stress. It is, after all, difficult for events to be off-schedule when there is no schedule in the first place. But people tend to create their own schedules or expectations of what may or may not happen to them at particular points in the life cycle, so that there remains ample opportunity for events to be off-schedule in the *individual's* scheme of things.

Another reason why increasing flexibility of social rules and expectations does not reduce stress is that it places much more responsibility on individuals for their life satisfaction. It also vastly increases the number of choices available to them, and they face more decisions than the people whose life is mapped out in advance. The rate of psychological disorders has often been observed to increase in those cultures where old social norms are breaking down—what we gain on the swings, we lose on the roundabouts.

Vulnerability to stress

If we see stress as an interaction between some aspects of the environment and the individual's coping skills, then it follows that we will be more or less vulnerable to stress at particular times. The middle-aged certainly do not have a monopoly on stress, but there are several reasons why they (and the elderly) are particularly interesting groups to study.

We know that chronic stress—a stressful situation, for example an unhappy marriage, which has continued for a long time—seems to make individuals more susceptible to small stresses, events which in other circumstances they would have taken in their stride. But it is not as simple as this. Continued or repeated stress can have the opposite effect and strengthen the ability to cope with future stresses. This tends, however, to be more true of less serious stresses which give people a chance of developing the coping skills which will stand them

What is stress?

Stress occurs when an individual is faced with pressures that make it difficult for him or her to cope. The stress-causing factors can occur in your physical or psychological circumstances or environment, and the manifestations of stress can be physical or psychological.

As the ability to cope with pressure varies from individual to individual, so does susceptibility to stress. That is, there are pressures that will provoke stress in some people but not in others (though obviously there are many events and circumstances, such as the death of someone close, that will cause some degree of stress in almost everyone).

There are many physical and mental conditions that may indicate that stress is building up—they should be taken as early warnings. While conditions such as insomnia, diarrhoea, headaches, and so on, are indications of stress, it is not enough to treat them alone—the underlying cause of the stress needs to be identified and, if possible, removed.

Early warning signs

Physical

Headaches
Insomnia and/or tiredness
Chest pains
Persistent diarrhoea
Indigestion
Palpitations

Mental

Inability to relax
Poor memory or
    bad concentration
Lack of will power
Over-reacting to small problems
Irritability
Inability to tolerate noise
Over-emotional reactions

Identifying factors that cause stress

Each individual should be aware of the potential stress-causing factors in his or her environment, so that actual stress can be avoided or minimized. The events and circumstances picked out in the "Counterstress checklist" on this page are simply examples of *possible* sources of stress.

When you are trying to identify the pressures on you, look methodically at all areas of your life: your physical environment; your personal relationships and social life; psychological strains at home and at work; pressures on your time and your pocket; and specific events.

Counterstress checklist

Do you live in a city?
Do you commute to work?
Is your place of work noisy?
Are your neighbours friendly?
Are your neighbours noisy?
Do you live in an area with social problems?
Is your home disturbed by outside noise (for example, from a busy road)?
Do you lack privacy in your home?
Do you have to travel either to work or on business more than you would like?
Do you watch more television than you think you should/would really like?
Is your normal day a rush?
Do you have not enough or too much responsibility?
Are you frustrated at work or because you are unemployed?
Do you regularly work late (or take work home with you)?
Do you respect those you work with/for?
Do you feel your work is not worthwhile?
Do you doubt whether you are up to your job?
Is your mortgage or tenancy tied to your work?
Are you short of money?
Do you smoke more than you should?
Do you often drink alone?

Do you have a weight problem?
Do you get out of breath when you run for a bus?
Have you got specific worries about your children's futures?
Do you sometimes go for a year without at least a fortnight's holiday away from home?
Do you only enjoy taking part in competitive sports?
Are you unable to relax if you take a day off?
Do you feel that your sexuality is abnormal in any way?
Would you say that you have a satisfactory sex life?
Do you worry that other people don't think too highly of you?
Have you got enough friends?
Do you feel that you have failed to make the most of your opportunities?
Are you a burden to your relatives?
Is any one of your relatives a burden to you?
Do you feel that your spouse does not understand you?
Do you feel that your spouse and children do not respect you?
Do you worry about illness in yourself or others close to you?

Assessing your stress level

Various "life events" can be identified as liable to cause stress. The following examples of such events have been given a stress weighting (by Dr Richard Rahe). If you score more than 150 points for the last year, you may be at risk from stress-related diseases.

Events	Score
Death of spouse	100
Divorce	73
Marital separation	65
Prison term	63
Death of close family member	63
Personal injury or illness	53
Marriage	50
Loss of job	47
Marital reconciliation	45
Retirement	45
Health problem in family	44
Pregnancy	40
Sex problems	39
Addition to family	39
Change at work/in business	39
Change in financial situation	38
Death of a close friend	37
Change in line of work	36
More arguments with spouse	35
Large mortgage contracted	31
Foreclosure of mortgage/loan	30
Son or daughter leaving home	29
Trouble with parents-in-law	29
Significant personal success	28
Wife starting/stopping work	26
Starting or leaving school	26
Change in living conditions	25
Change in personal habits	24
Trouble with superior at work	23
Change in working hours	20
Moving house/school	20
Change in leisure activities	19
Change in church activities	19
Change in social activities	18
Mortgage contracted	17
Change in sleeping habits	16
Change in eating pattern	15
Holiday	13
Christmas	12
Minor infringement of law	11

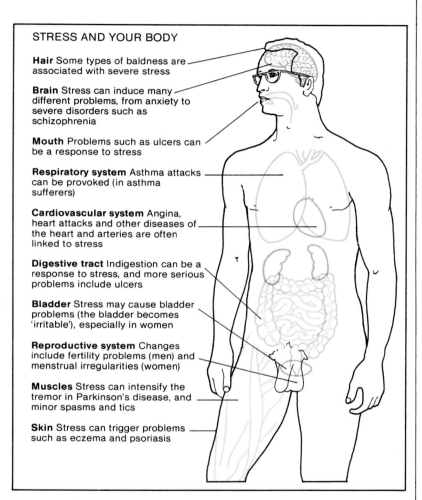

STRESS AND YOUR BODY

Hair Some types of baldness are associated with severe stress

Brain Stress can induce many different problems, from anxiety to severe disorders such as schizophrenia

Mouth Problems such as ulcers can be a response to stress

Respiratory system Asthma attacks can be provoked (in asthma sufferers)

Cardiovascular system Angina, heart attacks and other diseases of the heart and arteries are often linked to stress

Digestive tract Indigestion can be a response to stress, and more serious problems include ulcers

Bladder Stress may cause bladder problems (the bladder becomes 'irritable'), especially in women

Reproductive system Changes include fertility problems (men) and menstrual irregularities (women)

Muscles Stress can intensify the tremor in Parkinson's disease, and minor spasms and tics

Skin Stress can trigger problems such as eczema and psoriasis

Hypertension

It is normal (at least in Western nations) for blood pressure to rise with age, just as it is normal for it to vary at different times and in response to stress. However, if your blood pressure is consistently above a certain level, you can be said to suffer from high blood pressure (or hypertension).

Hypertension is a peculiarly Western problem. About 8 per cent of the population aged between 40 and 49 are affected, and that figure increases in older age groups. These high figures may be at least partly the result of some feature of Western dietary habits (such as an excess of salt or refined foods), or of an inherited tendency; but some experts suggest that stress is an important factor. Weight has an effect, with those who are overweight significantly more susceptible, and efforts should be made to reduce it.

Strokes and heart failure can be caused by hypertension. Other cardiovascular accidents, kidney damage and haemorrhage into the retina of the eye are also possible results if high blood pressure is not reduced.

in good stead in the face of future stresses. However, not everyone develops these skills. For some, this may be because they have experienced so little stress they have never had the chance to learn them. Others, however, seem to give up even in the face of mild stress. We will return to this point later, but we can see that by middle age many people may be experiencing chronic stress and that individual differences in coping skills will be very marked. Middle age is also a time when stresses in the form of uncontrollable losses—of health, of partners (by death), of jobs (by retirement), of looks, of social roles (such as motherhood) begin to accumulate.

Does the menopause increase vulnerability to stress?
The menopause, strictly speaking, means "cessation of the menses". For the majority of women, this occurs between the ages of 45 and 50, but the average age is rising. The more general term "climacterium" refers to changes in the ovaries and the various physiological and hormonal changes associated with the menopause—these happen over a period of time beginning perhaps as long as 10 years before and perhaps continuing for 10 years after the menopause itself. For some women, but by no means all, this process is accompanied by a variety of more or less distressing physical symptoms such as hot flushes and vaginal dryness. Various muscle and bone changes can also be detected, and the risk of coronary heart disease gradually increases.

Who says that the menopause produces stress?
Three lines of evidence are now challenging assumptions about the climacterium and the menopause as stressful events. Research which has looked at much more representative samples of women, rather than those attending clinics for depression, suggests that the menopause is rarely a crisis to them: there is more dread in the anticipation than difficulty in the experience. Bernice Neugarten found that while only 16 and 24 per cent of women in the age groups 21–30 and 31–44 agreed with the statement: "After the change of life a woman feels freer to do things for herself", 74 and 65 per cent of women aged 45–55 and 56–65 agreed. The post-menopausal women in this study also emerged as more self-confident and calmer than pre-menopausal women. It is not suggested that these differences are actually caused by the menopause, but this is a very different picture of the menopausal and post-menopausal woman than that derived from clinical samples.

A second line of evidence involves a comparison of the incidence of depression in women of different ages. In London, George Brown and his associates found a higher incidence of depression among women with children than among middle-aged women.

We can look more closely at those women who *do* report psychological distress around the time of the menopause to see if there seems to be a connection between the two. One study which did this found that life events—unrelated to the menopause—were much more strongly implicated in the women's distress than the menopause itself.

For some women, of course, the menopause *will* be a stressful event. But this will be because of its subjective meaning—loss of fertility, or decline in attractiveness as judged by society's standards, for example—rather than because the event itself is stressful. However, such widely held attitudes are hard to eradicate.

Hormone replacement therapy

For some women, the physical concomitants of the climacterium create very real psychological problems. Vaginal dryness, for example, may lead to painful intercourse, a decrease in sexual satisfaction or possibly the cessation of sexual relations altogether. Hot flushes may lead to avoidance of certain social situations, especially those from which a speedy escape is difficult. Concern about personal hygiene may increase, while sleep problems are also very common.

There is little doubt that oestrogen replacement therapy can considerably reduce or abolish these physical symptoms and, of course, the psychological problems which accompany them. HRT (hormone replacement therapy), however, has not been shown to be beneficial for the general psychological distress some women report.

Fears about HRT arise mainly from its possible connection with cancer of the cervix—the neck of the womb—and of the womb lining (endometrium). One study, for example, found that the risk of endometrial cancer was 4.5 times greater in those using HRT. In general, women who have high blood pressure, diabetes, or obesity and who have never been pregnant or given birth are more at risk from this type of cancer, and the administration of HRT does not seem to raise the risk further in this group. It is those who were originally "low risk" women who move into a higher risk category when given HRT.

There are some hopeful indications that the risk of cancer may be reduced by combining oestrogen and progesterone (although the effects of progesterone are not yet fully known), by administering the lowest possible dose which will control the physical symptoms, by using natural rather than synthetic hormones and by using them on a discontinuous basis so that the womb lining is shed monthly.

For many women the risks of HRT (which are still *relatively* small in terms of absolute numbers) will be far outweighed by its benefits. A woman whose requests for HRT are denied should try to ensure that this decision is based not on a sketchy knowledge of a few studies using only one type of HRT but on a balanced assessment of the possible risks of different types of HRT in her particular case.

Responses to stress

In her transitions study, Marjorie Fiske found little or no relationship between middle-aged people's current sense of wellbeing and whether they had recently experienced many or few of a number of "stressful" events as defined by the researchers. Her results showed that the group could be roughly divided into four categories: *overwhelmed, challenged, self-defeating* and *lucky*. When viewed in the light of these categories, then many of these people had "predictable" responses to stress—that is, they reacted badly to events which most of us would consider stressful or they realistically saw themselves as having experienced little stress and were glad of it.

A considerable number of the sample, however, were "deviants". They reacted well to severe stress (or even sought it out) or they gave up in the face of what seemed to be relatively mild stress; and whereas middle-aged men tended to be challenged by these events, in comparison with younger men, middle-aged women seem to lose their stress tolerance: the great majority of heavily stressed middle-aged and late-middle-aged women are overwhelmed.

When depression strikes

What happens to heavily stressed middle-aged women? We saw in the last chapter that, in comparison to their male counterparts, they have less contact with the world outside their families. Within this close, interpersonal context their family commitments are strengthened, while other kinds of commitments and opportunities for self-expression are neglected. Even those who work are strikingly family-centred. Whatever "ego-strengthening" positive feedback they experience is derived vicariously from the lives of their husbands and children. These women have denied themselves the opportunity to develop their inner resources and coping skills. They have also failed to establish networks of friendship and support. This factor—the existence of supportive relationships—has been shown to be crucial in coping with serious stress.

Why do women suffer most?

Research findings show that women of all ages experience a higher rate of depression than do men of comparable age. We can look at this difference in two ways. First, we can examine theories about what causes depression to see if there are good reasons for suspecting that women might actually be more vulnerable to depression. Secondly, we can question whether it is "real"—that is, are there reasons why men and women would show their distress in different ways and therefore be labelled differently?

Vulnerability

Two major (and not incompatible) theories of depression have been influential in psychology. The first relates depression to a low rate of positive reinforcement (pleasurable events) in a person's life. This state of affairs might come about in two ways. The individual might suffer losses in important life spheres, of, for example, job, health or partner. As we have seen, such losses, although they occur at all stages of the lifespan, may begin to accumulate in middle age for both men and women.

Unfortunately, most of these losses are not single events, but bring with them a series of secondary losses. The loss of a partner, for example, may mean the loss of a large segment of one's social life.

Can this formulation of depression help explain its common occurrence in middle age and the higher rates in women? It is not unreasonable to suggest that women, on the whole, actually suffer more losses in middle age than do men. They lose their fertility, while men retain theirs indefinitely, they are more often widowed, they lose the mothering role which our society insists is so important to them, they lose the "ideal" of youthful attractiveness so relentlessly pushed upon them—and not to the same extent on men—by the media.

Several studies have shown that physical attractiveness plays a more important role in happiness and adjustment for women than it does for men. It is not surprising, then, to find that women who were judged (from photographs) to have been very attractive in their youth should report themselves to be more unhappy in their forties than do women judged to have been less attractive in their youth. No such relationship was found for men.

A COMPARISON OF NORMAL AND DEPRESSED STATES

	Normal	Depressed
Stimulus	*Response*	
Loved person or object	Fondness and pleasure	Indifference, revulsion
Preferred activities	Enjoyment	Lack of enthusiasm
Changing opportunities	Eagerness	Indifference
Humorous events	Pleasure	Dullness
Unfamiliar stimuli	Curiosity	Apathy
Abuse	Indignation, anger	Acceptance, self-criticism
Goal/drive	*Direction*	
Gratification	Pleasure	Withdrawal
Wellbeing	Self-interest and care	Self neglect
Survival	Self-preservation	Apathy or suicide
Success	Progression	Retreat
Thinking	*Appraisal*	
Self assessment	Accepting	Highly self-critical
Hopes for the future	Optimistic	Pessimistic
Response to life events	Realistic	Defeated
Physical functions	*Symptom*	
Appetite	Appropriate hunger	Loss of appetite
Sexuality	Desire, responsiveness	Loss of desire
Sleep	Satisfying	Disturbed
Energy	Sufficient or high	Low or fatigued

Depression

Most of us at some time use the phrase "I feel depressed", indicating a disappointment, a low phase after illness or a temporary inability to cope. Real depression, as shown here, is a complete reversal from a positive to a negative state—the depressed person is apathetic and withdrawn, fails to respond to usual stimuli and cannot even follow a healthy pattern of eating and sleeping. Many factors may trigger depression in middle age— a bereavement; loss of home, money or important possessions; a sense of having failed to meet earlier ambitions; the onset of a disease that impairs capacities for work or pleasure. Depression becomes self-perpetuating; the person feels that no one can help. Self-esteem and confidence are non-existent.

This is not to say that every woman is worse off in middle age than every man, or that these events will constitute important losses for every woman. This is clearly not the case: men too suffer losses and become depressed while, as we have seen, many women actually welcome the loss of fertility or of their children's departure.

One important factor which influences how a person adjusts in the face of serious losses is the availability of alternative sources of reinforcement. We have already seen that those women most vulnerable to depression when their children leave home are the stereotypical housewives who have "put all their eggs in one basket".

If we examine, again in general terms, the relative availability of alternative reinforcers for men and women in middle age, then again women seem to lose out. The rate of remarriage among divorced and widowed men in middle age, for example, is much higher than the rate for women. Men tend to marry women younger than themselves. Middle-aged men can also start another family and, although many of them would not relish the prospect, at least they have the choice.

The importance of work as a source of pleasure is emphasized by research findings showing that working wives and single women tend to become less depressed than married women who stay at home. It may be, of course, that depression prevents these women from finding jobs. But if working women and housewives are equated for severity of depression, it seems' that women with jobs respond more quickly to therapy. Indeed, one study reported that women explicitly sought jobs to obtain a "new set of relationships and satisfactions which proved to be therapeutic".

Reinforcement and social skill

Not everyone who is depressed has suffered serious losses. Marjorie Fiske's "self-defeated" group, for example, seemed to have experienced relatively few adverse life events, but they still derived little pleasure from life and felt pessimistic about the future. A second reason why people may receive a low rate of reinforcement from their environment is that they are unskilled at constructing an environment which provides pleasure. A great deal of our pleasure in life comes through our interactions with others. Those people who behave in such a way that people do not wish to approach them or spend time with them or invite them to various social activities therefore lose out on a great many opportunities for reinforcement. Unfortunately, once individuals become depressed, people are even less likely to approach them, so that a vicious circle is set up.

There is no evidence to suggest that women are less socially skilled than men in terms of being liked or loved by others. But social skills involve more than this: they have to do with being able to achieve the kinds of outcomes one wants. This idea brings us to the second important formulation of depression.

Depression and helplessness

It has long been known that animals faced with adversive events which were uncontrollable and/or unpredictable reacted, after a time, by becoming what in human terms we would call apathetic. They gave up trying to control their environment. Martin Seligman, an American psychologist, noted many similarities between the behaviour of these animals and that of humans complaining of depression. In particular, he noted the apathy, the lack of interest in the environment and the lack of motivation to deal constructively with new problems.

On the basis of his experiments, Seligman suggested that depressed people had at some time been exposed to situations which they could not control, that is, where nothing they did produced the outcome they wanted. They had thus, according to Seligman, developed a belief in their powerlessness to control important aspects of their environment and had therefore abandoned attempts to do so.

But why should failure in one life sphere lead to the general belief that everything is pointless? Why, too, should depressed people so often refuse to accept evidence that they *are* effective and instead attribute their successes to other factors ("I only got the job because the other applicants were so badly qualified")? Perhaps most puzzling of all, why should some depressed people seem to hold two opposing sets of beliefs? On the one hand they claim that nothing they do makes any difference, while at the same time they blame themselves for adverse events.

Depression and alcohol

Both these formulations of depression give good grounds for suggesting that women are actually more vulnerable than men to depression at all stages of the lifespan and that these differences may be even more accentuated in middle age. But men too suffer stresses, perhaps of a different kind, and become distressed. For some men, this distress manifests itself as depression in the same way as it does in women. It has been suggested, however, that depression is a peculiarly female

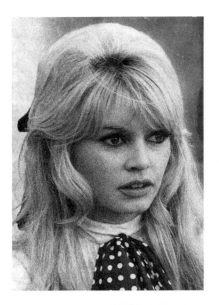

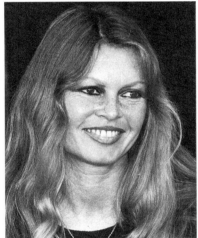

Physical attractiveness
In a culture that celebrates youth no one looks forward to the signs of ageing, and in Western society women are more vulnerable in this respect than men. While men are deemed to acquire "character" with their grey hairs and wrinkles, women are said to be "past it". But ageing produces different kinds of attractiveness for both sexes. A generation of female film stars are, in middle age, proving that intelligence, fitness, creativity and style are as much of an advantage as smooth skin.

style of responding to stress. If we consider depression as a set of behaviours rather than in terms of low mood, then it can be considered an intensification of "normal" female behaviours such as passivity, dependence, self-deprecation, self-sacrifice, naïveté, fearfulness and failure. We might then expect that depressed females would be considered less "abnormal" and be less rejected than depressed males. If it is indeed "easier" for women to become depressed and if they are less harshly judged for doing so, then it may be that men, rather than developing this kind of behaviour pattern, will express their distress in different ways.

Alcohol as a stress reliever

It has been suggested that depression and alcoholism are different but equivalent disorders, with heavy drinking being a male mechanism of dealing with stress and distress. But the gap in the figures for male and female alcoholism seems to be closing, with some studies showing that males and females seek treatment at equal rates from private sources. As we saw in "Adolescence", the incidence of alcohol use in various social situations is now virtually equal for males and females; a 1978 study of drinking amongst American university students, however, showed that almost five times as many males as females could be classified as "heavy drinkers".

Alcohol and tension reduction

The use of alcohol is a typical unconstructive response to stress—an artificial means of reducing anxiety, which neither changes the situation nor leads to the development of new coping skills.

Men and women with drinking problems give different reasons for resorting to alcohol. Men tend to attribute their drinking to internal states such as boredom, irritability, anxiety and shyness, while women see themselves as drinking in response to major life stress such as a divorce or an unhappy love affair. Such events presumably make the women feel anxious or depressed, but they do not seem to resort to alcohol as a habitual response to stress. In line with this, women with drinking problems usually report having their first drink and beginning to drink heavily at a significantly later age than male problem drinkers. A woman who drinks very heavily is also much more likely to be married to a man who also drinks heavily (if she is married at all) than is her male equivalent. These results are difficult to interpret, but they could indicate that women are more likely than men to develop their drinking problem by imitating their partner, rather than by using alcohol as a means of coping with stress.

These are the patterns found within a middle-aged population who grew up at a time when drinking was a much more likely male than female behaviour. The females, however, are now living through a time when alcohol is not only becoming much more acceptable amongst women, but is also much more widely available, for example in supermarkets. There is evidence that women are more likely than men to use tranquillizers to reduce anxiety; changing social attitudes to alcohol use and its increased availability and relative cheapness may lead the next generation of women to choose alcohol instead. Alternatively it may be that attempts to give women more active and wider social roles will make depression a less likely female response to stress.

Preparing for retirement

Retirement is a time when favourite activities can be extended, or it may be an opportunity to take up a sport, skill or occupation outside previous experience. How leisure time is to be spent should be given the same careful consideration as other aspects of retirement—how fit are you, what can you afford to spend on hobbies, do you prefer solitary activities or being involved with friends and new acquaintances? Isolation can be a problem of ageing, so it is as well to join an evening class, social or sports club that draws you into a group. To set unrealistic goals for retirement is to invite disappointment, but this is not to say ambition is out of place. Many people assume that they have no aptitude for a particular skill, when in reality they have only lacked the time and energy to acquire the aptitude. A retired person can take time to learn and enjoy new pursuits and to a large extent is relieved of the competitive atmosphere that caused a strict division between success and failure in earlier life.

Ideas for retirement activities
You may prefer to continue some kind of work after retirement, maybe part-time or voluntary. In recent years early retirement has been favoured to make way for a new workforce, so it may be difficult to find a paid job. But many charities, hospitals and prisons rely on voluntary workers for visiting and fund-raising activities and always welcome more help. If you have been interested in politics or active in the community, you might become involved in local government or serve on a committee dealing with community services.

Arts and crafts Many people shy away from trying to paint or draw, believing that it won't work unless they have innate talent. Millions prove them wrong every day by acquiring basic skills that lead to an enjoyable and productive pastime. The same applies to crafts such as carving, pottery, porcelain painting and enamelling. Once these techniques are understood it is surprising how much untapped creativity comes to the surface. All these skills can be learned at evening classes and day centres and a large number of books deal with artists' techniques. Printmaking and photography are also rewarding, but these activities require specialized equipment that can be expensive—though it is usually available from local societies and classes. Many women will already be accomplished in embroidery, knitting and sewing, but these skills are sometimes undervalued. They can be used to make clothes, toys or soft furnishings—or developed simply for the pleasure of the craft. Other useful and creative pursuits are carpentry, interior decorating and upholstery. Some investment in materials is needed for all arts and crafts. But it may be possible to sell some of the products to offset the costs.

Studying You may have an urge to study for its own sake, especially if you missed out on school or college. Many people take the chance to learn a lan-

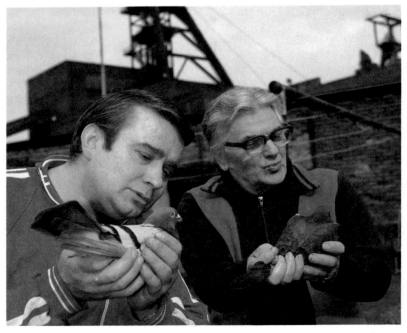

These pigeon fanciers have a hobby that demands some commitment, as the birds must be looked after, but this in itself can give plenty of pleasure. Other compensations may include getting out and about for races, and contact with like-minded enthusiasts.

guage or theoretical subject such as philosophy or economics. Those who prefer a more personal application of learning might like to study local history or genealogy, even creating a personal family tree. This can provide new contacts through letter-writing and visits to towns where there are family records. Art or music appreciation are popular subjects; the study of architecture also opens a new view of your neighbourhood.

Outdoor pursuits and sports To take real care of a garden requires much time and effort, and many people look forward to having more time for gardening after retirement. It is an added bonus if you grow fruit or vegetables, so saving a little on the food budget. Those with a keen interest in nature can extend their activities into joining a local conservation group, working to preserve the immediate environment and also contributing to broader debates and policies. If you enjoy fishing, birdwatching or exploring the countryside, it is wise to invest in camping or caravan equipment while you are still at work, to provide extra mobility and relatively cheap holidays during retirement. The same planning should be undertaken by sailing enthusiasts. Exercise and yoga classes are a good way of maintaining good health, as are cycling and jogging. Swimming, tennis, golf and walking improve fitness, and other sports, archery for example, are suitable for disabled people who might find it more difficult to exercise.

Hobbies and indoor pursuits There are plenty of pleasant ways to fill time at home—reading, board games, crosswords and jigsaws keep you mentally alert. Wine-making and cooking are creatively satisfying and their results can be highly appreciated. Collecting is popular—including stamps, cards, china, period pieces, coins and antiques. Darts, billiards, chess and bingo can be played at local clubs or meeting places. Keeping a manageable pet, such as a cat, bird or small dog provides absorbing and valuable company.

Getting out and about Join a club, church or voluntary organization and make full use of cheap rates provided by travel services, sports and recreation facilities, galleries, museums and so on.

Model making

With time to pursue new leisure activities, or to explore existing enthusiasms more fully, unexpected skills often emerge. Model railway and aeroplane enthusiasts cover the whole spectrum of age and are linked by magazines, national exhibitions and clubs. Making and flying your own model aeroplane provides much satisfaction as well as the opportunity to meet new people.

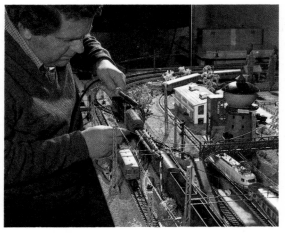

Many hobbies cross the generation boundaries, as these model aircraft aficionados demonstrate. The rewards of shared enthusiasm are great.

For this model railway enthusiast, the pleasure is as much in the gradual creation of his layout as in the final result.

Losing a partner

The loss, whether by death or divorce, of the man or woman who has shared a significant portion of one's life can be a devastating experience. Some people will receive advance notice of the event, but this may make little difference to the emotional reaction which follows. This reaction may be so strong that the person experiencing it, used to everyday worries, anxieties and unhappiness, may fear for his or her sanity.

It is only relatively recently that psychologists have begun to study such emotional reactions and to try to find ways of helping those who cannot cope with them.

Grieving or mourning?

In talking about bereavement and loss, it is important to distinguish between grief and mourning. "Grief" is the generic name given to the emotional responses to serious losses, while "mourning" refers to a set of behaviours which a particular culture decrees to be appropriate following such a loss. In our society, different patterns of mourning behaviour tend to be adopted by different religious groups, such as Jews or Catholics. Something like the Irish wake is found in different religious groups. What is important about these rituals is that they tend to set limits not only on the type of behaviour which may be shown, but also on the length of time for which it is deemed appropriate for the individual to display his or her grief reaction in public.

Rituals of grief

It is notable that Western society sanctions mourning displays only after losses by death. The idea that marriage should be for life, negative attitudes to divorce and the implication of failure have almost certainly prevented the development of a set of rituals which could accompany the grief after losses by separation. In societies where such losses are socially recognized, rituals for the expression of grief *do* exist. The Ashanti women of Ghana, for example, are often discarded by their husbands as they grow older, in favour of a younger partner. The husband transfers not only his love but also his possessions to the younger woman. The older wives may then enact the ritual of travelling in groups to religious shrines where they accuse themselves of witchcraft. This accusation justifies their feelings of failure and worthlessness. They are then able to be "cured"—again by a set of ritual procedures—before taking up the recognized and socially sanctioned role of rejected wife.

The value of rituals

It has been suggested that the grief response occurs in a series of stages which, if they are successfully worked through, end in a process of reintegration. This means that people are able to begin a new life, or continue their old one without undue "interference" from the lost object—the strong emotional reactions evoked by stimuli associated with the lost object are diminished or absent.

The problem with this approach is that although we can separate out various parts of the grief response, they rarely occur in an orderly fashion. It is perhaps better to think in terms of the grief response as

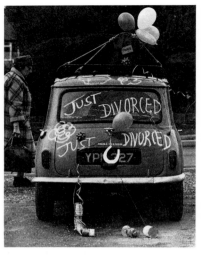

Losing a partner or regaining one's freedom? Such a positive response to divorce is rare, though some people report painless divorces even after forty years of marriage and others speak of feelings of relief, delight and even manic elation. For many people the actual divorce is a formality which occurs a considerable time after the trauma and grief of separation.

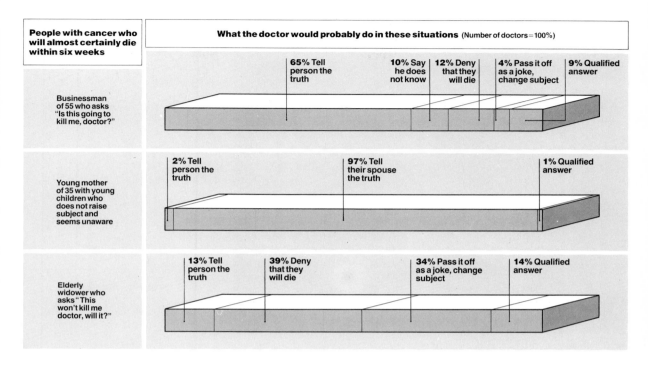

People with cancer who will almost certainly die within six weeks	What the doctor would probably do in these situations (Number of doctors=100%)					
Businessman of 55 who asks "Is this going to kill me, doctor?"	65% Tell person the truth	10% Say he does not know	12% Deny that they will die	4% Pass it off as a joke, change subject	9% Qualified answer	
Young mother of 35 with young children who does not raise subject and seems unaware	2% Tell person the truth	97% Tell their spouse the truth			1% Qualified answer	
Elderly widower who asks "This won't kill me doctor, will it?"	13% Tell person the truth	39% Deny that they will die	34% Pass it off as a joke, change subject		14% Qualified answer	

having several components. Some of these may be dominant immediately following the loss, and some later, but most people will feel a mixture of components at any one time, rather than experience them in orderly stages.

Unresolved grief

What is perhaps surprising about grief is not that some people do not cope with it, but that most people *do*. We still know very little about the mechanisms which underlie recovery from the effects of loss; it is therefore difficult to say with certainty when something has gone wrong with the process. If, however, someone is still very depressed many months—or years—after the loss, or if stimuli associated with the lost object continue to elicit strong emotional reactions, whether it be anxiety, fear, guilt or anger, or when the person shows little sign of rebuilding a life which does not "include" the lost object, then it seems reasonable to suggest that a problem exists.

Traditionally, such people would be treated either with anti-anxiety or anti-depressant drugs, they might be hospitalized because of the risk of suicide, or simply encouraged to take up new activities and interests. While these measures undoubtedly helped some people, they were not successful in many cases, particularly the more severe.

An Amsterdam clinical psychologist, Ron Ramsey, has recently suggested a new approach to the problem of unresolved grief. He has pointed out the similarities between this phenomenon and that of phobias, where a person shows an abnormally heightened fear response to, and avoidance of, objects or situations which most of us find relatively harmless. The grieving person reacts in a similar way to stimuli associated with the lost object—places, names, tunes and so on. Many of the people seen by Ramsey studiously avoided all contact

Illness and death

Heart disease and cancer are major causes of death amongst people of middle years or older. How medical staff deal with patients under such circumstances varies. But there is a growing feeling that dying people have the right to be given realistic information about their illness so that they can constructively plan the remainder of their lives. It appears that doctors tend to tell the truth to patients who ask questions about their condition rather than those who do not. So it may be the patient, and not the doctor, who determines what he or she is told.

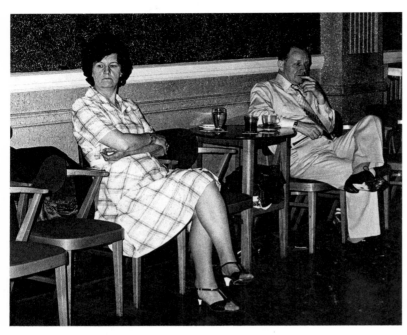

with such stimuli—often going to considerable trouble to do so—in much the same way as a phobic person might avoid spiders. The more people's lives are built around avoidance, the more depressed they become as they are constantly shutting themselves off.

Avoidence tactics

Ramsey has suggested that the person most likely to cope badly with grief is the one who avoids facing up to unpleasant situations or feelings. As we have seen, many of the feelings associated with grief are not only unpleasant, but frightening, so that it is not surprising that some people should choose to ignore or suppress them and avoid situations which elicit them. The problem with this tactic is that while the emotional reaction may be suppressed, it is not abolished and has an unfortunate tendency to resurface whenever people are unexpectedly confronted with stimuli which remind them of their loss.

Psychologists who deal with phobic clients recognize the importance of prolonged exposure to feared stimuli if emotional reactions towards them are to be abolished. In the face of such reactions, of course, most people respond by avoiding the source of fear.

Because psychologists have had such success in the treatment of phobias by prolonged exposure, Ramsey reasoned that a similar approach might be helpful for people showing "abnormal" grief responses. He therefore presented his clients with stimuli associated with their loss, either in the imagination ("think about the fact that you will never hear your husband's voice again") or in reality, using objects associated with the lost person such as photographs or articles of clothing. The person was also exposed to situations he or she had previously avoided, such as restaurants, or streets, or even perhaps the cemetery. In presenting these stimuli, the therapist attempts to evoke the whole range of emotional reactions associated with grief—depression, anxiety, guilt and anger.

The components of grief

Shock—Can take many forms. Individuals may be abnormally calm and seem apathetic, or they may complain of numbness or pain. Shock may also be experienced in the face of anticipated loss.

Denial—As shock recedes, it is common for the person to deny the loss, behaving as if the partner were present, or preserving the lost person's possessions. The strength of the reaction may be affected by sudden loss, or viewing the dead person.

Depression—As the loss is acknowledged, depression takes over, and the individual shows behaviours associated with depression: crying, social withdrawal, pessimism, and may be accompanied by anxiety. How anxious the bereaved becomes depends on the nature of the separation or bereavement. They may also feel anger or guilt, that they or the dead person could have prevented the death. These feelings gradually subside with time but may resurface on occasions such as birthdays or holidays.

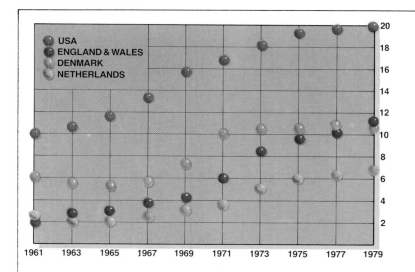

USA
ENGLAND & WALES
DENMARK
NETHERLANDS

1961 1963 1965 1967 1969 1971 1973 1975 1977 1979

20
18
16
14
12
10
8
6
4
2

Divorce rates

Divorce rates have risen steeply during the past decade and in some countries it is estimated that as many as one in three new marriages will end in divorce. There has been a change in social attitudes towards divorce—it still causes distress and disapproval, but no longer carries its previous social stigma. Correspondingly, divorce laws have been adjusted to deal with the situation. Rates for the USA are much higher than for other Western countries, although the UK divorce rate is climbing steeply.

Divorce and children

As the divorce rate has increased, so has the number of children affected. Divorces now involve more than a million children annually. In the late 1970s, about 45 per cent of divorcing couples had no children aged under 18, but 11 per cent involved three or more children. This compares with the mid-1960s, where the figures were 37 per cent and 20 per cent respectively. As a result, the number of children per divorce decree has declined slightly.

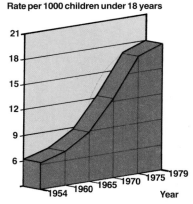

Rate per 1000 children under 18 years

21
18
15
12
9
6

1954 1960 1965 1970 1975 1979
Year

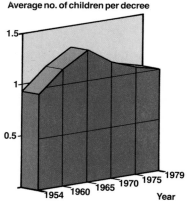

Average no. of children per decree

1.5

1

0.5

1954 1960 1965 1970 1975 1979
Year

Source: Social Trends 1983

This process is very painful, but the emotions must be evoked in order for them to be extinguished; the grieving person gradually finds that he or she can face an ever-widening range of stimuli associated with the lost person without experiencing strong negative emotions. This technique, like that used in the treatment of phobias, can obviously only be used by highly skilled therapists.

Ramsey's success with his clients suggests that "normal" recovery from grief is achieved by confronting the unpleasant emotions and by gradual re-exposure to stimuli associated with the loss. As we have seen, the process of recovery from depression is also facilitated by the availability of alternative sources of pleasure. In the initial stages of grieving, pleasure in these events or activities is usually lost, but is gradually regained with time. The person who does not have these alternative sources in the first place is likely to have far more difficulty in coping with grief than the one who has. It follows that the bereavement may be lessened by maintaining as active a social life as possible.

Work—the later years

The loss of a job produces all the symptoms described in the section on depression, and likewise involves a whole series of secondary losses. Surveys on employment show that, when questioned, most people enjoy their work, but that managers tend to enjoy it more than do unskilled workers. Presumably, not all those who give this answer are thinking of the actual work they do, but rather of the opportunities it gives them for social contact, of the status and identity it confers, or, although they may not have been able to articulate this, of the fact that work imposes a structure on our time and enables us to share goals with others. Those who have worked all their lives cannot imagine what it would be like not to. Small wonder that most people say that they would go on working even if they had no financial need to do so.

Unemployment, then, means the loss of these important aspects of life. There is nothing to stop the unemployed from providing all of these things for themselves, but the psychological and physical effort required to do so is enormous—especially if one is surrounded by people who do not have to make this effort.

There is good reason to believe that unemployment is a stressful experience, but we cannot account for individual differences in reactions to job loss. Nor can we explain why some people may be relatively unaffected by it, while others are driven to suicide.

The "unemployed" are a very heterogeneous group, and later studies of the effects of job loss have tried to clarify the influence of various personal characteristics on reactions to unemployment. As we would expect, these studies produce a more complicated picture of the effects of job loss.

A study carried out in the early 1970s examined the psychological concomitants of unemployment in a sample of professionals and executives. There was very little evidence in this group of the expected effects—boredom, feelings of alienation or reduction in sociability. This sample of unemployed people seemed to have countered boredom by engaging in hobbies or home improvement. An American study conducted a few years later produced similar results, again using a professional sample. Many of these people saw job loss as an opportunity to build new skills or expand old interests, as well as a welcome relief from the demands of work.

A consistent and not unexpected result of studies of the unemployed is that those who are most ambitious or work-oriented are more negatively affected. More specifically, the belief that one is competent at a job makes the loss of it more difficult to bear.

The age group which seems to suffer most following job loss is the 40 to 54-year-olds. This is easy to understand: younger people are more optimistic about changing direction and eventually finding a job, while those approaching retirement may welcome unemployment, especially if the financial loss is not severe. It is the middle-aged who feel they have been "thrown on the scrap heap"—possibly at the peak of their career—and who see least hope of starting again.

One of the most important predictors of how individuals will react to unemployment seems to be whether or not they can occupy their time. This, in turn, tends to be related to occupational status:

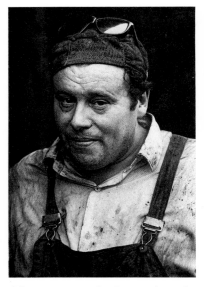

The routine involved in work can be more important than we realize— only when we are without a job may we experience the depression associated with being unemployed— that lack of stimulation and motivation that keeps us going.

Unemployment in middle age

Unemployment in middle age may be the result of early or enforced retirement or of redundancy. People's reactions to it reflect their differing attitudes to the importance of work (apart from financial considerations). Whereas early retirement is often seen as a positive step, sudden redundancy is traumatic; optimism, which many people feel after the initial shock, is short-lived. Even those who looked forward to retirement at the usual age are profoundly shocked by the loss of work.

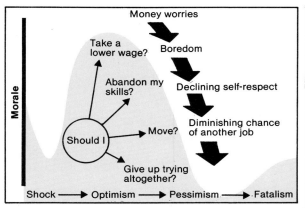

from Understanding the Unemployed by John Hayes and Peter Nutman, Tavistock Publications

Above: the experience of unemployment. The first phase is shock, which often turns to optimism when people contemplate their new freedom. However, boredom, the lack of fresh job prospects and money worries lead to pessimism and then defeatism. But morale can recover, on coming to terms with the new status.

The columns on the right show attitudes to job loss through retirement. Most men saw attachment and gain when contemplating retirement, but some talked of detachment and loss. Attachment refers to continuing or new activities or processes, either favourable or otherwise, whereas detachment refers to cessation.

Attachment	%	Detachment	%
FAVOURABLE		**FAVOURABLE**	
1 Increased leisure time	86	1 Less pressure and frustration with work	26
2 More time with family	44	2 Less routine	12
3 A new life style	28	3 Less responsibility	4
4 New work opportunities	23	4 Less travel	3
5 More time for own needs	21	5 Fewer social relations	1
6 More time for new and existing friendships	16	**UNFAVOURABLE**	
7 Opportunity to move	10	1 Less income	43
8 Increased relaxation	9	2 Fewer social relations	34
9 New financial situation	7	3 Less mental stimulation	21
10 Awareness of ageing	5	4 Less status	8
11 Increased time	5	5 Less routine	6
		6 Less fitness and health	5
UNFAVOURABLE		7 Less responsibility	4
1 A new life style	24	8 Less travel	4
2 Increased financial problems	22	9 No company car	4
3 Awareness of ageing	13	10 Less pressure associated with work	2
4 Increased time	5		
5 More time with family	4		
6 Car purchase problems	3		
7 Pressure to move house	3		
8 Increased leisure time	1		
9 New work opportunities	1		

With unemployment rising, more people are retiring early, but very few receive any guidance about the future. Plans for retirement should be made as early as possible so that problems of adjustment will be minimized. Finances, whether or not to move, or take another job, planning an expansion of leisure activities can all be usefully explored well in advance.

This unemployment line is in Miami, Florida. In Western nations, unemployment now hits all age groups and all types of workers.

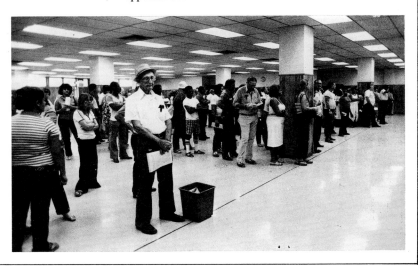

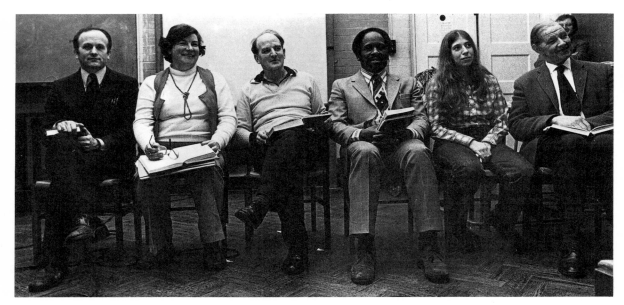

those in high-status occupations seem better able to fill their free time with other activities during unemployment than do those who once held unskilled jobs. It is this latter group who score lowest on measures of life satisfaction and certain indices of mental health—depression and anxiety, for example—when compared to the professional and managerial unemployed. This finding goes against the suggestion that it is high-status workers who will suffer most from unemployment, because in our society personal value is measured in terms of money earned.

Recent research certainly presents a more complex picture of the effects of unemployment than did earlier, more global, studies. The research, however, is mainly the study of individual reactions to the event of job loss, without reference to wider social and economic factors· or to the moderating influence of the individual's social networks. To what extent, for example, are the negative effects of unemployment caused by financial stress? Or by the prevalent attitude in Western society that the only meaningful work is that for which we are paid? What effects does the attitude of family or friends have on reactions to unemployment?

Finally, there is a dearth of research into sex difference in reactions to unemployment. This would seem to be a particularly important area to study, given the increased pressures, in times of recession, for married women to remain at home and given the still prevalent, but principally unsupported, idea that paid work is somehow less important for women.

Retirement—the gateway to old age?

The fact that our society requires many people to give up their main employment at a certain age, and obliges them to provide financially for this event, can be looked at from two viewpoints. We can look at retirement as an event which will overtake most of us sooner or later and examine how individuals prepare for and cope with it. This information can then be used to advise those approaching retirement.

Not everyone finds the transition from an active working life to retirement a difficult one, but those who encounter problems may be helped by group therapy sessions, where experiences and opinions,can be shared and discussed to mutual benefit.

We can also, however, look at retirement in a wider, more abstract way. What are the assumptions which underlie the event? What does it tell us about society's attitudes to the middle-aged and elderly? How valid are these assumptions? We will deal with these issues first.

Step aside—the forces of exclusion

The awareness of being well integrated into society can bestow a feeling of deep security. Integrated people know they are "somebody" because they are treated as such. They take part in at least some of the decision-making and have access to many privileges and opportunities.

Social integration, however, can be experienced as burdensome and oppressive. A person may feel there are too many obligations to meet, too much time pressure, too many expectations. This of course, can make one determined to have a break, to take a holiday, to "get away from it all". As we age, we seem to have a tendency to opt out— to let it all get away from us. We may find ourselves less socially integrated. We have vacated our place in life, although we would not describe ourselves as on vacation. Some social scientists regard this as a process of *disengagement*. This is one of the ideas incorporated in the disengagement theory, formulated and introduced in the United States, mainly by sociologist Elaine Cumming and psychologist William Henry. They examined the results of a study of normal, community-dwelling elders in Kansas City. It seemed to Cumming and Henry that the transition from adulthood to old age involves a natural withdrawal from activities and obligations that previously linked individual and society so closely together.

Think of a ritualistic dance. One partner (the ageing adult) takes a step back. The other partner (society) takes the cue, returns the bow and also takes a backward step. The dance continues, but at a slower pace and with the partners gradually moving further apart. Soon society is whirling round with a new partner, while the old person settles into a chair next to the wall. Then these old people occasionally smile and nod to the active dancers and tap time with their fingers, but their thoughts and feelings are turned ever inward. They have become—both by their choice and society's—rather more private people who are willing to leave the high-stepping to others.

A new stability

When the disengagement process goes smoothly, both partners get what they need. The old people have time to pursue interests and activities that had to be set aside during the peak years of social integration. They can dress, speak and act just as they prefer, rather than having to please a boss or clients, or fit into general expectations. The old people continue to age. Ill health and other life changes usually lead to further extremes of disengagement, with death the final move. Society, meanwhile, has had time to teach its new partners their intricate steps of mutual obligation and to prepare itself for the final departure of its former partners. The disengagement theory tells us that it is natural for the distance between society and the individual to increase with advancing age.

In one sense, disengagement is kinder to women. There is always a need for people who can relate well to others, who are sensitive to

---

PREPARING FOR OLD AGE

Health

The best preparation for health in the later years is simply to keep active physically, mentally and socially. It is wise to have a regular check-up at your doctor's and to seek his or her advice about your general health.

Exercise is probably the most valuable way of keeping yourself fit and of guarding against later problems. A word of warning, though. If you are not used to very much physical activity, begin slowly. If you have difficulties consult your doctor at once.

Exercise does not have to entail following a rigid plan of strenuous push-ups and knee-bends. But if you do favour this type of exercise, there is plenty of information available in books and libraries. Or you can attend fitness, dance or yoga classes.

There are many other methods of exercise: walking is both easy and enjoyable, and many people in retirement get a dog to ensure that they walk regularly. Cycling, swimming and golf are good exercise, as are most sports.

The beneficial effects of exercise will be increased by learning to relax and avoid stress, by careful attention to diet and by reducing alcohol and tobacco consumption (better still, stop smoking altogether). A regular, healthy pattern of eating can combat many diseases of middle age.

feelings and emotions. A woman does not necessarily lose this kind of "employment" with age; a man, however, may find himself at a loss—no job to go to in the morning and not much skill in the finer points of interpersonal relationships and expressive activities.

Emotional superiority?

Many other researchers have looked into the disengagement theory, however, and found that it does *not* hold up well as a firm general statement about how and why people age in the social sphere. There is, first of all, the highly questionable assumption that women are "superior" in the area of emotional relationships. There is, in fact, no empirical evidence to support this view. The difficulty which some men may experience in this sphere after retirement (as compared to women) may have more to do with the fact that their relationships centred round work rather than the home or community. It is well known that proximity and frequency of contact are crucial factors in the establishment and maintenance of relationships; women whose relationships centre on work are likely to experience similar difficulties in remaining socially engaged to those experienced by men.

A number of studies have also found that the active and engaged old person tends to have a higher morale than the person who has withdrawn from the mainstream, and this is taken by some investigators as disproof of the theory's main implications. The original propositions also did not give much attention to individual differences, and this has further weakened its case.

Pushing the old aside

There is a quality in the disengagement theory that one might almost call "polite". It emphasizes that society and the individual take leave of each other with mutual consent. But other social scientists see the situation differently. They agree with the broad conclusion drawn by the disengagement theory: the ageing person tends to remove himself or herself from the core of a society's life. However, these social scientists are more apt to use such terms as "discrimination", "segregation" and "political expedience". They do not see it as a gracious dance. Society steers or pushes the ageing person to the sideline, most explicitly through the process of retirement. These writers see disengagement not as a natural process, but as society's solution to a variety of economic, social and political problems.

In the past, young and old generally worked as they could on the many tasks that had to be done to keep family and community afloat. The young worked as early in life as they were able and the old as long as they were able. It was biological capacity or functional status that determined when a person entered and departed from the workforce. Today, both young and old are increasingly excluded from the producer's role. The basis is not biological, for children and the aged are stronger than in the past. The basis is cultural: people are defined as "too young" or "too old" for longer periods of time than ever before.

Competing generations

Education and retirement, of course, are spheres of activity to which people can be assigned when they are not welcome in the workforce. Middle-aged people are able to enforce such assignments because they manoeuvre shifting age *coalitions*. Sometimes the middle-aged join

PLANNING YOUR POST-RETIREMENT BUDGET

A common worry when approaching retirement is how to adjust to living, on a reduced, fixed income which is vulnerable to inflation.

The best way to plan ahead realistically is to consider the differences in your life style pre- and post-retirement, and here you should begin with two major items: travel and domestic spending. There will be no daily travel to work but increased leisure time may mean more holiday travel. The loss of a company car means increased expenditure (it may be possible to purchase your company car cheaply) and you should calculate the advantage of having your own car against concessions available on public transport and the occasional use of a hired car. Being at home all day will mean an increase in consumption of heating, lighting and food. It may also mean that you can save by growing your own vegetables. More time to cook usually means less use of expensive convenience foods.

For a realistic guide to your post-retirement budget, draw up two schedules. The first should compare pre- -and post-retirement domestic spending, including the following items: food, transport, entertainment, leisure (including newspapers, magazines, garden tools, holidays), personal (clothes, and so on), gifts, donations, the house (repairs, bills and the like), savings/insurance payments and pets. Check to see if you are entitled to rate or rent rebates and remember concessions are available on travel, meals on wheels, welfare services, prescriptions, and that there are reduced prices at the cinema, hairdresser, evening class and swimming pool. These totals should be incorporated into the second schedule as expenditure to be deducted from your total net annual income (that is, salary, pensions, investment and other income *less* income tax and other employee contributions).

You now have a guide to the differences in your budget and can consider new ways of increasing income and decreasing expenditure.

It is never too early to plan ahead for retirement.

with the aged to exclude the young; at other times they are in collusion with the young to expel the old. The results of this power display by the middle-aged can be seen in economic discrimination, age stereotyping and territorial segregation.

Economic discrimination appears not only in employment, but also in barriers to obtaining credit, negligent or even criminal mishandling of pension plans and so on. Age stereotyping is a way of rationalizing the exclusion of young and old from positions of opportunity and power. The young may be dismissed as irresponsible and frivolous, the old as burnt-out or inflexible. Looked at from this point of view, age stereotyping takes on a sinister character. More than just carelessness and insensitivity, it emerges as part of an unspoken policy of discrediting those who might be competitors for social power.

There is a glow of constructive possibility here that seems to be absent from the disengagement theory. If society has created definitions that set people apart from each other, then society may also have the ability to redefine and integrate. There is more than one way to retain power, and sharing it is not necessarily the worst. As people become more aware of the power aspects of age-based exclusions, of which retirement is one of the most obvious, there should be more opportunity to develop alternatives. Young and old could stand together on more issues. The middle-aged would appreciate more keenly the benefits they might gain by allowing their juniors and seniors to shoulder part of the burden.

Retirement and the individual

There are many people who look forward avidly to retirement and appreciate every minute of it; others, for a variety of reasons, do not enjoy it so well. In one study of men who had retired, the researchers identified five kinds of general reaction to the processes of ageing and disengagement, ranging from the passive, withdrawing from unwelcome responsibilities, to angry, feeling that life had been unfair to them.

The kind of reaction most often seen among the elderly men was described by the researchers as *mature*. These men acknowledged the realities of ageing both in themselves and in their relationship with society. They were neither surprised nor embittered to find themselves growing old—it was just what they had expected. They enjoyed both personal relationships and their favourite activities.

One regrettable aspect of this, and indeed of many studies, is its assignment of value-laden labels to people, when in fact it is simply describing a variety of behaviour patterns. Why should people who are happy to give up jobs they never liked or responsibilities they never enjoyed be labelled "passive"? Or others who (possibly quite justifiably) feel they have had a raw deal be called "maladjusted"? And why should only those who accept the "realities" of ageing be called "mature"? These realities, as we have seen (and will explore in greater detail later) are often only the concrete reflection of the needs and opinions of those who have power over the aged.

The concept of "adjustment" is a dangerous one. It carries the implicit assumption that the environment is all right and that it is the individuals' task to come to terms with it. If they cannot or will not, they are maladjusted or immature. Were we to try and increase the level of "maturity" in this group of men, we would immediately rush to the individual and try to change him, rather than recognizing, firstly, that there are many ways of being "mature" and that fighting vigorously against encroaching age may be one of them. Better still, we could abolish subjective concepts such as being well-adjusted or mature and concentrate instead on simply increasing people's senses of wellbeing. In dealing with or labelling the individual we would also be missing the fact that "ageing" is largely part of a set of environmental contingencies: it is these which are reacted to and may be in need of change.

Preparing for retirement

The practical problem of retirement often centres for most people on a reduction in income. People prepare for this eventuality in a number of ways. Some organize their savings so that their income is reduced as little as possible. Others try to arrange things so that their outgoings will be reduced after retirement. They do this by, for example, moving to a more economical house, or by purchasing or upgrading major items such as car or washing machine. These solutions will not suit everyone, but it is as well to recognize that the problem exists.

How will you fill your time? We can see retirement as a kind of socially sanctioned unemployment. Those who coped best with unemployment (or who even saw it as a positive experience) were, as we saw, those who were able to fill their time with other activities. In thinking about this problem, those approaching retirement should be careful to avoid two common errors. One is to underestimate the actual amount of time to be filled. Overtime and travelling time, which once ate into their days, must also be taken into account.

Look for variety

Getting up late, relaxing over a drink or a book are all the more enjoyable because we do not do them too often and because they are contrasted with periods of activity which we may not enjoy so much. This is not to say that retirement must consist mostly of unpleasant activities, just so that pleasant activities will be more enjoyable. It does mean, however, that no one should expect to enjoy unlimited amounts of any activity, no matter how pleasant it appears.

What retired people need is a wide variety of enjoyable activities. The problem here is that, unlikely as it sounds, many people have no real idea of what they actually enjoy doing. A working life spent in the service of others, doing things because they have to be done, can blunt people's appreciation of activities they enjoy for their own sake.

Some people approaching retirement will claim that what they most enjoy is their work. For these people, the solution may be to continue working on a different basis. We take it for granted that when sportsmen and women retire they should move into coaching or management. With a bit of imagination, many retired people could (and do) find alternative ways of using their skills, perhaps in combination with others with similar or complementary skills.

Marriage and retirement

How will your marriage stand up to your or your partner's retirement? Couples are often unprepared for the extra amount of time they will spend together after one or both retire. They may have overestimated the number of interests they share (not including their family), or underestimated the extent to which their conversation is about work. It is very easy, subject to the demands of home, family and work, for couples to grow apart, so that retirement finds two strangers facing each other across the breakfast table. Unfortunately, their interpersonal skills may have fallen into disuse, so that it seems impossible to discuss what is happening and find constructive solutions to the problem. Middle-aged couples would be well advised to face these issues long before retirement, so that the extra time spent together becomes a source of pleasure rather than resentment.

Retirement in perspective

Is it necessary that our lives and our theories place so much emphasis on employment, productivity and earnings? The achievements and social status associated with occupation are major ingredients in the way we judge ourselves and others. When asked who we are, don't we often answer in terms of our work? As long as values associated with work remain dominant in our society, they are important for the ageing person.

However, the barren thought that there really is no life worth mentioning after work has been disproved many times. Increasingly, studies of the retirement years reveal diversity of "afterlives". Not all retired people stay retired. Many continue to be active in fields related to their lifelong interests, others cultivate new interests or return to interests they could not find the time for earlier.

Middle age myths

Some thoughts on ageing:

"For the last 20 years I have known what happiness means. I have the good fortune to be married to a wonderful wife. I wish I could write more about this, but it involves love, and perfect love is the most beautiful of all frustrations because it is more than one can express"—Charlie Chaplin talking about his wife Oona O'Neill whom he married in 1943. He was then 54 and she was 20. They had eight children.

"Aging is natural and the changes in us are natural. My wrinkles and my arthritis are a part of my testimony of change" —Margaret Kuhn, who at 64 (in 1970) founded the Gray Panthers, an organization of older people dedicated to fighting the ageing process.

"There is beauty in sincere and honest aging. I guess people who concentrated on themselves are most afraid of age. If they would think of the purpose of our being here, they wouldn't stop to worry if their teeth were crumbling or if a bit of gray appeared in their hair . . . To be helpful to others makes the world so much brighter, keeps one youthful and active . . . There is simply no time to worry about growing old. It's such a wasted effort to try to turn back the clock when there's so much to be done"—Helen Hayes, American actress, when aged 60.

"Some people tend to resign—to retire or to withdraw too early. Others may not recognize the necessity of switching their function to one that is less active and more advisory. I don't believe in retiring from life. Retirement from business is an artificial, technical thing, simply from a certain responsibility to a certain group. It's true that some older people become too inflexible, too habituated to certain ruts and reactions they can't get out of. But then there are some people of 40 to whom this also happens and some to whom it does not happen even at 80"— Karl Menninger, founder of the Menninger Clinic and Foundation in Texas for the treatment of mental illness, at the age of 77. And consider the following people:

★ Charles De Gaulle was 68 when he was returned to power in 1958
★ Gandhi was 60 when he led the 200-mile march of non-violent disobedience against the salt tax in 1930
★ Sonia Delaunay was 65 when her painting first began to be exhibited internationally
★ The Irish poet W. B. Yeats produced some of his best work after the age of 60

★ Helen Bradley, illustrator, began to paint when over 60 to show her grandchildren her own childhood.

Myths of middle age

1 *After 65 everyone goes steadily downhill.* There is no truth in this at all: in fact, some people's health improves after retirement. Many of the problems connected with this period are due to illness, not ageing.

2 *People should retire because their capabilities decline.* The age for retirement is an outdated convention. The many artists, musicians, writers and politicians active over this age prove the point.

3 *Middle age is a time for settling down.* On the contrary, many people make fresh starts in their lives at this time.

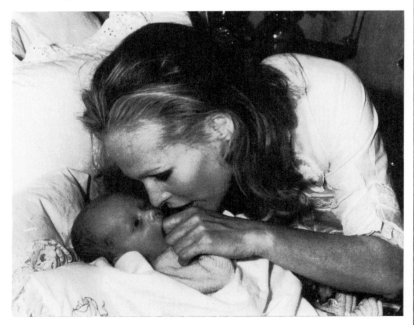

Film star Ursula Andress was 43 when she gave birth to her first child, Dmitri. Her acting career has continued despite the demands of motherhood.

Health problems in middle age

One of the major hazards of middle age is coronary artery disease. Several contributory factors have now been isolated, and suggested ways of maintaining health through prevention rather than cure are given on page 217. It is important to note "early warning signs", both mental and physical, that indicate that all is not well — for example, chest pains, headaches, persistent diarrhoea, indigestion and palpitations; inability to relax, remember or concentrate, or habitual over-reacting.

ILLNESS	SYMPTOMS	TREATMENT/ACTION
Angina pectoris	The arteries harden with age and become clogged up so that blood circulation is impaired. Can result in stroke or heart attack.	For prevention: diet carefully to avoid cholesterol. Treatment: diet, as above.
Bronchitis	Can cause permanent lung damage.	For prevention: lose weight; stop smoking; have an influenza injection each autumn. Treatment: antibiotic drugs; "postural drainage"; change sleeping posture.
Coronary thrombosis (myocardial infarction)	A coronary artery becomes blocked by a blood clot (thrombus) and the heart muscle is deprived of its blood supply. Symptoms: chest pain radiating out towards the left shoulder and sometimes down the left arm.	For prevention: lose weight; stop smoking; decrease anxiety and tension. Treatment: complete rest until circulation is restored; the heart muscle has to be re-educated back to full activity. Gradual exercise.
Diabetes	The pancreas secretes insufficient insulin to control the blood sugar. Sufferer feels extremely unwell (weight loss, fainting, excessive thirst, low energy) until the disease is diagnosed and treated.	Cannot be cured but is controlled by doses (in tablet form or, more often, by injection) of insulin.
Duodenal ulcers	Sufferers complain of "chronic indigestion".	For prevention: balanced diet, reduction of stress. Treatment: diet; sometimes an operation is necessary.
High blood pressure (hypertension)	Known as the "silent killer" because it is rarely accompanied by any symptoms. It is estimated that one in every five people is hypertensive and one-third of those are not aware of it. Can lead to strokes, kidney failure, heart disease and a haemorrhage into the retina.	For prevention: reduce stress; lose weight; have regular checks on blood pressure. Treatment: may need hospital observation; drugs can reduce blood pressure and reduce strain on the heart and arteries.
Strokes	A blood vessel in the brain either gives way suddenly thereby allowing blood to leak out into the brain tissue, or it becomes blocked by a clot of blood so that part of the brain is deprived of essential blood supplies. A small clot can cause temporary interference with speech; a large clot can cause unconsciousness or even death.	For prevention: lose weight; take proper exercise. Treatment: physiotherapy; "re-education" of affected muscles.

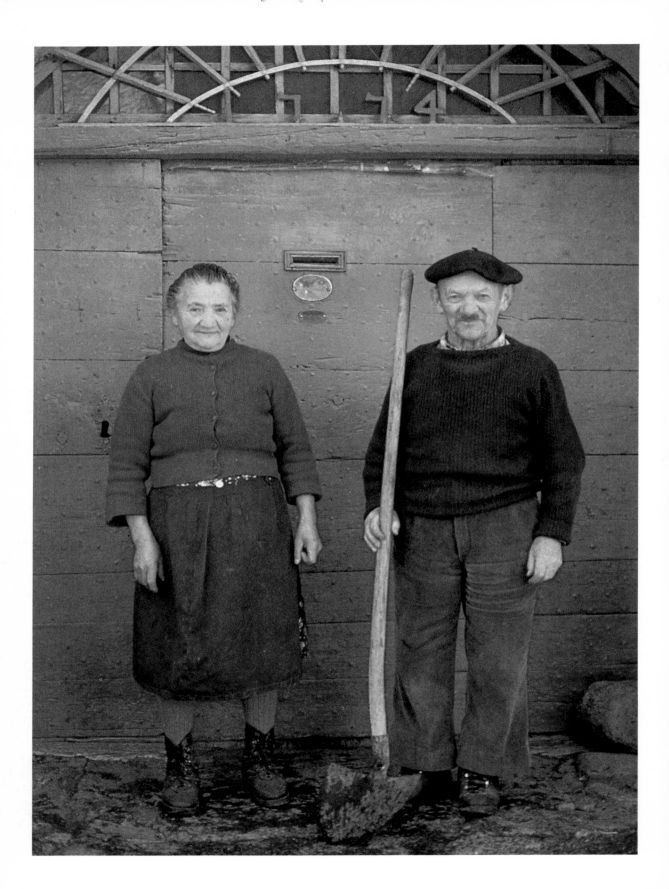

Old Age

What is "old age" and how do we define it? There is no simple answer. In our society, chronological age seems to have pride of place in defining old age. We have strong expectations about what people should look like and how they should behave at certain ages. "Carrying on like that at her age" or "You'd never think he was 70" and similar phrases indicate that, in the face of evidence to the contrary, we rarely change our expectations: instead we regard those who violate them as abnormal or deviant. This emphasis on chronological age raises many problems, not least of which is that age is a very unhelpful predictor of many of the skills and abilities we regard as important. There is also the problem that there is often little correspondence between chronological age and the age which people *feel* themselves to be. Not only that, but people feel themselves to be different ages in different areas of their lives. Thus, two people at the same chronological age may behave differently and make different life decisions if they have different private versions of their age.

It will help, in reading this section, to bear in mind the difference between ageing and being old. As we will see, ageing can be looked upon as a process or set of processes. We go on ageing for years and years. Oldness, however, is a state of mind. It is defined for us, or imposed on us, by outer standards or by our own judgement. We can set "oldness" relatively late in life; we can choose to regard it as a desirable or dreadful condition. Here, we will use the word "old" to refer to men and women in their 70s and beyond. No disrespect is intended by this usage, nor does it involve any assumptions about the person's quality of life or value as a human being. "Ageing" will be used to refer to the process that accompanies us throughout our lives, starting well before old age.

Left: Days of peace and tranquillity, or unending toil?

Changing bodies and minds

Old age as illness?

We often associate being old with being ill. There is undoubtedly more physical impairment and illness among 80-year-olds than among men and women half a century younger. It is easy but not accurate to conclude that old age itself is a kind of generalized illness. Let us see why this conclusion is off the mark and whether there is an alternative view.

Results of an official national survey in the United States actually show a decreased incidence of certain illnesses among adults aged 45 and over. Asthma, hay fever and peptic ulcers, for example, are conditions that afflict young and old equally, while older people are strikingly less vulnerable than the young and middle-aged to a variety of diseases caused by certain infections or parasites.

Loss in various capacities may begin fairly early in adult life and without being caused by disease. Fitness and agility are good examples of abilities which have far more to do with life styles than with actual chronological age.

What then are the effects of old age on its own, apart from physical illness and the effects of an unhealthy life style? Is there a biological process that could be known as normal ageing, a process partly hidden by additional deficits brought on by disease, accidents and unhealthy life habits? This is the view of many gerontologists. It is

Music, whether pursued as career or pastime, can be a lifelong pleasure and one that is not diminished in old age. Many performers and composers have produced their most accomplished and even innovative work in their seventies and eighties. Some have refused to allow failing faculties, poor eyesight or advancing deafness, to restrict their work.

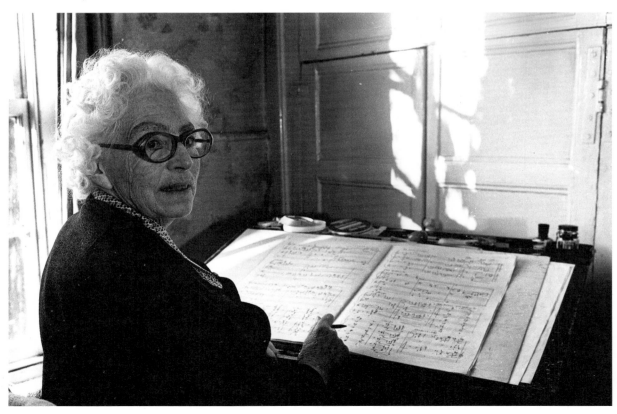

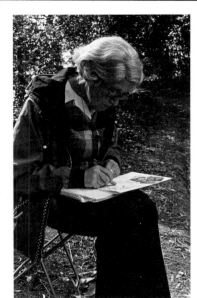

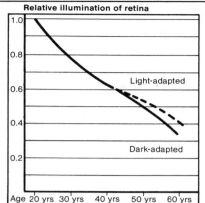

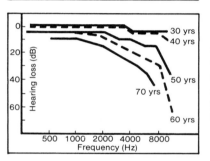

Adapting to changes is a key to continued activity. Drawing is easier than painting if eyesight and colour sense are impaired.

Sight and hearing
Age usually brings a decline in the powers of vision and hearing, even when no illness is present.

The decline in sight seems to be attributable to changes in the pupil and the lens of the eye. One major change is that the lens "yellows" (becoming more opaque) with age, with the result that less light reaches the retina.

Hearing declines as a result of a variety of physical changes in the ear and brain. The graph shows how the decline in older people is significantly greater at higher frequencies, whereas for younger people it is relatively constant throughout the frequency range.

difficult to put to the test, especially with humans. It is very important that we do test it, however, because those who care for or live with the elderly (and the elderly themselves) usually have a set of more or less explicit beliefs about the standards of health or cognitive functioning we would expect to find in the elderly. Thus, many physical states and "mental" behaviours which are changeable or preventable may be put down to ageing' As we shall see later when talking about dementia, the danger in having such an easily available label with which to "explain" an old person's state is that it distracts attention from social, psychological or other physical variables which are actually responsible.

Healthy old age
There have been some carefully designed studies that help to establish the distinction between being old and being ill. Psychologist James Birren recruited a group of elderly men who were free from illness, as determined by both clinical and laboratory examinations. These men willingly cooperated in extensive studies of their physical, psychological and social functioning. Although all the men (average age 71) were in good health, the researchers were still able to' distinguish between the healthiest and the less healthy.

The very healthy old men functioned as well in various physical tests as did a comparable group of healthy young men. Altogether, the old men showed less impairment when compared with healthy young men than would ordinarily have been expected. There were no differences between old and young in blood levels of white blood cells, haemoglobin, the basic level of blood sugar and serum cholesterol, or in the type of electrical brain function. The very healthy old men were similar to the young men in blood pressure, in the utilization of oxygen and the flow of blood in brain tissue.

There were, however, a few clear-cut differences between even the healthiest old men and the young men. For example, electroencephalographic readings indicated that the brain waves of the older men were slower. However, the apparent reduction in the tempo of brain waves is not a sign of disease, nor was it obviously associated with observable changes in thought or behaviour.

When the researchers looked at the complete set of findings, they were impressed by the negative effect on an older person of even a small "touch" of disease. An older man who would be considered quite healthy by ordinary standards would show a loss in measures of brain functioning with even a small degree of arteriosclerosis. It was concluded that decreased oxygen consumption and blood flow in the brain were not signs of ageing as such, but had resulted from a specific disease.

In everyday life, however, all too often old *is* ill. Apart from the fact that certain chronic conditions are more common in later life, there is the additional consideration that many older people suffer from several physical problems at the same time. Multiple illness can greatly complicate both diagnosis and treatment. Also, the over-readiness to take old for ill sometimes prevents the elderly themselves as well as their families and doctors from making efforts to restore health. Studies of this kind emphasize the importance of prevention and early treatment of diseases in the elderly.

How the body changes

It could be said that when a person stops growing, he or she begins to age. Some of our bodily functioning may have passed its peak before we have reached peak functioning in other areas. For example, the adolescent who has not yet completely matured physically may start losing a little visual aeuity and the ability to respond to changes in illumination.

This means that different aspects of our body begin the downhill run—often aided and abetted by our life style—at different times. It is one reason why the concept of biological age is not satisfactory: we have many different biological ages within us.

The general process of biological ageing can be compared to a long, slow tide that moves upon us so gradually that it might be quite a while before we are aware of its presence. We learn to adjust to many of the changes so gradually and naturally that we may not be clearly aware of their taking place. There may come a particular point when we define ourselves as "old" or when others make this definition, but the process will have been going on for a long time. And it is entirely possible to enjoy a long life without ever being faced directly with this redefinition.

There are some exceptions to this. Illness and enforced retirement are among the life circumstances that can suddenly focus attention on physical changes that have been going on for some time. It is also likely that the rate of ageing may itself be accelerated in some circumstances. Emotional stress or an inhospitable environment—say, a very noisy one—can have this effect.

Changes in old age

There are many changes—both physical and mental—associated with old age. While some of these are undoubtedly a normal and natural part of ageing, others are less inevitable.

Tell-tale signs of ageing

1 Eyes—look dimmer and mucus tends to collect in the corners.
2 Hair—on the head becomes grey or white and thinner. In women more hair grows on the upper lip and chin, while men's facial hair grows less thickly.
3 Teeth—become yellow and may be lost.
4 Skin—becomes more wrinkled and rougher, and sags, with the dark circles and bags under the eyes becoming more prominent. Bluish red patches may appear on the ankles and lower legs.
5 Muscles—become flabby around the chin, abdomen and upper arms.
6 Limbs and joints—may become stiff, and movements awkward.
7 Body fat—accumulates around the stomach and hips.
8 Posture—the spine contracts slightly, leading to a loss in height, and the shoulders tend to become more rounded.

Other common changes in appearance

1 The nails on hands and feet may become thicker and more brittle.
2 The feet can become larger (as a result of sagging muscles) and blemishes may appear.
3 The nose may become less fleshy and appear to lengthen.
4 Moles, warts and dark spots may appear on the skin.
5 The shape of the mouth may change (as a result of the loss of teeth).
6 The veins can become more prominent on the legs (especially around the ankles) and on the backs of the hands.
7 In a woman, the breasts may become flabby and sag.

Changes in sensory functioning

1 Vision—the eyes adapt less quickly to changes in lighting, the field of vision shrinks, spots may appear before the eyes and basic visual sharpness declines.
2 Hearing—sensitivity diminishes, especially at the higher frequencies.
3 Appetite—the taste buds in the tongue and inner surface of the cheeks function less efficiently, as do the sensory cells in the nose, so that the sensual appeal of food decreases, often contributing to a loss of appetite. (Increased hair in the nostrils can also contribute to a diminished sense of smell.)
4 Touch—drier and rougher skin makes the sense of touch less acute.
5 Sensitivity to pain—declines.

Mental changes in old age

1 Reasoning—old people seem to "think more slowly". This may be because their daily lives give them less "practice" in speedy problem-solving, rather than because of an organic decline in mental powers.
2 Learning—old people are expected to find learning more difficult. This may to a significant extent be because of deficient hearing, vision, and so on, and lack of confidence and motivation.
3 Creativity—old people are generally seen as past their creative peak, but this may be culturally determined (that is different, expectations might produce a different pattern).
4 Memory—old people tend to remember very recent and remote events better than those in between. Physiological changes may partly explain this, as may lack of attentiveness or motivation.
5 Mental rigidity—old people often seem to have very set ideas. This can be related to the apparent decline in learning ability and creative powers (it may be partly culturally determined).

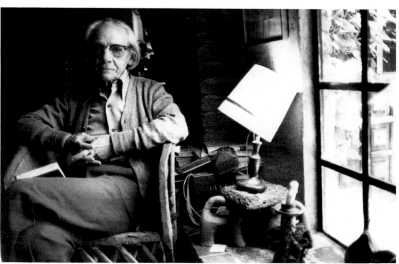

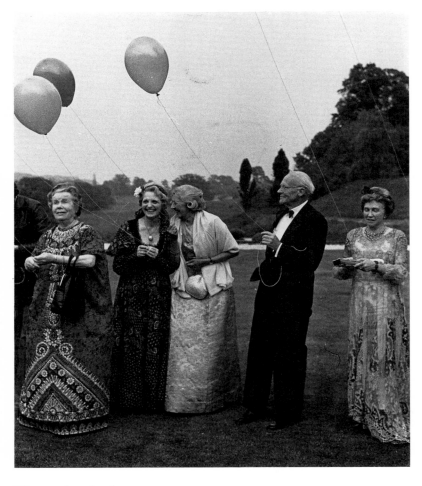

Second childhood setting in? More likely these people are making use of the prerogative of age to disregard other people's standards of 'proper' behaviour—to enjoy a little fun and nostalgia without self-consciousness.

The ageing body

Older is shorter, for both sexes and all racial groups. In the largest single study of this theory, involving 23 000 Canadians, the old men were, on average, three inches shorter than the young, and older women 2.2 inches. Some of this difference may be attributed to improved nutrition in the last decade or two, so that each generation is slightly taller than the last, but some of it has an anatomical basis. The discs between our spinal vertebrae shrink with age, and so do the muscles that support erect posture. However, some of us develop a slumped bearing while still young, and this is exaggerated by ageing. Detectable loss in height usually does not occur until the age of 50 or later.

Both skin and hair thin with age. Wrinkling and sagging of skin result from a loss of the underlayer of fatty tissue, and from exposure to decades of sunlight. The skin's functions are also affected by age. It is brittle and less flexible and does not offer as much protection from disease and infection.

Changes in muscles and bones are far-reaching. The bones themselves tend to lose calcium and become thinner and more brittle. This results in heightened risk of injury, along with a more limited capacity to make a quick and full recovery. One of the more familiar misfortunes of old age involves the person who falls, breaks a hip and who from that point on is bedridden or crippled. Depression, susceptibility to infection and a loss of the will to live may follow if sensitive and effective care is not provided.

It has been well established that collagen, one of the connective tissues which holds our body frame together, loses much of its ability to give and stretch with advancing age—rather like a piece of worn elastic. This is the source of much of the old person's difficulty with smooth and rapid movement. Along with the wear and tear that has affected our joints (notably the knees), the impairment in function of connective tissue can bring about an aches-and-pains feeling which discourages old people from using their bodies. They are caught in a vicious circle, for the less they use their bodies, the more effortful and painful every movement becomes.

However, the muscles themselves often remain in basically good condition well into advanced age, given adequate nutrition and circulation. If muscle weakness does occur, it may have more to do with the integration of muscular activity and sensory information than with failure of the muscles themselves.

The vital functions

All bodily functions are vital—as we discover when something goes wrong. Otherwise, we tend to take them for granted—we eat, we digest, we eliminate wastes. So simple. As we grow older, we are less able to take these functions for granted. Breathing becomes more difficult. Lung movement is less complete, so that there is more air left in the lungs of an old person when he or she breathes out. This reduction in efficiency can have serious consequences for other bodily functions. Cells throughout our body rely on the oxygen we breathe in and the removal of the carbon dioxide as we breathe out. Oxygen starvation or the slow removal of carbon dioxide threatens the very survival of our cells.

The danger is most critical in the brain, which needs a plentiful supply of oxygen. When the supply is reduced through poor respiration or circulation, brain functioning deteriorates. Many old people tend to have intermittent periods of difficulty in breathing. They may have a confused episode because not enough oxygen is getting through to the brain, but recover mental and physical functioning without permanent damage having been done. Unfortunately, there is a tendency to conclude that an old person is "senile" whenever such a lapse in functioning is observed. In fact, many younger adults show similar lapses for a variety of reasons.

The cardiovascular system is another critical link in our survival apparatus. For a long time it has been said that "a man is as old as his arteries". This cliché has gained much support from research. With advancing age, our arteries tend to become narrower, less flexible and obstructed with various substances that interfere with circulation. These changes often lead to a rise in blood pressure. Increased blood pressure in narrower and less efficient arteries increases the risk of strokes and cerebral-vascular accidents.

Increased blood pressure with age is the rule in Western societies. This is not an inevitable concomitant of ageing as different societies show different patterns of blood pressure change.

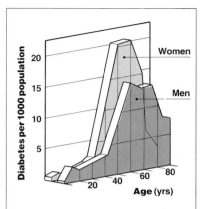

This graph shows the rates of newly diagnosed cases of diabetes at different ages. Sixty to seventy years is a prime time for this disease to set in. It appears that hormonal changes brought on by ageing can lead to a failure by the insulin produced by the body to perform adequately its functions of controlling blood sugar and promoting the storage of glycogen.

Diet and debility

Adequate nutrition depends both upon what we eat and drink and on how our body utilizes these substances. Some of the problems in the digestive process that people encounter later in life reflect more upon bad habits of eating and drinking than upon changes that can be blamed directly on the ageing process.

Generally, older people take in fewer calories than younger people, probably because their activity level is lower and their basal metabolic rate slower. The tendency is made worse by poverty (and in Western societies the poor include a disproportionate number of aged people). This may result in eating habits which deprive people of some of the essentials for good nutrition. The elderly person who has an incomplete diet becomes more vulnerable to a variety of diseases and shows a reduction in vigour.

The digestive system does not seem particularly vulnerable to the ageing process. Research in this field has not been extensive, but it has been established that nutrients are still well absorbed and digested. Our small intestines have a remarkable reserve capacity, and the liver, with its vital detoxifying function, seems to hold up well with age.

The kidneys fare less well: they take longer to concentrate waste products into urine and are not as effective in helping the body retain its fluid balance (a critical, if less familiar, vital function). Even people in good health show these changes, which seem to be an intrinsic part of the ageing process.

Bladder capacity also decreases with age, and there may be less awareness of the need to urinate until the bladder is almost full. These changes make the old more vulnerable to kidney and bladder infections. There is also the challenge to self-esteem when people discover, for the first time in their adult life, that they do not have complete control over their bladder. It is possible to help some people to regain control and so make it easier for them to maintain a normal personal and social life.

The central nervous system

Biochemical and electrical messages crackle through the central nervous system (CNS) almost as rapidly in old age as they do in youth. As we have seen, blood flow and utilization of oxygen are unimpaired in healthy old men. These are among the more reassuring facts that have been established recently.

However, some degenerative changes have also been observed. The cells of the CNS, unlike other body cells, grow old along with us and, when they die, are not replaced. Fortunately, the CNS is not short of cells, and a great deal of this loss will go unnoticed. The brains of both old people and animals, however, tend to show a reduction in weight and many other changes in cellular composition.

The loss in functional neurons may be responsible for the slowdown in electrical activity of the brain observed even in very healthy old men. It also seems to be more difficult for the appropriate signal to get through. This could lead to a longer reaction-time to events in the outer world and more difficulty in coordinating the activities of various bodily systems that require "commands" and "fine tuning" from the brain.

There are, however, two factors to bear in mind. Because of the fine distinction between simple ageing and the effects of disease, it is possible that people who remain free of high blood pressure (hypertension), arteriosclerosis and other common disorders might also remain free of many of the negative changes observed in the typical aged brain.

The other factor concerns our body's ability to compensate for deficiencies. For example, when problems in blood flow arise in later life, the number of small vessels which serve specific parts of the body tends to increase. The brain also has its compensatory mechanisms. We seem to possess a considerable reserve capacity and an ability to shift some CNS functions from one pattern of operation to another. The fact that some people make an almost complete recovery following a stroke attests to the compensatory powers of the brain.

The senses

Vision is usually the first sensory system to show appreciable changes, even in the absence of disease. The lens and cornea become less transparent, the eyes adapt less quickly to changes in lighting, we are more apt to see spots before our eyes as the vitreous humour (the jelly inside the eyeballs) deteriorates. The field of vision shrinks (this is particularly important for crossing streets or driving) and our basic visual sharpness diminishes. We are also likely to be beset by cataracts and to lose some of the colour that made our eyes so beguilingly blue or brown.

Hearing sensitivity decreases, especially in the higher frequencies. While this is a common finding in industrialized societies, there is evidence that, in quieter places, people show less impairment of hearing with age. The fact that greater hearing loss is also found in men might also be related to their exposure to industrial noise.

In practical terms, increased difficulty in hearing human speech, especially if it must be picked out from a background of other sounds, is one of the major auditory problems experienced by many people from middle age onwards. The old man who seems to be frowning severely at you across a room brimming with conversation and noise is probably not expressing disapproval of your words—he is simply trying to hear them.

Appetite senses diminish with age. Many foods become less attractive in aroma and taste (a process aided by a lifetime's smoking). This can contribute to undernutrition and argues for the careful preparation of meals and the establishment of a social atmosphere conducive to their enjoyment.

Body senses—perception of motion, vibration, feedback of body positioning and activity—also become less acute with age. Some of this can be attributed to the ageing process, but much is probably due to a more sedentary life style.

A good night's sleep often does wonders to restore not only body functioning, but also a sense of zest and optimism. Unfortunately, research suggests that we do not sleep as deeply or as well in old age. The time spent in the deepest phase of sleep (the delta-wave phase) shows the greatest decline, along with time spent in the rapid eye movement phase, when dreaming occurs. Old people who half-sleep during the day may be trying to compensate for the fact that they only half-slept during the night. On the other hand, old people may actually need less sleep (but of the right kind) than the young. Many old people go to bed early, and rise late, simply for want of something

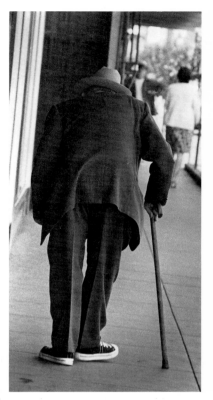

Outwardly, the effects of age take their toll. For some, this may mean major illnesses or hospitalization, but for others, it is simply a matter of slowing down.

better to do. Many who complain of sleeping problems may be suffering from boredom and underactivity. It is important to check the amount of sleep an old person is actually getting, rather than accepting that "lying awake for hours" constitutes a sleep problem, because of the deleterious effects which sleeping tablets may have on their functioning.

Mental functioning in later life

According to the "standard brand" theories of mental development and the most common methods for assessing intellectual functioning, people will have reached their peak in adolescence or the early twenties. They might be expected to remain at a plateau of intellectual competence for a while and then slide downhill.

However, this picture has proved too simple. The use of more sophisticated research techniques shows that patterns of mental functioning from early to later life are more complex and interesting than was originally thought.

First, it is important to recognize the multidimensional nature of what we call "intelligence". One person, for example, may be especially gifted in mathematics, but be nearer the average in his or her comprehension and use of language. Another may show just the opposite pattern. In addition, the relationship between all the dimensions of intellectual functioning may change from childhood to old age. Intelligence, then, is a living and complex function of a living and complex person, not a single attribute or dimension.

As people age, they may well improve in some aspects of mental functioning. They will know more about many subjects and become even more skilled in the use of their talents. Verbal comprehension scores, for example, do not flatten out and then decline after the twenties: 30- and 40-year-olds show better comprehension than 20-year-olds, and 50- and 60-year-olds even better.

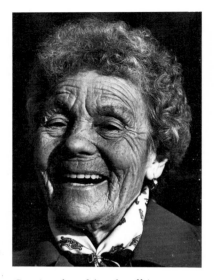

Staying cheerful and well is important to all of us. But as we grow old, and our bodies begin to let us down, it may help to keep our minds active, to derive a sense of purpose from some project however small.

The challenge of immediate tasks

Sometimes, however, individuals' stored-up knowledge is not enough to master the task before them. They must figure things out, solve the particular problem on its own terms instead of plucking the right answer out of their knowledge repertoire. Most people show a decline in this ability over the second half of life. If we wanted to put people into the old-age category as soon as the ability to master new and unusual problems goes into decline, however, we would have to be lying in ambush between the school and the office or factory.

We must be careful not to fall into the trap of using phrases such as "decline in intelligence" or "loss of ability to solve complex problems" to explain any changes in mental functioning we observe in the elderly. Intelligence, as we have emphasized in earlier chapters, is simply a word used to describe how individuals behave on certain tasks relative to others of the same age group. We can never, then, use this term to "explain" any changes in this behaviour. Likewise, since "ability" is often wrongly inferred from performance (we can never, in fact, know what ability someone has), we cannot use this concept in an explanatory way.

What we are actually talking about when we talk about changes in mental functioning with age are changes in behaviour. If we see problem-solving behaviour as similar to other skills, and as dependent on practice, then we can look much more constructively at age changes. It is not over-cynical to suggest, for example, that the kinds of abstract problems which psychologists include in intelligence tests are much more likely to be presented on an everyday basis to schoolchildren and adolescents than to the middle-aged and elderly. Until we can find some way of equating recent practice on such tasks across age groups, it seems premature to talk about a "decline" in intellectual functioning.

Learning new things

Virtually everyone remains capable of learning throughout his or her life. Illness and other factors, however, may make it more difficult for old people to learn new things. And when it may look as if old people have failed to grasp something, this is not always because they have not learned, but because they choose not to risk making a mistake (a caution which the old share with many younger people). At other times old people may have impairments that interfere with demonstrating what they have learned. One external "impairment" may be the presence of people who do not expect the old to learn and who never bother to ask their opinion on important topics.

Learning requires the accurate perception of information. For the old person, sensory deficits—in hearing and vision, for example—can impede this process. Again, many younger people suffer in the same way. Similarly, people who feel slighted, isolated or unwanted in a social situation—as do many elderly people—may be too preoccupied with inner distress to pay attention to what is going on around them. Small wonder that they subsequently cannot remember much of it.

Just how much an old person can achieve given the chance to learn something new was shown in a study where the researchers were struck by the great differences in mental decline and survival among different people as they aged. One study of personnel on the French railway system, for example, found that 20 per cent of the workforce showed virtually no decline, and that these people were those whose jobs provided a mental challenge.

The former study was conducted with a group of 80 old people, with an average age of 70 (the youngest was 63 and the eldest 91) and taught them German. The average IQ score for the group was 118. But although their intelligence level was above average, their experience of schooling was well below. Half the group had only primary schooling and only a quarter had completed secondary school.

After only three months of having one lesson a week, more than half the old people passed a formal exam at a level which schoolchildren normally take three *years* to reach. And after another three months, just under half the group passed at the 16-year-old matriculation standard. Just as striking as their actual achievement was the effect it had on the old people. The researchers comment:

> It is no exaggeration to say that the attitude of the majority of our students underwent a revolution before a few weeks had passed. So widespread and deep-rooted has the "old age" stereotype become in our society that it had been widely accepted by the elderly themselves. Those of them who had smiled disbelievingly at assurances of their capacity to succeed . . . could not escape the impact of their progress.

I remember . . .

The shape of memory changes for many people in later life. If our typical old people have one real complaint about their own mental functioning, it is likely to concern their memory for recent events. What happened in the distant past is clear in their minds (or they think it is), but not what happened a week ago last Monday.

The picture is even more complicated than this. Research shows that another type of memory must be distinguished: recall of immediate events. Old people in good health do not appear to suffer any particular problems in this area: they can remember what has just happened, can remember what happened decades ago, but have difficulty with the time in between.

Why these differences in memory? Current research suggests that several processes must function well if we are to have a sound memory. The experience has to register on us in the first place. Next, it must be entered into a sort of storage system where it is coded and becomes part of our personal data bank. We must also have an effective retrieval system, a way of searching through all that we have on file and coming up with the particular information we need at the moment.

Old people recalling events of 50 years ago are likely to remember those which were important to them and which by now are well rehearsed. It is also worth noting that they may not actually be very accurate—few listeners take the trouble to check! Some of our more recent experiences, however, may fail to "take". If we are distracted for psychological reasons or undergo a weakening in the physiological processes that support memory formation, then incoming information may not make a clear enough impression to become part of the long-term storage system.

Unfortunately, some of the ways in which the elderly try to cope with memory problems can create additional problems in everyday life. One person may withdraw from social interaction or a favourite activity because he is afraid that his memory problems will show. Another may develop habits that make life more complicated (changing the subject or picking an argument when she fears that her memory will be tested). Others borrow, bend or simply invent facts to replace those that do not come easily to mind. The problem with worrying about memory is that it becomes a self-fulfilling prophecy: preoccupied with anxiety about memory lapses, elderly people pay less attention to what is going on around them and therefore remember less. More satisfactory adjustments are usually made by those who acknowledge their memory problems—which, after all, are by no means confined to the elderly—and neither surrender to them nor try to cover them up.

Keeping a keen mind

In youth and middle age, some people are more mentally alert and vigorous than others. Keeping a keen mind tends to be habit-forming, a combination of fortunate genetic endowment and a life style that keeps the intellect well honed. Evidence suggests that those who start off with strong mental assets are more likely to preserve them throughout the lifespan. It is not just that their functioning remains high because it started high; the rate and amount of falling-off in old age appears to be smaller. In fact, studies of very bright people

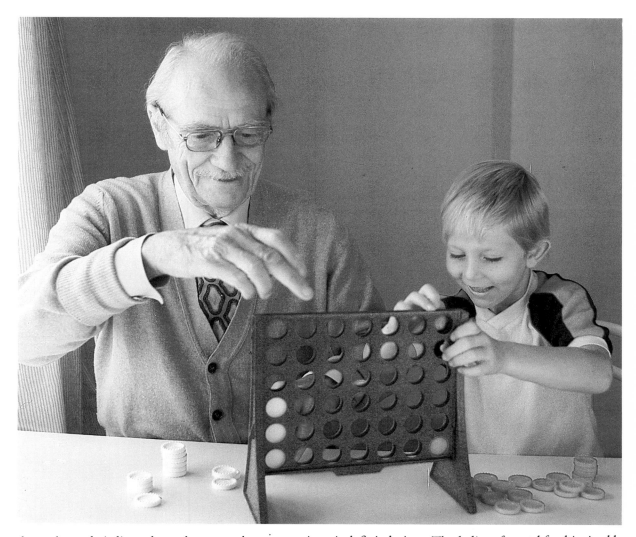

throughout their lives show that growth may continue indefinitely in some areas and show little, if any, decline in others. How we make use of what we have seems to be as important in the mental as the physical sphere.

Attitude and expectation play important roles here. Our society usually calls upon children to live up to expectations, but upon old people to live down to them. Old people can become the victims of the expectations they have absorbed earlier in life. It is the rare individual who can transcend the climate of such attitudes.

However, there is no reason to suppose that this process starts in old age: how many people continue to expect creative thoughts from themselves and others in middle age? Does our family life, our work, our culture in general reward us for reflective or innovative thinking? Looking back even further, do we leave school more interested in learning than when we entered? It is possible that the mentally inert old people are the victims of experiences throughout their lives rather than the products of any new problems encountered during old age.

The decline of mental faculties in old age is yet another of those myths which have been scientifically exploded but which remain in the people's minds as a "fact". Patterns of mental functioning, as we have seen, vary throughout life and are really changes in behaviour rather than in "intelligence" and "ability". Age does not diminish the capacity or the appetite to learn.

Keeping fit

The benefits of keeping fit are both physical and mental. For an elderly person fitness means maintaining mobility, greater resistance to disease and a better standard of general health. It also increases mental alertness and the ability to cope with stress or emotional problems. Because older people expect to become less active or more vulnerable to illness, many signs that only mean lack of fitness are put down to age and are not countered by positive action. But old age is not a disease, nor should illness and immobility be accepted as a necessary state.

Several basic points should be remembered in keeping fit. First and foremost, forget your age and don't let it become an excuse to retire from life. Watch your weight and keep up a diet that includes proteins, vitamins and carbohydrates for energy. Get some exercise every day and resist the temptation to take long naps in the daytime. Cut out or cut down on alcohol and cigarettes. Keep busy with a job, hobbies or chores at home. Visit a doctor if any health problem arises that signals a definite or sudden change.

Exercising keeps joints and muscles working smoothly and improves the functioning of the heart and circulatory system. Exercising the spine is important, to avoid backache or a stooping posture. When you start a sport or exercise routine, take it slowly and work into it naturally. Have a medical check-up before you start and follow a doctor's advice if you are disabled or have been ill.

Highly competitive sports and team games are stressful; choose an activity where you can set your own pace and enjoy its physical demands. Swimming uses most of the body muscles, tennis can be paced to the abilities of the players. Walking, jogging and cycling are good for keeping fit, or a gentle sport such as golf or bowling. Yoga and dancing classes offer exercise and pleasant social contact. If you prefer to be on your own there are many books that show routines to do at home.

There is no need to be over-ambitious—even a small amount of regular exercise is beneficial. Start walking short journeys instead of using car or bus; take stairs instead of lifts.

Keeping fit becomes a fashionable activity from time to time; its more dedicated proponents prove over a period of time how it helps them to age gracefully.

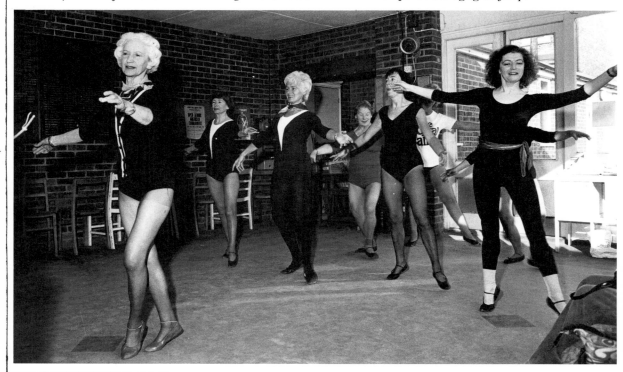

Exercising for mobility

These exercises are designed to mobilize the spine and hip joints and give the body practice in bending and stretching. This should become a daily routine, but exercise is not meant to be a form of self-punishment and the beneficial effects are cumulative. Don't force the body to do something it cannot or continue with actions that cause pain. After a few days of routine exercising, the joints gradually become flexible and the body more supple and these signs of improved fitness are the best incentive for continuing. If you are under medical care, ask your doctor before starting an exercise routine. Learn to monitor your pulse rate to avoid overdoing it.

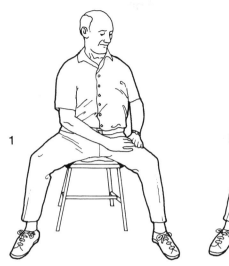

*Turning and stretching. Sit in a chair with feet apart and hands on thigh (**1**). Start to bend from the waist.*

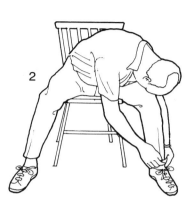

*Bend right over, sliding hands towards the ankle (**2**). Alternate left and right leg, 20 times in all.*

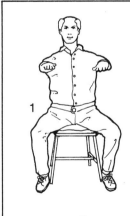
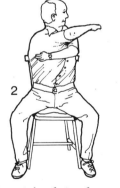
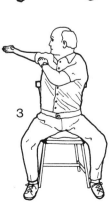

*Sit upright, facing forward with feet wide apart and arms outstretched (**1**). Turn head, shoulders and arms to the left (**2**), bending the right arm across the body. Turn slowly so movement is felt in trunk and spine only and keep the lower half of the body still. Repeat the exercise turning to the right with left arm bent (**3**). Repeat ten times each side.*

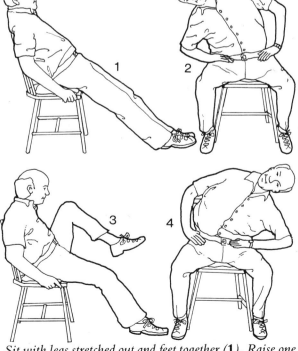

*Sit with legs stretched out and feet together (**1**). Raise one knee, bringing your head down (**2**). Repeat ten times. With hands on hips bend right (**3**) then left (**4**), ten times.*

Reacting to problems

How do old people cope with the problems that beset them? An inconvenience for one person may be a disaster for another. One person may accept a setback such as enforced retirement or a hip fracture as a challenge, another may be completely demoralized. The individual who can bear up well against one source of threat or loss may be extremely vulnerable to some other problem, even if "objectively" the other problem does not appear so important to an outsider.

The suffering of old people is sometimes unrecognized, because we assume it is natural for old age to be a time of low spirits. We often mistake old people's quiet withdrawal and lack of complaint as philosophical acceptance when, in fact, they are putting the best possible face on a bitterly disappointing, humiliating or frightening situation.

Either assumption—that it is normal to be unhappy or that old people are somehow content about, or resigned to, being unhappy—obstructs our view of the person's true state of mind. Signs of distress deserve attention in old age as much as at any point in the lifespan.

Loss and depression

Depression is one of the most common expressions of emotional distress in old men and women. We have seen that the two major psychological theories of depression emphasize the role of serious loss and individuals' belief that they no longer have control over important aspects of their environment.

If we apply these ideas to the lot of many old people, then it is not difficult to see why depression should be such a common reaction. Take, for example, two fairly common physical problems which face the elderly. A person may have an episode of incontinence. This can generate self-doubt, perhaps even shame. He or she may become reluctant to participate in social life out of fear of embarrassment, even after the episode has passed. The person would rather withdraw from human relationships than face possible rejection, avoidance, pity or ridicule. The trigger need not be incontinence. It can be skin changes, problems with hearing or vision—anything that threatens to reduce the person's status and functioning in society.

Limitations on physical mobility may spell disaster for other old people. This can involve a loss of control over one's environment—a loss so extensive it can be difficult for the healthy and mobile to imagine it. Old people too, for financial reasons, may be less able to take advantage of mobility aids: they may never have learned to drive or have sensory impairments which make driving impossible; they may live alone. All of this increases their dependence on other people or, in other words, decreases the amount of control they have over their environment.

Anxiety

It does not necessarily take the experience of loss or of loss of control to trigger depression. The anticipation of such losses can have the same effect. Anxiety is, in fact, the more common response to the anticipation of loss and, as we have seen, anxiety and depression tend

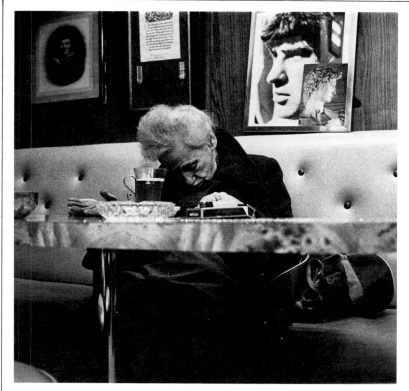

Loneliness

Loneliness is a problem of old age and though more people expect to be lonely than actually are when they become old, studies show that loneliness increases after retirement age. There are now more elderly people as a proportion of total population and more of them live alone. In an increasingly mobile society many live far from younger family members, and in old age a person may have outlived his or her spouse, contemporaries and friends by some years. Most would like to stay in their own homes and can be supplied with some services such as meals and health care—but not with the type or amount of companionship they would really like. Day centres, homes for the elderly and sheltered accommodation sometimes offer a greater degree of physical and emotional security although a certain amount of independence is lost.

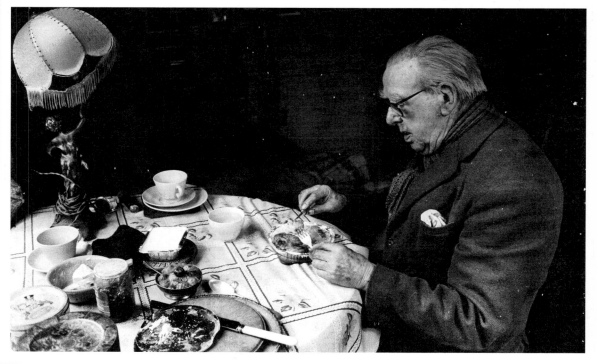

to go hand-in-hand. One mechanism whereby the anticipation of loss is heightened is through vicarious learning: we learn what may happen to us by observing what happens to others. Obviously, anyone can look around and see impending disaster everywhere, quoting examples of others' misfortune. But we can also look around and see a great deal of good fortune. Whether these observations make us happy or anxious depends partly on the probability we attach to events happening to us.

The mechanisms by which people attach (and distort) such probabilities are a fascinating area of psychology which is only beginning to be researched. For the old person, however, two factors are likely to be important in this process. One is the amount of similarity which is perceived between the observer and the observed. If a 25-year-old man sees someone being knocked down by a car or being committed to hospital and later discovers that the person was also 25, he is very unlikely to use this information to adjust his estimates of whether these events will happen to him. But so ready are we to use age as a spurious causal factor in talking about the elderly that an old person could be forgiven for assuming that when such events happen to another old person, then age itself has something to do with it. Thus, the probability that the event will happen to him or her may seem to increase.

The second factor is that the real rate of occurrence of positive and negative events is probably weighted towards the negative end for many of the elderly. To make things worse, when positive events *do* occur—remarriage at 80, fathering a child at 70, obtaining a degree at 75—we tend to talk about such things being achieved *in spite of* the person's age, as if to emphasize to old people that they need not get distorted ideas about what *they* might look forward to. Small wonder that the elderly are often anxious and depressed about the future.

What do the signs of depression mean?

An added problem is that although depression tends to show itself in similar ways throughout adult life, in old age it can be difficult to know where a physical difficulty ends and depression begins. Reduced appetite and an inability to get a good night's sleep, for example, are among the clues that suggest depression. But old people may choose to eat less and have sleep difficulties for reasons other than depression. It is when an entire pattern begins to emerge that we should seriously consider the possibility of a depressive reaction.

The pattern is likely to include reduced and slowed-down speech; the person may also seem to be thinking more slowly. There is less attention to personal grooming. Energy is lacking for even routine activities. A general feeling of pessimism prevails and life appears increasingly grim and hopeless. There may be talk of feeling empty inside and of being a useless, worthless person. The future holds nothing; the past is no source of comfort; the present moment is intolerable. Depressed individuals usually turn their feelings against themselves; sometimes they also lash out in anger at other people.

In such a condition, there is a heightened risk to survival. Suicide is one possibility—and the suicide rate in old age is high, especially among white males. But there are also other ways in which old people may endanger their own lives. They may neglect a medical regime that is necessary to control an illness such as diabetes. They may limit

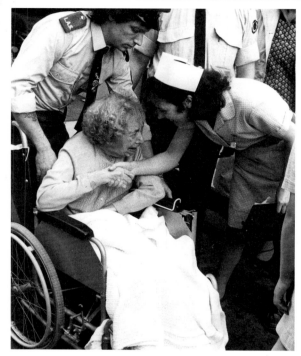

A hospital becomes home for some in old age. This old lady cries from the pain of parting, on being transferred from a hospital that is closing down.

PHYSICAL HAZARDS OF OLD AGE

Disease and chronic ailments In old age people are susceptible to illnesses causing accompanying disability—rheumatism and arthritis, impaired sight and hearing are relatively common, as are diseases of the heart and circulatory system.

Malnutrition Some old people feel they cannot afford to eat properly and a greater number lose appetite through illness, anxiety or depression. Poor diet undermines health, lowering resistance to disease. In addition, chronic digestive disorders may reduce the value of food intake. Decaying teeth or ill-fitting dentures interfere with chewing, often causing the person to prefer low protein foods because they are easy to swallow.

Loss of fitness Some muscles and joints are more used than others through life and those that have been neglected stiffen or weaken with age. Most people expect to slow down and fail to realize the importance of continuing to exercise and keep fit.

Accidents All the above factors put old people at greater risk of accidents, such as falls and collisions. The damage from a fall may aggravate other health problems.

Sexual deprivation There is evidence that a happy sexual relationship helps prolong life.

themselves to bed and chair, becoming increasingly inactive and thus vulnerable to degenerative processes and infections. Unsociable behaviour, often characteristic of depression, may also drive away the people who would otherwise shield them from a number of life-threatening circumstances.

Perturbed old people may also show their distress in other ways, either along with or alternating with depression. They may be agitated, confused, paranoid, go through episodes of keyed-up manic behaviour. Some people express their distress indirectly through physical complaints, intensifying existing physical problems and developing new problems by emotional upset. It requires a wise person as well as a competent clinician to respond to the true distress that is represented by this mixture of physical and psychological complaints.

The intimate connection between psychological and physical distress in the elderly can reveal itself in many ways. An episode of mental confusion, for example, might be interpreted as "just old age", "going a little crazy" or being upset about some personal situation. In fact, it may instead be a symptom of a myocardial infarction or congestive heart failure. Emotional distress and mental confusion in old age can be, at the same time, a response to psychosocial problems and to serious physical disease processes. Such possibilities should not be dismissed out of hand.

Jumping to conclusions

Though the physical problems of the elderly are sometimes wrongly interpreted as psychological, the opposite danger is just as great. Episodes of mental confusion or memory difficulties can easily be interpreted as signs of "senility". And not only is the lay person at fault here: an international mental health team found that many elderly patients are diagnosed as suffering from "senility" when their problems are actually functional.

Few of us are at our best mentally when our bodies are beset by illness, distress or fatigue. We tend to be more charitable to ourselves than we are to old people. ("I'm not feeling well, he's senile.") Malnutrition is a common cause of mental confusion, whether from a bad or an inadequate diet. So too is tiredness, possibly due to worry, depression and fearfulness. Drugs administered to treat a physical condition may also result in mental confusion.

The psychosocial effects of hospitalization can be deeply disturbing for people of all ages. An individual who has always been a rather private person and who now finds herself among strangers in a hospital ward may withdraw socially and lose some contact with the world around her. If treatment is carried out in a way that strips her of her identity and self-respect, this too can precipitate a mental flight that closely resembles senility.

There is now a considerable body of research which shows that "normal", much younger people are severely stressed by the experience of hospitalization. Most patients, for example, remember very little of what they are told by doctors and nurses; many deny ever having received any information at all about their illness—this is particularly the case when people are told about terminal illness. These memory lapses are probably partly caused by the way in which the information is given, but the stress of hospitalization is also to blame. It is not uncommon for patients of any age to forget what day it is, because one day is just like another, but we do not bother to apply the label "disoriented in time" to young people.

Old people in hospital are likely to be doubly stressed. Not only are conditions in geriatric wards often inferior to those in other wards, but patients have the added worry of whether they will ever go home again. Surrounded by similarly stressed and possibly senile patients, there is ample opportunity for vicarious learning which heightens anxiety even more.

Answering distress

No single principle of mental health can guarantee that a person will pass through the challenges and perils of a long life without experiencing distress. Indeed, he or she would probably be a less complex and fulfilled person for having done so. However, it is within our abilities to reduce the depth and frequency of suffering and to help each other when our own resources are temporarily overrun.

In old age, distress can be more acute, because immediate problems bring to mind earlier difficulties. Old people may be haunted by memories of stressful events as far back as early childhood. Tormented by both past and present, they may feel helpless. At the same time, there may be fewer resources available to cope with problems in the immediate situation—fewer people to share experiences with, less physical control over the environment and so on.

We can help such people by encouraging them to use all the control they still have and by supporting them in all their remaining areas of vigour and competence. Unfortunately, the opposite often happens: old people who lose control over one area of their lives may be placed in an institution which, perhaps with the best of intentions, deprives them of control even in areas where they still remain competent.

We can also hear out distressed old people, listening carefully to their sorrows and alarms. This sharing is not only useful in itself, but can also help old people to realize that problems of the past need not continue to weigh upon them today. We can help each other by giving support and security without asking a high psychological price for it. An impaired or emotionally upset old person should be helped without asking for anything in return, and without unnecessary invasion of privacy or deprivation of rights in the name of welfare.

Old people who face difficult life situations or have emotional problems often benefit from psychological consultations. This possibility, however, seldom presents itself to them, for many grew up in the pre-psychotherapy era. It must also be said that there are relatively few counsellors and therapists who appreciate the contribution they could make in this area. Fortunately, however, some clinicians have opened themselves to the challenge and discovered that psychotherapy can prove effective with the old as well as with the young. It is to be hoped that individual and group therapy will become increasingly available and acceptable to the elderly.

There is general agreement that there is a higher percentage of people suffering emotional distress in old age than at any other time in adult life. Yet the provision of mental health services for the elderly is much below the average. The gap between need and suitable care is all too often filled by dubious measures, such as heavy-handed prescription of drugs.

The shadow of senility

We have mentioned several times the dangers of glibly attributing an old person's memory lapses or temporary mental confusion to "senility". What exactly is this condition so often mistakenly invoked to account for the behaviour of the elderly?

The word "senile" is used by physicians and gerontologists in connection with a cluster of genuine brain diseases and disorders. Senile dementia and senile psychosis, too, are regarded by some physicians and psychologists as separate conditions, while others believe that senile brain disease is one basic disorder that simply shows up in a variety of ways.

What are the characteristics of the type of old person most clinicians would consider "senile"? Among the most obvious are those in the realm of thought. One of our most valuable assets is our ability to develop and grasp abstractions. People who are accurately classified as senile have often lost this type of cognitive ability. They think concretely. In other words, they miss the relationships and implications that both give richer meaning to experience and help to solve problems. If, for example, a senile person is asked how an apple and an orange are alike, he or she may reply, "Oranges don't grow around here," and then repeat this answer several times—an accurate statement, though it fails to answer the question.

Senility may also include serious difficulties with memory. The memory impairment is greatest for recent events. Yesterday may draw a blank. The person may not even recall something that happened 10 minutes ago. Problems with memory are also experienced by many people who are old, but not senile. However, memory loss is more radical and extensive in senility. Isolated memories may remain accessible, but memory is lost as a general resource for coping with life.

Another very important problem is lack of attention. The alertness and concentration needed to register new experience seems to be missing or is undependable. A senile man may not remember what you said a moment ago, because he could not summon up the kind of sustained attention necessary for the information to take hold in his mind in the first place.

So it is not surprising that senile people often have great difficulty in coping with even the routine tasks and challenges of life, let alone with situations that arouse special anxiety or make special demands. Senility may therefore show itself in other aspects of behaviour. The senile individual may withdraw from interaction with others, have difficulty in keeping himself or herself clean and groomed, suffer accidents related to forgetfulness or misunderstanding and so on.

Overcoming difficulties

Although there is as yet no "cure" for senile brain disease, we must realize that the comfort and wellbeing of an afflicted person can be improved even when a progressive disease process does exist. Environments can be adapted to allow for a measure of independence together with safety. Instead of isolation the person with senile brain disease can be given the opportunity of continued social contact in a warm and friendly setting. Research has demonstrated improvements in mental and physical functioning when the senile aged are moved to a socially enriched environment. Damaged brain cells have not been repaired, but the individual becomes motivated to make better use of his remaining function.

Good nutrition and careful use of medication and exercise can also dramatically improve the condition of those with brain disease. There is great satisfaction in seeing serenity, dignity and self-esteem return to an old man or woman who has been treated with respect. We may find ourselves with a person whose strong character or gentle radiance remains intact despite the ravages of illness, instead of a stranger for the person we once knew.

We must also understand the continual effort of a jeopardized and stressed old person to cope with his difficulties and to make the best he can of the situation. Although he may "confabulate", reporting incidents that never happened, this in itself is a creative though impaired action. It is an attempt to compensate for the gaps carved in a failing memory.

Is she not paying attention to what is happening in this room? Perhaps this is because she is deeply engrossed in events taking place within her own mind and body, problems to be met or resources to be salvaged out of the range of all perception but hers. Even when senile-type behaviour appears quite bizarre and ineffective, it often has the same goals as our own behaviour: to understand, to relieve anxiety, to achieve safety, to feel like a person.

Changes in the central nervous system

Cerebral arteriosclerosis—the hardening and narrowing of blood vessels serving the brain. The resulting inadequate supply of nutrients and oxygen leads to deterioration or death of the afflicted brain cells. The process begins at 50 in some, with men being more vulnerable. Heredity, environmental pollution and cholesterol have been implicated as influences. Other common vascular problems include "little strokes"—they produce temporary confusion, dizziness and nausea, often causing residual damage. Ischaemic attacks (temporary reduction of oxygen to the brain) can have lasting effects, showing in a fitful or episodic pattern, although the person improves to some extent after the episode.

Senile dementia—Surprisingly little is known about this condition. The most striking feature is the widespread atrophy (wasting) of cells in the cerebral cortex, as distinguished from the patchy effects of cerebral arterio-sclerosis. The damage is also independent of changes in blood vessels. Heredity is thought to play a part, along with certain psychological traits; and the environment also contributes. The disease usually expresses itself in the form of steady and gradual deterioration.

Unfortunately, both types of brain damage are progressive and there is little in the way of treatment or cures—both progressively disable the afflicted and shorten their lives.

Leisure activities

Leisure is all too often defined as the absence of work, surely a hangover from the Protestant work ethic and the days when unemployed people were popularly branded as "shirkers" or "work-shy". With high unemployment in many Western countries and the advent of new technology which will replace whole sections of the workforce with machines, new definitions of the concept of leisure are being explored.

Most men retiring in the 1980s will have worked all their adult lives with only short holiday breaks. Women are likely to have had long periods away from paid employment working in the home bringing up a family, but they too will have had little opportunity to pursue leisure activities. Research has shown that there are three main patterns of leisure and work. There is the 'opposition' pattern where leisure activities are deliberately different from those at work (e.g. a factory worker might race motor cycles); the second pattern is one where work extends into leisure (e.g. a teacher may volunteer for a literacy scheme); and third, a matching of passive work (e.g. a sedentary office job) with passive leisure (e.g. watching television).

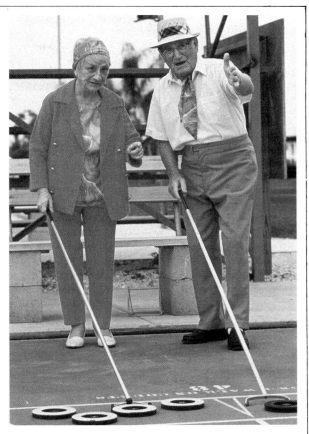

A competitive sport need not be arduous. A gentle game of curling or golf can be great fun, and a way of keeping fit and meeting people.

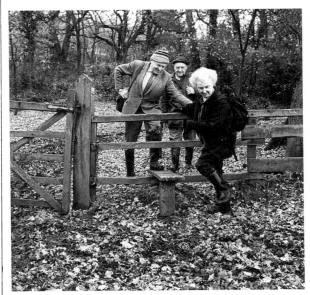

Though much else has changed, there is still some new countryside to be explored, its flora and fauna observed, at a leisurely, rambling pace.

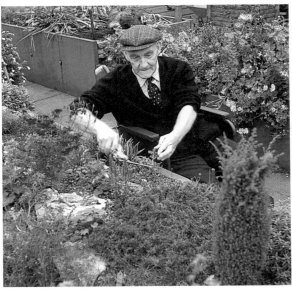

A gardener's world can be scaled to fit ability, if not ambition. Both the fit and the disabled can enjoy the pleasure of making things grow.

Love and intimacy in later life

Studies of sexual interest through the lifespan show that it remains, if somewhat less strongly, in both elderly men and women. These studies also confirm what is true for middle age—that active young lovers are more likely to become active old lovers.

Physical responses

The problems faced by elderly men or women attempting to retain their sexuality are similar to those faced by the middle-aged—only more so. The gradual "slowing down" of the male physical response, first noticed in middle age, may become more marked. But the brain remains the major sexual organ, and in any individual it is almost impossible to separate out the physical from the psychological factors involved in sexual functioning. Physical excitement, performance and enjoyment follow naturally when we think ourselves into passion. By the same token, the physical side of loving can be disconnected through a negative mental state. It is most likely that the major barriers to sexual intimacy in later life are to be found in the mind. This is true even when physical problems *do* exist: many of us (including the elderly themselves) assume that old people do not have much of a sex life. Why? Because they *cannot*. But if they could? Well, then, they shouldn't!

Preparing for courtship

To maintain a sexual relationship, or to start new ones, elderly people must overcome strong expectations and admonitions to the contrary. Families and neighbours sometimes act as though the intimate relationships of an old person needed their approval. Their grown children may behave as though the old person were in fact an inexperienced, impulsive adolescent who could embarrass them by "doing something foolish", such as falling in love or sprucing up as a candidate for romance. It is easy to surrender to subtle and not so subtle pressures and declare oneself no longer a sexual being.

It is not only the negative attitudes of society that must be overcome. Unfortunately, the general life styles of many old people are a long way from anyone's romantic ideal. Their immediate physical environment, the clothes they wear, the activities they can share—many of the elements that contribute to the "feel" of everyday life—are often limited by finances. Even basic requirements may be lacking. The old man may lack the hearing aid that would help natural, intimate dialogue; the old woman may be wearing glasses that have needed replacing for a long time. He might feel more like a live man if he had a smart addition to his wardrobe and the means to take his partner somewhere special. She might feel more special herself if she could afford a beauty treatment now and then. Both might feel more ready for sexual intimacy if they lived in a less noisy and dingy neighbourhood. Lusty, healthy young adults can more easily overcome the distractions, inconveniences and even ugliness that surrounds them. Nevertheless, most young lovers will prefer certain settings that make them feel "right". Old lovers could benefit even more from an environment conducive to ease, stimulation and pleasure.

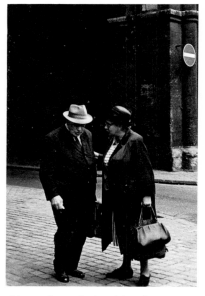

Above: In a relationship of many years standing, a sense of intimacy runs through day-to-day behaviour as well as the peaks and troughs of shared emotions. The very set of people's bodies can announce a connection, whatever the subject of their discussion may be.

Below: Contrary to popular belief, there is no basic reason why physical intimacy need decline in later years, although practical reasons, such as loss of a partner or illness, may prevent it.

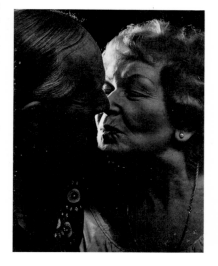

Sex in later years

In spite of all these barriers, there are hopeful indications that the elderly *do* manage to maintain sexual intimacy. For instance, in some longitudinal studies conducted at Duke University (North Carolina) it was found that at 68 years of age, about 70 per cent of men still regularly enjoyed sexual activity, while 25 per cent still did so at 78. Kinsey, who collected his data some 30 years earlier, reported that about 80 per cent of 60-year-olds and 20 per cent of 80-year-olds were still having sexual intercourse. Similar figures were found for women.

In the absence of any data, we can only speculate about the reasons for the rather large drop in those engaging in sexual intercourse between the ages of 70 and 80. Some of it is almost certainly accounted for by serious illness which would prevent sexual activity, or by the loss of a partner by death. The Duke studies reported, however, that in marriages which remained intact, it was the husband who was usually responsible for the cessation of sexual activity. Again, we do not know for certain why this should be so, but it may be because changes in what is mistakenly called "sexual prowess" can be more marked in men than in women. Indeed, it could be argued that the concept of sexual prowess is distinctly male. It was stressed in "Middle age" that these changes by no means signal the end of sexual activity, although they are interpreted by many men in this way. If we add real physical problems, or just aches and pains and psychological pressures to this natural slowing down, then it is not surprising that many old men see sexual intercourse as a daunting, rather than a pleasurable activity.

Sex as reassurance

The importance of a sustained love relationship in old age is hard to overestimate. Sex brings more than direct physical gratification, although this itself is not to be slighted. It also reaffirms each partner's identity as a person who can offer something worthwhile, who can *be* someone worthwhile to another person. The body is still a means of giving and receiving pleasure. Old lovers like their bodies better than those who have closed this chapter of their lives.

There is another important function of sexual intimacy in old age. Old people are all too often "typecast" by the outside world. They are the secondary characters, belonging on the fringe of the real action. We tend to remain at an emotional distance from them. Every day we walk past, almost *through* old people on the street, without clearly registering them as individuals.

How and where are old people to find reassurance that they are truly individuals? That their distinctive personality has not been forgotten? That they mean something to somebody? Surely, they cannot rely on the sad image of themselves that is reflected back to them by society.

The intimacy of two people who have shared joys and sorrows or even who just met a short time ago and have found each other lovable is an excellent buffer against a world that looks at old people, but does not really see them. In each other's arms, even if their intimacy does not conclude in intercourse, they continue to be themselves rather than society's impoverished image of the aged. The small intimacies, the quiet conversation, the sense of togetherness remain both precious and life-affirming.

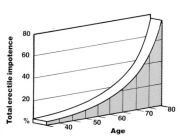

Erectile impotence

Although men do not experience a phenomenon equivalent to the menopause—there is no abrupt cessation of hormonal activity— they may experience a gradual decline in potency. This is manifested as erectile impotence. However elderly couples need not be deprived of a happy sexual relationship. With understanding, the problem is not insuperable.

It's never too late to love. Hector Hughes was married at the age of 79 to Elsa Lillian, aged a mere 70 years. This picture shows the pride, pleasure and sense of occasion in both of them as they walk out together after the marriage ceremony.

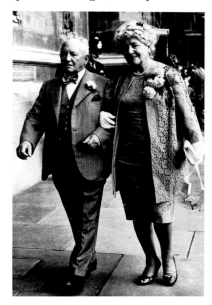

Making a will

It may be appropriate to draw up a will at any time in adulthood, but many people put off the moment. They may think they have little of value to leave, or find it morbid to contemplate disposal of their property after death. Making a will, however, is a simple procedure that will relieve some of your own anxieties and make matters easier for friends and relatives.

Why make a will? Your property is the measure of your investment of time and money throughout life, so it is only right that you wish to choose how it is handed on after your death. It enables you to provide for your family or give them a little extra, or to leave small items or sums of money to specially close friends.

Even if you want to leave everything to your spouse and children, it is advisable to make a will that expresses that purpose in precise and unambiguous language. If you die intestate then your property will be distributed under the intestate succession statutes.

In the United States, the capacity to make a will is defined by the laws of each state. In general, however, the legal age for making a will is usually twenty-one, and the testator has the relative freedom to bequeath or devise his property as he chooses.

Within certain boundaries you are at liberty to dispose of your interests in any legal manner. For instance, you may

choose to disinherit one who might otherwise have had an intestate claim; or you might pass property to a person or an institution. This freedom for distribution is not so unlimited in France and other civil law countries.

Drawing up the will Having made the decision to draw up a will it is best to consult a lawyer. Wills can be drawn up on any writing material, but, to be valid, they must be executed strictly in accordance with statutory formalities and signed by the testator with the signature of two or sometimes three witnesses. The witnesses should *not* be beneficiaries under the will.

Amendments to the will may be made at any time. This is known as a codicil, a postscript to the will, and it must be signed by you as the testator and witnessed in the same manner as the original will.

Obviously, British law provides its own rules for drawing up a will, and again, it is best to enlist the services of a solicitor to sort out the ambiguities of legal jargon. In brief, a valid will must be in writing, signed by you, or a proxy, and signed or acknowledged in the presence of two or more witnesses. An executor will be appointed to ensure that the terms of the will are carried out.

A Living Will — a document enabling a person of sound mind to ensure that their wishes are carried out if they are overtaken by a disability which deems them unfit to make decisions.

To My Family, My Physician, My Lawyer and All Others Whom It May Concern

Death is as much a reality as birth, growth, maturity and old age—it is the one certainty of life. If the time comes when I can no longer take part in decisions for my own future, let this statement stand as an expression of my wishes and directions, while I am still of sound mind.

If at such a time the situation should arise in which there is no reasonable expectation of my recovery from extreme physical or mental disability, I direct that I be allowed to die and not be kept alive by medications, artificial means or "heroic measures" I do, however, ask that medication be mercifully administered to me to alleviate suffering even though this may shorten my remaining life.

This statement is made after careful consideration and is in accordance with my strong convictions and beliefs. I want the wishes and directions here expressed carried out to the extent permitted by law. Insofar as they are not legally enforceable, I hope that those to whom this Will is addressed will regard themselves as morally bound by these provisions.

(Optional specific provisions to be made in this space — see other side)

Optional proxy statement I hereby designate _____
to make treatment decisions for me in the event I am comatose or otherwise unable to make such decisions for myself.

Optional Notarization   Signed_____

"Sworn and subscribed to   Date _____
before me this _____ day
of _____, 19_____"   Witness _____

                                                                    Witness _____

Notary Public
(seal)

Copies of this request have been given to _____

_____

(Optional) My Living Will is registered with Concern for Dying (No. _____)

A home full of strangers

Weathering the storms of old age sometimes needs the kind of shelter that an institutional setting can provide. Generally, it is the older person who is institutionalized. In the United States, for example, the average age of those in nursing homes is about 82. The shift in the population balance towards the old means that, like it or not, the old-age "home" will be with us for years to come.

The process of "institutionalization"
This word suggests something heavy and massive. And it does mean something far more than simply moving someone from one place to another. During the settling–in period, the old people have to come to terms with all aspects of their new environment. Perhaps the fact that the process is known as institutionalization rather than "individualization" makes it clear that the people must adjust more to the home than the home will to them. It is a difficult process, at any age.

The upheaval often begins before the old man or woman even arrives at the new home. Something has already gone wrong, otherwise he or she would not be moving. It may be illness; it may be the loss of a protective person or a place to live. This means that the old person and the family are both vulnerable and perturbed. Although institutionalization is seen as the solution, it can make the family feel guilty and the old person feel abandoned. Although this may not be objectively true, it would be unwise to ignore the very serious problems which can arise when the elderly are cared for in their own or their relatives' homes. In "Middle age" we discussed research showing that the burden of care most often falls on women, whether or not the old person is their parent. Recent, and disturbing, reports suggest that violence against the elderly by their relatives is not uncommon. Not surprisingly, the victims are reluctant to report such incidents and indeed may have no opportunity to do so.

Moving out of reluctance
Thus, the move to an institution may be made in desperation on both sides. But even if this is not the case, after years of living as an integral part of the family, the old person now faces a wrenching separation. Added to this anxiety is the dread of what the institution will be like.

Many studies of institutionalization show how many psychological changes can occur beforehand. Sheldon Tobin and Morton Lieberman studied 100 people on a waiting list for entry to a home for the aged in a large metropolitan area. There was one comparison group of 35 old people living in the community and not anticipating institutionalization, and another comparison group of 37 who were already residents of institutions. The researchers found that the psychological characteristics of the institutionalized aged were already shown by those on the waiting list. Amongst these, Tobin and Lieberman found ". . . a tendency towards apathy, condoning or passively accepting what life has brought, somewhat negative feelings about having accomplished what is regarded as important, plus tendencies towards self-criticism, depression, bitterness or irritability".

There are at least two possible overlapping explanations. Deterio-

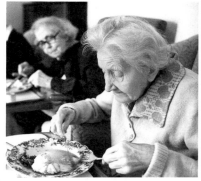

Wherever you are, sooner or later you must eat. Is this a sign of settling in, accepting a new home? For some, regular meals are a welcome symbol of care and security; for others, one more ordeal to be faced in a strange environment.

ration of the old person's life situation can cause the kind of feelings described, and also adds to the likelihood of institutionalization. The prospect of the move can also be depressing in itself.

The study also found that those on the waiting list had more problems and limitations than those who had been living in institutions for more than a year. Those who had settled in for an extended stay were found to be more emotionally responsive, less anxious and more efficient in mental functioning than old people still waiting to move in.

Threats to identity

Anxiety and dread sometimes reach new heights as a person actually enters the institution, even if a brave face is shown to the world. Weeping in private, staring at the wall, loss of appetite and other signs of distress may follow later, despite best intentions to be content with the move.

The impact of the move can be softened in many ways. In some places, staff members visit the old person's own home several times before admission to get to know them and answer questions. Sometimes, the prospective resident visits the institution.

The person may bring his or her cherished possessions, which help give a sense of continuity and identity. Staff members may make special efforts to reassure the newcomer, and other residents are actively welcoming and friendly.

Unfortunately, well-meaning staff sometimes add to a newcomer's distress by an inappropriate show of familiarity. They are not fully aware of the crisis of identity that the old person is experiencing. Individuals have already lost some of the components of their usual life style, and one of the few remaining firm clues to their identity is their name. Yet a perfect stranger may bypass the newcomer's proper name and proceed immediately to a first-name greeting. Mrs Donaldson is transformed into Elizabeth, or more likely, into Beth or Bessy. She may even be reduced to an all-purpose "dearie" or "love". This may seem a small matter, but it exemplifies many of the little-big ways in which institutionalization makes its inroads. The name is detached from the person and replaced with a generalized term that does not acknowledge the individual's unique self. The message is clear: "Who you were before does not count for much here. Just slip into the identity we give you and we'll get along fine."

The older person entering an institution for the first time—and knowing it may be his or her last dwelling place on earth—may naturally experience these and other aspects of institutional life, such as loss of privacy or the right to choose when one eats or sleeps, as personal onslaughts against his or her integrity. But it is just the way the system works. The staff may have the wellbeing of the residents very much at heart, but still function along the mechanical channels of a "total" institution.

Settling in—the need for caution

Research by social gerontologists has found that newcomers to institutions receive very little help in making a compromise between their previous life habits and the structure of the institution. The rules are often not made explicit at the start. It appears to newcomers that there is very little the residents are expected to do, very few roles that

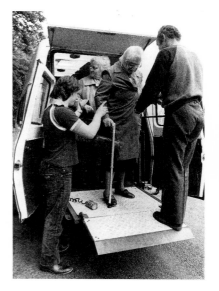

As the average age of the population increases, more and more old people live in institutions. For some they are havens and for others a prison. The period of adjustment to new surroundings and loss of independence is crucial. Schemes to improve facilities and to introduce smaller residential units are being explored, but far more assistance needs to be offered to people who prefer to live in their own homes.

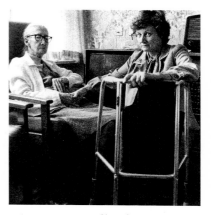

The experience of loneliness is a common one, but there are now neighbourhood schemes which aim to ensure that old people who live alone are visited regularly. Sharing past experiences breaks down the barriers of age.

can bring personal satisfaction and gain social approval. In all too many settings, the less the person does the better. This is a very difficult situation in which to learn and adapt at any age. It is exactly the kind of setting which produces the apathy, social withdrawal and mental inefficiency which, to add insult to injury, is wrongly labelled "senility" and then used to justify the nothingness in which the old person is expected to function.

The early days of institutionalization may be marked by excessive caution ("What if I do something wrong and make them angry?"), and by little incidents that unfairly establish a reputation that sticks ("She's a stubborn one", "He's confused"). Some old people take more readily to living in groups, preferring others to run things for them. It gives them a sense of security and helps them to relax. People like this have often had earlier experience of living in institutional settings and know how to "learn the ropes" and make the best of things. But those who have lived much more private lives are ill-prepared by experience or temperament for this type of arrangement.

The early days of institutionalization are critical. An old person's anxiety about separation from home, and dread of what awaits him or her, may intensify any existing physical, psychological and social problems. It is a time when "home" should provide the most sensitive and comprehensive care. Thus when the possibility of institutionaliz-

CARING FOR OLD PEOPLE AT HOME

Surveys show that a significant number of elderly people who cannot cope alone live with or rely upon their family, despite some state provision of services and accommodation for old people. This may mean staying in their own homes with frequent visits from relatives, or living with a daughter or son and younger family members. Both parties must adjust to rearrangement of living space and the resumption of closeness in a relationship that may have become quite distant.

Roles and relationships When an elderly person moves into the home, the earlier parent-child relationship is effectively reversed. The senior parent, giving up the autonomy and authority of living alone, must learn to accept dependence on his or her child. A middle-aged person looking after a parent may already have young or still dependent children—there are considerable demands on his or her time and energy and probably increased financial burdens. The day-to-day responsibility falls more heavily on women—a daughter or daughter-in-law, since they are usually the ones running the home or may themselves be coping alone. When the old person is a woman used to having control of a household, there can be awkward clashes even over quite trivial aspects of everyday life. Resent-

ment tends to be more noticeable between in-laws than among blood relatives, but this depends greatly on the nature of the parent-child relationship in earlier years. If there is a history of loving care in the family no problems need arise; but many elderly parents and adult children are forced to live together although they have never got on well. A lot of give and take is needed among people who may all be set in their ways.

Physical and psychological needs Privacy is extremely important and it is vital that the old person has a separate room or flat that is a private domain. It is best if it is quiet and on one level of the house to save stair climbing, and independence is increased if it is large enough to be equipped with cooking facilities and, if possible, a bathroom. Warmth and good lighting are necessary. The person should have storage space and shelving for personal possessions, and a comfortable chair. A television may also be a good idea. If the old person is disabled, special equipment for washing and cooking can be installed, in the private apartment or in the family bathroom and kitchen. If he or she is still quite mobile, it is an advantage if shops and local facilities are nearby so that outside interests and social life can be independent of the family at least part of the time.

ing an old person arises, it is vital that the most suitable institution is chosen. There must also be ample social and emotional support during the critical period after admission.

A new-found family

Those who settle into long stays at homes for the aged often find friends among other residents and staff and eventually come to regard them as family. This is an interesting phenomenon. It seems most likely to happen when family visits become infrequent or cease altogether, or when stability amongst institutional staff allows good relationships to develop. Residents are genuinely comforted by the presence of their new family, and staff may also go well beyond mere job requirements in caring for the "grandmother" or "uncle" they have come to love. The situation sometimes seems to represent the triumph of humanity over the impersonal institutional process.

Nevertheless, loneliness, isolation and the tedium of having nothing to do characterize the lives of many old people during extended stays in institutions. This is more likely to be true in large homes, and seems to happen when the institution gets beyond the size of a large private house. The difference between a 100-resident and a 500-resident home in terms of psychological adaptation may be less than the difference between a 25- and 50-resident home. This is now well known to many administrators, and more attempts are being made to establish smaller residential settings in which everyone has a greater opportunity to feel at home.

New outlooks on institutions

Institutions for the aged are changing. Staff are better qualified, facilities are more varied. The best also respect the individual life styles of the residents, as far as any institution allows. Some even attempt to introduce elements of life outside, such as sheltered workshops, congenial pubs and clubs for people with common interests.

There are also signs that thought is being given to alternatives to institutionalization. Home care organizations are helping aged people to remain in the community, looking after people where they live, without requiring them to move into a home. These services can be as simple as assistance with shopping, or meals-on-wheels. Old people who live in large houses can have them converted to provide homes for a small number of elderly people, while the "owner" retains his or her home. Specially adapted group homes with a resident caretaker are becoming more popular.

The possibilities of such means of helping old people to maintain their style of life and their all-important control over their environment have not yet been fully explored. There are many parallels here with our attitudes to the disabled and the mentally retarded: we cannot seem to resist taking control from them in the name of care, rather than providing an environment which would enable them to help themselves.

However, there comes a point in the lives of some old people when physical disability increases beyond the reach of either individual or social coping. The very old and very frail will probably always need to be admitted to institutions, indeed it is in their best interests. Long-term homes will probably become increasingly committed to people who need total care.

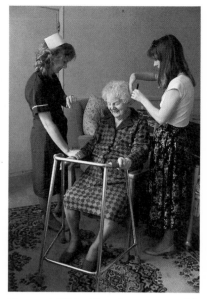

Once established in a home, some old people enjoy the benefits of the new environment—company, attention, security, warmth, and nourishing, regular meals.

Prodigies and myths

Some commonly held beliefs about ageing

★ Most old people are senile
★ Most old people have no interest in or capacity for sexual relations
★ At least one-tenth of the aged live in institutions
★ Older people do not work as effectively as young people
★ Old people cannot learn anything
★ Older people become more religious
★ Old people are set in their ways

These are all fallacies. The myths of decline and decay in ageing are amply discredited by a look at a few of the most well-known examples of remarkable old people.

★ Florie Ball undertook a 200-mile journey by motorcycle aged 77.
★ Coco Chanel retired in 1938 but returned in 1954 aged 71 to run her Paris salon for 17 years.
★ Eamon De Valera was President of Ireland until the age of 91.
★ Sigmund Freud wrote *Moses and Monotheism* at 83.
★ Goethe completed *Faust* at 83.
★ Victor Hugo was 81 when he published his last novel.
★ Dr Malley Kachel, at 94, was the oldest practising doctor in Germany.
★ Duncan Maclean, the "Tartan Flash" sprinted 100 yds almost daily at 91.
★ Margaret Mead the anthropologist made a field trip to New Guinea aged 72.

How many people would care to run a marathon at any age? Yet there are always a surprising number of elderly participants ready to face one more athletic challenge.

★ Claude Monet was painting until shortly before his death at 86.
★ Anna Mary Moses—"Grandma" Moses—began painting in oils aged 78.
★ Bertrand Russell chose to go to prison aged 89 in his protest against nuclear weapons.
★ Giuseppe Verdi composed *Falstaff* at 80 and *Te Deum* at 85.

There are also the politicians Golda Meir, Gandhi, Mao-tse Tung; musicians—Pablo Casals, Artur Rubinstein; painters—Titian, Picasso; writers—Tolstoy, George Bernard Shaw, Sophocles; and actors—George Burns, John Wayne, Sir Ralph Richardson and Lord Olivier. The list goes on and on.

Some thoughts about old age:

'I thought [old age] attractive because old people were interesting and experienced and, sometimes, since character has shaped the lines on their faces, very beautiful'—Baroness Mary Stocks, 80.

'An individual human existence should be like a river—small at first, narrowly contained within its banks, and rushing passionately past boulders and over waterfalls. Gradually, the river grows wider, the banks recede, the waters flow more quietly, and in the end, without any visible break, they become merged in the sea and painlessly lose their individual being'—Bertrand Russell, at 80.

Casals, asked the secret of his "good old age", replied, "I live. Very few people live."

"Young and old for me are meaningless words except as we use them to denote where we are in this process of this stage of being. Would I wish to be 'young' again? No, I have learned too much to wish to lose it"—Pearl Buck, 79.

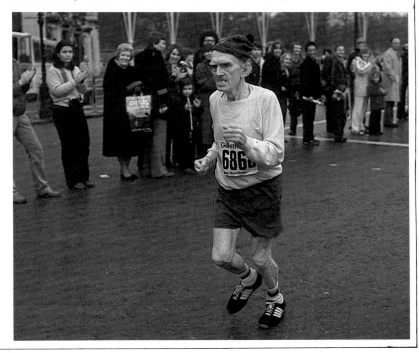

Taking our leave

Will it be a "good death"? Scientists prefer to avoid terms such as "good" or "bad". Avery D. Weisman, who is involved in terminal care, has offered the concept of an "appropriate" death. By this he means the kind of death individuals would have chosen for themselves, given the option. They are allowed to depart from life in a manner consistent with their own values and style. An "appropriated" death, on the other hand, would have meant that their death had been taken away from them by force of circumstances.

Most deaths occur in some kind of institutional setting. More than four out of every five people who die in old age spend their last days in a hospital, nursing home, or other type of institution. Their lives tend to become part of the institution's workings, rather than a continued expression of their own distinctive patterns.

Terminal illness often brings about a loss of function and strength which intensifies the dependence on the socio-physical environment. It has been said that "we die the death of our diseases", referring to the specific physical and psychological changes caused by diseases such as kidney failure, coronary diseases, pneumonia, lung cancer and so on.

However, we also die the death that follows most naturally the contours of the environment. Two old people approaching death with the same physical problems will have completely different experiences if one is in an impersonal institution and the other in an institution with a shared life style. The second person may be a nun who lives and dies in the same convent school–retirement home complex, or an orthodox Jew, dying amongst companions who faithfully carry out the prescribed rituals and practices. These contrast sharply with routine care-giving in an environment that offers no special attention to the values of the individual terminally ill person.

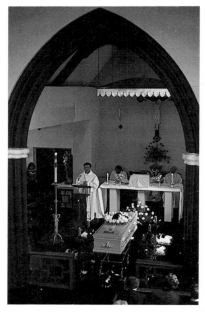

A funeral in a Roman Catholic church usually includes a Requiem Mass. God is petitioned to look favourably on the soul of the dead person. The service is a reaffirmation of belief and, although sympathetic to the feelings of the bereaved, mourning is tempered by the confidence that the soul has been released and is going to heaven.

Treat a person, not a disease

An old person's death may be "appropriated" from him or her outside institution walls as well. Some doctors treat diseases, yet bypass the individual. Information about his or her condition is shared only with one or two family members. Decisions are made with little or no consultation, and actions are carried out with a minimum of preparation and explanation. In taking away the responsibility, credibility and control of the old people themselves, we also set up a situation in which much of their life has become the property of others long before the process of dying begins.

Terminally ill old people deserve to live and die as they themselves would choose. Simple though it may seem, this concept runs counter to much in our social and health care network. It is easier to treat "diseases" and to look after "geriatric patients" than to work intimately with each person's individual needs.

The need to be open

There are many other factors that make it difficult to achieve what we shall continue to call (for want of a better term) an "appropriate" death in old age.

Health care of the aged has become a major budget item in many countries. There is reluctance to spend any more than is "necessary", and the definition of "necessary" is seldom in the hands of the elderly themselves. Any new programme of improved care for terminally ill elderly people that threatens to cost more is likely to run into determined opposition.

Many of us (including health care providers) assume that we *know* what old people and dying people want. This assumption is often a projection of our own thoughts and feelings upon the other person. "When I get to that age, I'll be ready to die," a young person may think. This assumption may also be constructed out of bits and pieces of observation. "I don't want to go on like this," may be interpreted as a desire for death, when the person is actually lamenting the poor quality of his or her current existence. "I won't be around long," may be interpreted as a plea for attention or a "morbid preoccupation", when it is a simple acknowledgement and notification. Whatever the source of our assumption, it provides an excuse to avoid close contact with terminally ill old people.

Ignoring the signs

"He doesn't know" and "It's better that way" are both assumptions that interfere with the achievement of an "appropriate death." The first is based on the premise that the old man is too confused or senile to be aware of his situation. Yet research has shown that awareness of impending death is common, even if it is expressed in ways that escape our notice. Communication between a dying person and others is subject to extraordinary omissions and distortions. Even direct statements may be "not heard" or "forgotten" or reinterpreted by the listener.

The idea that a dying old person should be "protected" from knowledge of his or her condition often serves to protect others from the uncomfortable prospect of a conversation about dying and death. Since many terminally ill people know or suspect the truth, this evasion does not accomplish a protective function. Instead it leads to increased isolation and gives dying people the feeling that it is best to keep their knowledge and suspicions to themselves. An opportunity to discuss the situation, clear up misunderstandings and express preferences is lost.

Making our wishes known

Our deaths, as well as our lives, affect other people. An "appropriate" death for a person may depend upon the actions of other people, and the nature of the death may influence their lives for a long time to come.

It is not unusual, for example, for one close family member to believe that life-sustaining efforts should be restricted at a certain point, while another person believes that everything possible should be done to keep the person alive. Both may believe they are advocating precisely the kind of action the dying person himself or herself would prefer, when the old person's wishes are not consulted or not taken seriously. The likelihood of the dying person achieving an "appropriate" death is greater when there has been a pattern of continued, open communication among patient, family and professional care-givers.

General theories, no matter how firmly based, cannot take the place of direct contact with particular people. We put the books away

Life expectancy

The average life expectancy has increased dramatically over the last 2000 years. Despite the Bible's "three score years and ten", in New Testament times most people lived for only 20 to 30 years. The sharp increase recorded this century is partly due to a fall in the rate of infant mortality, and partly to the development of new techniques in medicine and surgery which save lives which earlier would have been lost, and the control of many communicable diseases. In addition, health care (in Britain) is now available for everyone; public health programmes have improved hygiene at work and at home; better nutrition is more widely available.

However, the general rise in the standard of living has had a negative effect as well. Children now survive to become adults but they are then prone to the diseases created by affluence—over-indulgence in food and alcohol, lack of exercise and smoking.

Various factors contribute to longevity, such as heredity (other members of the family living long or having suffered serious illness), life style (type of job, type of home environment, income, stress, and so on), health habits (smoking, weight, exercise) and attitudes (a happy, easy-going person tends to live longer). In studies carried out in America it was shown that doctors and lawyers on average lived longest, followed by administrators and managers; at the other end of the scale were skilled and unskilled labourers.

Catherine Bramwell Booth, great granddaughter of the Salvation Army founder, is an active centenarian.

Life expectancy at birth in selected developed nations

Country	Year	Life expectancy at birth (years)	
		Males	*Females*
Canada	1970–2	69.3	76.4
Denmark	1975–6	71.1	76.8
Iceland	1971–5	71.6	77.5
Netherlands	1971–5	71.2	77.2
Norway	1975–6	71.9	78.1
Sweden	1976	72.1	77.9
United States	1976	69.0	76.7
Great Britain	1974–6	69.6	75.8

Above: a chart showing the average life expectancy at birth during the early to mid seventies in various nations. In the US, a female born in 1976 can expect to live to be 77 and a male to be 69. This represents an increased life expectancy of 5 years for women and 3 years for men since 1950. But a comparison with similar figures for many African nations shows a sharp decrease in life expectancy. For example, in 1960 in Burundi, a man could expect to live to 35 and a woman to 38, and in Ghana the average was 37.

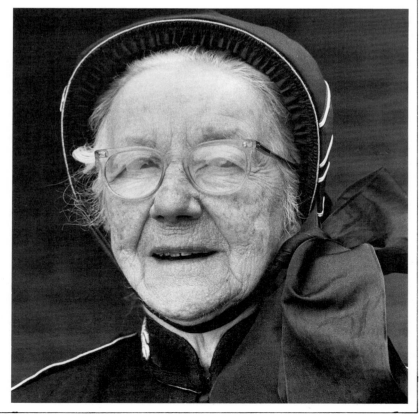

when we approach this unique person whose life is drawing to an end. Guidelines drawn from clinical experience and research are only useful if they supplement the good sense and emotional honesty that a helping person can bring to the situation.

Suicide and euthanasia

It is easy to accept the idea that the elderly person—or anyone approaching death—deserves to die with dignity in a manner consistent with his or her wishes or preferences. What we do not find so easy to accept is that the concept of an "appropriate" death may include the individual having control over the *timing* as well as the place or manner of his or her death. Why do we find this idea so unacceptable? One obvious reason is the belief that the taking of life is in the hands of God. Yet many who subscribe to this belief would acknowledge that the taking of life is appropriate in certain circumstances. Perhaps the real difficulty in accepting this idea is part of the wider inability to come to terms with death as a fact of life. If it happens to us, well, that can't be helped. But to encourage it, positively to bring it about, is an action we can only accommodate with phrases such as "while the balance of mind was disturbed".

In that case, we must accept that the balance of mind is disturbed in a great many old people. In England and Wales and in the United States, the group with the highest suicide rate is aged 65–74, with the rate for men being almost 50 per cent higher than that for women. The available figures almost certainly underestimate the true rates, as many old people may deliberately hasten their deaths by neglecting important medical regimes.

The rituals and social events surrounding death—which vary greatly from country to country— help the bereaved to adjust to the changed circumstances of his or her life. In the Western world, graveyard memorials range from a simple plaque or headstone like the one above, to the massive, highly decorated family mausoleums of the rich.

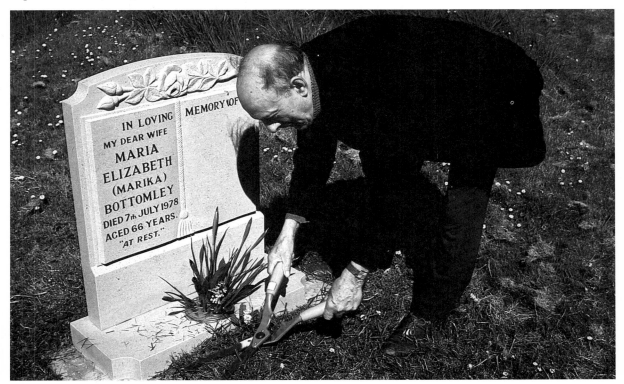

Common causes of death in the elderly (UK, 1980) as a percentage of all deaths for particular age groups	General hospital			Geriatric unit		
	65-69 yrs	70-74 yrs	75-79 yrs	Over 80 yrs	80-89 yrs	Over 90 yrs
	%	%	%	%	%	%
Cancer	29	27	27	24	10	7
Cardiovascular	25	25	32	36	40	40
Respiratory system	14	12	13	10	24	25
Digestive system	12	9	13	16	—	—
Nervous system	11	9	8	6	9	—
Renal tract	4	7	5	3	—	—
Other	5	1	2	5	16	28

Causes of death in the elderly

Left: chart showing the most common causes of death among elderly people based on the experience of a general hospital and a geriatric unit. While deaths from cardiovascular disease increased with age, the incidence of cancer and death from diseases of the nervous system (with the exception of cerebral thrombosis) decreased.

This is not to suggest that the answer to the very high suicide rates of the elderly is simply to accept that people have the right to decide when they will die. There is no doubt that some of the misery which precedes suicide is preventable, but this is not always so. If we *listen* to old people, rather than imposing our own values and standards on them, we will hear that what many of them dread is not being able to end their lives, or to arrange for others to do so, not only *as* but *when* they wish. We do not, and perhaps cannot, provide for the elderly the high quality of life which we seem to expect for other age groups. It is therefore important that we seek ways of resolving the conflict between recognizing the right of an individual to decide rationally when he or she will die and appearing to encourage such an action when other measures would be more appropriate.

Dealing with a unique person

Any prolonged illness is apt to influence our mental functioning. Sheer fatigue is one important element. Efforts to remain at least partially self-sufficient drain our energy and almost everything becomes harder to do. Pain and other physical discomforts also reduce the available mental energy.

The mental changes are often seen as indications of senility or "how dying people think". In fact, most people show mental changes when their bodies are depleted and not functioning well. If we simply accept that negative mental changes are an inevitable part of the dying process, we are less likely to seek ways of preventing or alleviating them. We are also less persistent in our efforts to maintain good communication with dying people. This lack of support increases the probability that they will continue to drift away, and the downhill process is accelerated.

Reduced stimulation from other people deprives individuals of here-and-now reality for their minds to work on. At a time when their inner bodily signals are distressing and their outer senses are diminishing, they have an increased need for significant interactions to help maintain mental functioning.

When a dying person feels that he or she is being abandoned and that he or she is no longer worth time and effort, he or she is likely to show very understandable mental and emotional reactions. Such individuals become demanding and agitated, or more depressed and withdrawn. They think and talk in ways that may come across as peculiar to others. Unfortunately, reactions of this type often provoke responses that compound the misery. Depressed because he or she feels abandoned, an old person may stop eating. Sensitive care-givers may recognize what is happening and increase their efforts to provide a sense of affection and security. Less sensitive people, however, may immediately resort to forced feeding by intravenous means or through a gastro-intestinal tube. Or they may decide the person is ready to die and let them perish of malnutrition.

There is another fairly common reaction to the distress expressed by terminally ill old people. Depressed, fearful, trying to find some way to counter the loss of a normal human environment, they may behave in a way that makes them, in some people's eyes, candidates for mind-influencing drugs. Instead of receiving a human response to their distinctly human needs and distress, they may be pacified by drugs. This approach reduces some of the expressions of distress (especially those that disturb other people on the scene), but gives little true comfort to the individuals. Drug treatment can be part of an effective, comprehensive approach to caring for terminally ill old people—but it can also be misused and become a further obstacle to meaningful communication.

Signs in advance
Mental changes in old people are sometimes the first signs of terminal decline. Awareness of this can help us provide more appropriate care for individuals and encourage sensitivity to their needs and wishes.

Two people of the same age may function at the same intellectual level. Six months later, one shows a decline, while the other holds steady. Research shows that the person whose mental functioning has declined is more likely to die soon.

A quality of agitation may appear in speech and manner. Behaviour may be inappropriate to the situation. Mental contact with the environment may become disarranged. Premonitions of death are often expressed indirectly.

Professionals as well as lay people have made the mistake of regarding those who show this kind of behaviour as senile. Terminally ill old people have been misdiagnosed as mentally ill and shunted away into closed custodial wards, where they have spent their final days without sensitive medical or nursing care and away from the people and places who have been part of their lives. They are left alone with their sense of disintegration. We respond only to the changes in thought and behaviour, using perhaps the good old stand-bys: "senile", "confused", "stubborn" and so forth, missing the opportunity to comfort and to share one of the most intimate human experiences.

Some chronically ill old people show a dramatic improvement in mental functioning shortly before death. A person who has seemed confused and out of contact for a long time suddenly becomes lucid and in control of his or her life shortly before death.

The tendency for mental functioning to decline does not mean that dying old people are without thought and feeling. Research with geriatrics indicates that most people retain a significant degree of mental functioning, or continue to be alert until the very end of life, unless put under heavy sedation.

Dying old people are usually more alert and responsive to those with whom they have a special relationship. They are also likely to be more alert on some occasions than on others. It is not unusual for such people to be in two realms, either alternately or at the same time. They can be in contact with the world around them and with their practical needs. At the same time, they may also be engrossed in another reality in which past meanings dominate without the rules and logic of everyday life. Their inner world is, in many respects, more meaningful for them than the institutions or "sick rooms" that comprise their immediate environment. A sensitive companion will respect the dying person's presence in both the world we all share and his or her own world.

What does a dying person need?

Each person has his or her own specific personal resources and needs. We do not relate to an abstract "old" or "dying" person, but to a very special individual who deserves consideration on his or her own unique terms. As death approaches, the person may be flooded with feelings and experiences from the past. Some memories can be painful. The person may recall how somebody else died many years ago and hope that some of those conditions do not exist for him or her. There may be memories of disagreements, rivalries, petty misdeeds and good deeds left undone. Helping the person to share some of these concerns can provide a useful release. Such people may need the chance to explain why they did or did not do something. There may be a request for forgiveness—or perhaps a family secret that must now be passed on to somebody else. Even if we know a person fairly well, we may not recognize what situation from the past is troubling him or her most at a certain time.

Leaving their lives in proper order

Dying people may have simple requests to make which allow them to feel that they can leave their lives in proper order. Sometimes this involves messages and the distribution of small items to certain people. Sometimes it involves certain aspects of the funeral arrangements. Dying people may be concerned about the welfare, of the survivors: "Look in every once in a while on George; he's so absent-minded"; "Fanny's never learned much about handling money; would you give her some help with the bank and the insurance?" Most messages and·requests are either practical or sentimental. Dying people do not ask to be made young or immortal. They simply want to round off their lives.

People are sometimes afraid to enter into conversations with the terminally ill, especially if the topics of dying, death and funerals come up. Part of this hesitation is based on the concern that such talk will only depress or frighten the dying person. Yet often it is our own apprehension or difficulty in facing death and acknowledging the plight of the dying person that interferes with communication.

People's functioning during terminal illness depends on who they have been throughout their life, the type of condition afflicting them, the treatment being received, the special characteristics of their present environment and many other factors. We can relate better to terminally ill old people if we do not load ourselves with expectations and assumptions, but approach them as the individuals they are.

Health problems in old age

Old age is not synonymous with poor health; in fact, older people are less vulnerable to certain diseases. The universal process of ageing leads to reduced abilities at all stages of life. However, certain conditions are more common in later life and an injury considered minor in a younger person could prove serious. The most common problem is degeneration of the heart and arteries. For more information about this and other diseases, see "Health problems in middle age".

ILLNESS	SYMPTOMS	TREATMENT/ACTION
1. General health Nutrition	Bad eating habits can cause problems later in life. An inadequate diet leaves the elderly person more vulnerable to a variety of diseases. A few old people suffer from malnutrition because of deficiencies in their diet, often due less to economic factors than to psychological ones (e.g. loss of appetite due to anxiety and depression).	Emphasis should be placed on green vegetables, milk, eggs, meat and wholewheat bread. Fried food is best avoided and rich highly spiced food is not easy to digest. Salt intake should be reduced. Hot meals are more easily digested than cold.
Sleep	Research suggests that we sleep less as we grow older and that sleep is less deep. Many people half-sleep during the day to compensate for a disturbed night.	
Accidents	Older people are more accident-prone. Men are more likely to be involved in a motor accident, either as driver or pedestrian. Women are more prone to falls. Poor eyesight, reduction in leg-lift when walking, and temporary dizziness are the usual causes.	
2. Physical illness Hypothermia	It usually means that the body temperature has dropped to below 95°F. It may be caused by a disease which causes a failure of the body's temperature regulating system or by environmental/economic factors which lead to cold living conditions.	Relatively little is known about the numbers of old people who die from this condition. The environmental/economic factors should be improved.
Osteo-arthrosis	Affected joints are painful and sometimes deformed but there is no inflammation. It usually affects the knee, hip and spine. The elderly are particularly vulnerable to all forms of arthritis.	Pain relief through analgesics; the strain is reduced by losing weight; exercises improve joint mobility and strengthen muscles. In some cases joints may be replaced by surgery.
Rheumatoid arthritis	Joints become swollen, stiff and painful, with limited movement, and are eventually destroyed. Occasionally fever and weight loss.	Physiotherapy and exercise are recommended to prevent joints from becoming deformed, with painkillers or anti-inflammatory drugs.
Pneumonia	Inflammation of the lung. Old people often suffer from hypostatic pneumonia due to staying in one position for long periods of time.	Can be eased by drugs and rest, but often occurs at the same time as other chronic illnesses.

Glossary

accommodation A term coined by Piaget to describe the act of altering our thinking when a new idea or object does not conform with our existing concepts. Also, a cessation in the transmission of nerve impulses when there is continuous or unvarying stimulation.

adaptation A term used by Piaget to describe infant behavioural change resulting from repeated experience of the same situation.

adolescence The period between puberty and maturity. *See also* puberty, identity crisis.

affective disorder A term used to denote extreme disturbances of mood, or affect.

ageism The widespread social attitude that overvalues youth and discriminates against the elderly.

aggression Strictly speaking, hostile behaviour intended to injure; but the word is often used for behaviour that is merely self-assertive, e.g. the "hard sell" of the dedicated salesman. Aggression in the strict sense can be divided into three categories: instrumental aggression, the aim of which is to obtain something; hostile aggression, which is aroused by hatred or cruelty; and defensive aggression, which is prompted by fear, or by the desire to escape from an unpleasant stimulus or a source of danger.

amnesia The partial or total loss of areas of memory; usually temporary. It may be caused by ECT, injury, sensile brain disease or trauma. *See also* repression.

amniocentesis The removal of a small amount of amniotic fluid in order to test for chromosome abnormalities.

amnion The membrane enclosing the foetus.

amniotic fluid The liquid contained within the amnion.

amniotic sac *See* amnion.

amphetamines Stimulant drugs, such as Benzedrine and Dexedrine, that act on the nervous system to increase alertness, concentration and level of activity. They can also reduce appetite, and cause wakefulness, irritability and anxiety. At one time they were widely prescribed for depression and as an aid to slimming.

analgesics Pain-relieving drugs.

androgens The collective term for male sex hormones. *See also* testosterone.

androgyny A concept of personality incorporating elements of both traditionally masculine and traditionally feminine characteristics and behaviour.

antidepressants Drugs used to combat depression, such as imipramine (Tofranil) and tranylcypromine (Parnate).

anxiety A feeling of general uneasiness and apprehension, sometimes without any conscious cause, sometimes related to anticipation of some event, real or imagined. *See also* neurosis, stress.

aptitude The capacity to learn new skills.

assertive behaviour Firm, direct but non-aggressive behaviour aimed at obtaining one's rights in relation to others.

associative learning Learning the connection between one event and another.

attachment The bond that grows between a child and another (usually adult) individual, particularly a parent. This first bond is usually one of strong emotional interdependence.

attribution The process by which we try to account for the behaviour of others. Attribution theorists are particularly interested in the ways in which we are biased in our interpretation of behaviour.

authoritarian Favouring obedience to authority rather than initiative or individualism. An authoritarian parent or teacher is strict, inflexible, domineering and punitive, and does not encourage the development of a child's own conscience or evaluative powers.

autosome A chromosome which does not determine sex.

behaviour genetics The study of the inheritance of behaviour.

behaviour therapy A learning-based method of psychotherapy which attempts to change behaviour by such techniques as counter-conditioning and reinforcement of desired responses.

birth control The planned prevention of unwanted pregnancy, by technique, operation or contraceptive drugs or device. Abstinence during the fertile phase—the 'rhythm method'—is one alternative to using a contraceptive device. In this method, sex may take place only during the first eight days and from day eighteen to day twenty-eight, assuming a twenty-eight-day cycle. It is also possible for a woman to work out her fertile phase by taking her temperature daily in order to establish when she is ovulating. Male withdrawal is another alternative to using a device, but it is unreliable and can be frustrating. Surgical sterilization remains an option for both men and women, but should be considered permanent.

The only device used by men is the sheath, or condom, sometimes used in conjunction with a spermicidal pessary. Devices used by women include: the occlusive diaphragm (the 'Dutch cap') a rubber dome which prevents sperm from gaining direct access to the cervix; the cervical cap, similar to the occlusive diaphragm offering more sensitivity and comfort, but more difficult for a women to learn to use, and not suitable for everyone; intrauterine devices, of metal or plastic, positioned in the uterus by a physician; and the oral contraceptive pill.

blastocyst The collection of cells that develops from the fertilized ovum, later to become an embryo.

breech presentation A baby positioned in the uterus presenting buttocks first. About 3 to 4 per cent of babies are breech presentations.

Caesarian section Surgical removal of a baby from the uterus through the abdomen. (According to popular history Caesar was delivered in this way.)

cardiovascular disease Diseases of the heart and blood vessels, including arteriosclerosis (hardening and thickening of the walls of the arteries), leading to hypertension (high blood pressure) often caused in part by a combination of stress, lack of exercise and bad diet.

chorion The embryo's outer layer.

chromosome A thread-shaped body consisting of DNA in the form of a single long helix. Chromosomes are found in pairs in all body cells and carry the genes transmitted from parent to child. A human cell has forty-six chromosomes in twenty-three pairs, one chromosome from each pair coming from each parent. *See also* DNA; genes.

circadian compliance The compliance of the body in terms of temperature, excretion, wakefulness, etc., to a cycle of roughly twenty-four hours.

classical conditioning *See* conditioning.

climacteric The range of physical and emotional symptoms accompanying reproductive changes in middle age. *See also* menopause, mid-life crisis.

cognition The process of knowing: perception, imagination, reasoning, memory, judgement, etc. Also the result or product of the act of knowing, e.g. a thought.

colostrum The nutritious liquid produced by a mother's breasts before the arrival of true milk.

concept formation Comprehending an abstract idea; forming a general thought.

concrete operations period The third stage of cognitive development postulated by Piaget, during which seven to eleven-year-olds are usually said to become able to think logically, to classify, to arrange objects in serial order and to conserve—i.e. to grasp that an object's qualities (e.g. quantity, volume) are unaltered by changes in appearance.

conditioned response (CR) In classical conditioning, the learned or acquired response that is elicited by a previously neutral stimulus, e.g. the salivation response of a dog to a buzzer sounded at feeding time. *See also* conditioning.

conditioned stimulus (CS) In classical conditioning, a previously neutral stimulus that elicits a conditioned response by association with an unconditioned stimulus or with another conditioned stimulus.

conditioning The process of learning or acquiring new conditioned responses. In classical conditioning, introduced by the Russian physiologist I. P. Pavlov, the subject apparently cannot influence the conditioning, although there is controversy over the extent to which this is the cause. In operant conditioning, studied extensively by the American psychologist B. F. Skinner, the subject can influence the conditioning by altering its response to stimuli.

conscious processes Events, such as perceptions, thoughts and dreams, of which only the individual is aware, accessible to others only by some form of communication between them and the individual. *See also* subconscious, unconscious.

conservation The ability to grasp that an object's qualities (quantity, volume, etc.) are not altered by changes in appearance—e.g. a pint of water in a tall, thin glass is the same as a pint of water in a short, fat one.

contraception Commonly used synonymously with 'birth control', though strictly speaking applies only to those methods of preventing conception that employ a contraceptive device. *See also* birth control.

control group In an experiment, a group that is similar to the experimental group in all important respects, but is not exposed to the variable whose effect is being studied.

crossover During meiosis, a process by which individual genes on a chromosome cross over to the opposite chromosome, thus increasing the random assortment of genes carried by offspring. *See also* meiosis.

dependent variable In an experiment, the variable whose measured changes occur as a result of manipulating the independent variable. In psychology this is often a response to a measured stimulus. *See also* independent variable.

depressants Drugs which reduce arousal.

development The series of changes that take place in an organism from conception to death.

developmental task An achievement or ability that, at any given age, is deemed necessary for socially acceptable functioning.

dizygotic (DZ) twins Twins developed from different zygotes (fertilized ova) no more similar genetically than ordinary siblings.

DNA (deoxyribonucleic acid) Large, complex molecules found in the nuclei of cells or organisms; thought to be the basis of genetic inheritance. They produce ribonucleic acid (RNA). *See also* RNA.

dominant gene One of a gene pair, the presence of which determines that an individual will possess the trait determined by that gene, whether the other member is the same or is a recessive gene.

ectoderm In an embryo, the outer layer of cells, which eventually becomes skin, sense organs and the nervous system.

ectomorph In Sheldon's type theory, the third of the three physical types, characterized by a thin, bony build and by delicate skin, fine hair and a hypersensitive nervous system.

ego In Freudian psychoanalytic theory, that part of the personality which is rational and controls the impulses of the id until they can be gratified in socially acceptable ways. *See also* id, superego.

egocentrism The inability to distinguish between one's own perceptions and the perceptions of others; also, the inability to see the world from another's perspective.

electroencephalogram (EEG) An ink-on-paper recording of the brain's electrical activity, obtained by attaching electrodes either to the scalp or, less often, the brain itself. Used, among other things, for detecting epilepsy.

embryo The developing organism in the womb between approximately the third to the eighth week after conception (the 'embryonic period') during which all major organs of the body are formed.

endoderm The inner layer of cells in the embryo, which becomes the gut and other internal organs.

endomorph In Sheldon's type theory, the first of the three physical types, characterized by prominence of internal organs, fatty tissue and obesity. *See also* ectomorph, mesomorph.

ethology The study of animal behaviour specific to particular species, particularly in the natural environment. Notable in the field are Konrad Lorenz and Nikolaas Tinbergen.

euthanasia The bringing about or hastening of gentle and easy death, often by drugs or the withholding of life-support systems, especially in cases of incurable disease.

extended family A family with many relatives living near to each other and to some extent cooperating with one another. Sometimes taken to mean simply the aunts, uncles, grandparents, etc., of a nuclear family (usually composed of two parents and their children) whether in close contact or not.

extravert In Jungian psychology, the type of person who is more concerned with social life and the external world than with inner experience.

fallopian tube The tube that connects an ovary to the uterus.

foetal period The last period of prenatal development, from the beginning of the third month after conception until birth, during which all organs, limbs, muscles and systems become functional.

foetus The baby while in the uterus.

forceps delivery Delivery of a baby by applying obstetric forceps, which fit around its head, to assist its passage through the birth canal. Forceps are used in cases where there is delay in the second stage of labour, foetal distress or maternal distress.

formal operations period The fourth and final stage of cognitive development postulated by Piaget, usually beginning after the age of twelve, in which the child/adolescent is said to learn to deal with abstract concepts.

fraternal twins *See* dizygotic twins

frustration The thwarting of the achievement of a goal, together with the consequent feelings of anger and exasperation.

full-term Born at the correct stage of development, rather than prematurely. This does not necessarily mean an exact nine months from conception.

genes The units within chromosomes that carry and transmit hereditary traits.

genetics The study of heredity.

genitalia The external sexual organs.

Gestalt A system of psychological theory that began in Germany in the 1920s, founded by Wolfgang Kohler, Max Werheimer and Kurt Koffka. Gestalt therapy, originated by Fritz Perls, often takes place in groups, though emphasizing the importance of the individual. Individuals are encouraged to recognize and accept previously denied elements of their personalities, in pursuit of a new wholeness.

gestation period The period of time from conception to birth—in humans about 266 days.

gonorrhoea A sexually transmitted disease, now curable with antibiotics.

gynaecologist A physician who specializes in medical problems peculiar to women.

habituation The process of becoming used to particular stimuli and ceasing to respond to them.

hallucinogens Drugs that produce hallucinations, e.g. LSD.

heterosexuality Sexual attraction towards members of the opposite sex.

homosexuality Sexual attraction towards members of one's own sex.

hormone A substance secreted by the endocrine glands that is distributed via the bloodstream and affects behaviour and physical condition.

id In Freudian psychoanalytic theory, that part of the personality reflecting unorganized, instinctual impulses that demand immediate gratification. *See also* ego, superego.

identical twins *See* monozygotic twins.

identification Assuming the attitudes, values, beliefs and behaviour of an admired or respected person. In children this is normally a 'significant' adult, especially the like-sex parent. In adolescents it is often a popular 'hero', e.g. a pop star, or an older pupil or teacher at school.

identity crisis A state of emotional confusion, usually accompanied by anxiety, that occurs to an individual when a prescribed social role is confused or withdrawn, particularly in adolescence, but also in widowhood, redundancy, etc.

identity diffusion A concept originated by Erik Erickson to describe the problems experienced by adolescents and young adults in striving towards integration of the personality.

implantation The embedding of the embryo in the wall of the uterus after it has descended through the fallopian tube.

imprinting A term used by ethologists, e.g. Konrad Lorenz, for the instinctual process whereby newly-born animals (especially birds) form a fairly permanent bond with the parent within a few days or even hours of birth.

independent variable In an experiment, the variable that it manipulated to produce measurable changes in the dependent variable.

instincts Non-learned, patterned, species-specific behaviour.

intelligence A hypothetical, abstract concept that is said to comprise the sum of all the different areas of mental ability, particularly the ability to think abstractly, to learn and to master new situations. Measurable, with varying degrees of success, by standardized intelligence tests. *See also* intelligence quotient (IQ).

intelligence quotient (IQ) An estimate of an individual's intelligence obtained by dividing mental age (according to an IQ test) by chronological age and multiplying the result by 100. The average IQ for any age is therefore always 100.

intermittent reinforcement Reinforcing a particular response to a stimulus, but only for some set proportion of the total number of times it occurs.

intrinsic motivation Motivation for behaviour that is rewarding or pleasurable in itself, rather than goal-directed.

introvert In Jungian psychology, the sort of people who, especially when under emotional stress, tend to withdraw into themselves and avoid social contact.

Klinefelter's syndrome A rare condition of the sex chromosomes (XXY instead of XX or XY) in which the individual has male genitalia, but coupled with pronounced feminine characteristics.

lactation Maternal milk production; also the period for which milk production lasts.

language acquisition devices In psycholinguistics, the mechanisms said to be possessed by all normal children, which enables them to learn to understand and use their native language.

learning A relatively enduring change in behaviour resulting from change in the organism's environment; contrasted with maturation, which is an internally initiated process.

learning disability Difficulty in a child's learning, especially of skills such as reading and writing, without apparent physiological cause.

longitudinal study A method of research that studies individuals through time, taking measurements at regular intervals.

low-birth-weight infant An infant whose birth weight is markedly below the average for full-term infants. Premature babies usually have low birth weights.

mean The arithmetical average of a series of numbers.

median The middle score in a series above and below which there is an equal number of cases.

meiosis The process of division in reproductive cell nuclei whereby the paired number of chromosomes is halved, to be combined with another half-set at fertilization, resulting in an infinite number of possible chromosome arrangements.

menarche The onset of menstruation.

menopause The permanent cessation of menstruation, occurring in middle age; may be accompanied by physical symptoms.

mental age A scale unit proposed by Alfred Binet for use in IQ testing. A child, irrespective of chronological age, with a mental age of nine is one who has achieved the same score as the average of a cross-section of nine-year-olds.

mesomorph In Sheldon's type theory, the second of the three physical types, characterized by a muscular, well-proportioned, athletic build. *See also* ectomorph, mesomorph.

mid-life crisis A transitional period, occurring in middle age, where individuals assess and confront their changing roles and limitations.

minimal brain dysfunction A postulated physiological cause of some learning disabilities.

mitosis The process of division in non-reproductive cell nuclei resulting in two cells identical to the parent cell.

mode The most frequently occurring score in a distribution, or the class interval in which the largest number of cases fall.

modelling In social learning theory, the process by which a child learns behaviour by observing and imitating others—usually adults with whom the child identifies

monozygotic (MZ) twins Twins resulting from the division of a single zygote (fertilized ovum) and who are thus genetically identical.

motivation The combination of need or desire in an individual, and the object of that need or desire, leading to need-satisfying and goal-seeking behaviour.

motor control The ability to control the muscles that cause different parts of the body to move.

mutation A random genetic alteration transmitted to offspring and producing a variation; an essential factor in evolution, as successful mutants survive to reproduce and spread the mutation.

nativism The theory that behaviour is innately determined.

nature/nurture issue The debate on the relative importance of heredity (nature) and social/physical environment (nurture) on character and ability.

neonate A new-born baby—loosely, during the first month of life.

neurosis A term applied to problems such as vague and irrational fears, tension, phobias and insomnia. In Freudian terms, these problems result from inability to reconcile the opposing demands of the three parts of the psyche, the id, ego and superego, usually dating from childhood. But it is now generally accepted that such problems can also result from social stresses arising in adult life.

norm The average performance under specified conditions. Also, commonly held values.

nucleus The central part of a cell, containing the chromosomes.

object permanence Piaget's term for a child's realization that an object still exists when hidden.

obsession A persistently intrusive irrational thought that cannot be willed away.

obstetrician A physician specializing in pregnancy, delivery and post-natal care.

operant conditioning *See* conditioning.

oral stage In Freudian psychoanalytical theory, the first stage of psychosexual development, in which pleasure is focused on sucking, biting and chewing.

oviduct The tube traversed by the ovum on its way from ovary to womb.

ovulation The release of the ovum by the ovaries into one of the two Fallopian tubes, normally occurring fourteen days before the start of the next menstrual period.

ovum The female reproductive cell.

paediatrician A physician specializing in children's physical development and illness.

peer group A group of children who regularly interact and who are of roughly the same age and social status.

perception The process whereby the brain makes sense of sensory stimuli.

performance Active behaviour, as opposed to knowledge possessed but not acted upon.

perinatology The branch of medicine dealing with the period from conception to the first few years of life.

personality The sum total of the individual's characteristic ways of responding to his or her own environment.

phallic stage In Freudian psychoanalytic theory, the stage of psychological development from about age three to five when the child's sensual pleasures are primarily genital-based.

phenotype In genetics, a characteristic that is obviously displayed, e.g. hair colour, intelligence, as opposed to one that is carried but not displayed, which is called a genotype.

phobia Extreme fear of particular objects or situations in the absence of any rationally perceived danger.

pituitary gland An endocrine gland that joins the brain just below the hypothalamus. It has an important role in regulating growth and it also controls other endocrine glands.

placenta It transfers the baby's essential requirements from the mother to the baby in the uterus and transfers the baby's waste products to the mother; the afterbirth.

preconceptual stage In Piaget's theory of child development, the first part of the preoperational period, lasting roughly from ages two to four, in which there is a new use of symbolic play. *See also* preoperational thought.

premature Born before the gestation period is completed. *See also* low-birth-weight infant.

preoperational thought The second stage of cognitive development postulated by Piaget, during which two to seven-year-old children begin to use language and to think symbolically. *See also* conversation.

projection A defence mechanism postulated by Freud whereby people are said to avoid recognizing undesirable traits in themselves by attributing them to others.

psychopharmacology The study of the way drugs affect behaviour.

psychosexual stages In Freudian psychoanalytical theory, the various stages of personality development (oral, anal, phallic, latent, genital) as characterized by particular pleasure zones and appropriate objects of sexual attachment.

puberty The point at which adolescents become capable of sexual reproduction.

quickening The point at which the pregnant mother first becomes conscious of the child's movements.

range The 'distance' between lowest and highest scores in a frequency distribution.

rationalization A Freudian defence mechanism whereby an individual is said to maintain self-esteem by inventing plausible and socially acceptable reasons for his own undesirable behaviour.

reaction formation A Freudian defence mechanism whereby an individual is said to dissociate himself from undesirable motives or desires by behaving in a way that contradicts them—e.g. someone who secretly hates children but is overtly adoring towards them and solicitous to their needs.

recessive gene A member of a gene pair that determines a trait only if its partner is also recessive, rather than dominant. *See also* dominant gene.

reflex action An innate, involuntary response to a stimulus.

regression Coping with anxiety by returning to an earlier, now superseded, mode of response.

reinforcement In operant conditioning, a consequence or set of consequences which strengthen the response they follow. *See also* conditioning.

reliability The extent to which an experiment or measuring device produces consistent results when repeated.

REM (rapid eye movement) sleep A stage of sleep, detectable by eye movement and characterized by dreaming; occurs in everyone.

renunciation A developmental task of old age in which individuals must adjust to changing roles and relinquish some of their powers.

repression A Freudian defence mechanism whereby an impulse or memory that evokes guilt, pain or anxiety is said to be forced into the unconscious mind. *See also* amnesia, unconscious.

respondent (classical) conditioning *See* conditioning.

reversibility The ability to return to a previous stage in a series of actions in complex problem-solving.

RNA (ribonucleic acid) Complex molecules similar to, and formed from, deoxyribonucleic acid (DNA), determining the structure and functioning of cells. Believed by some to be the chemical basis of memory. *See also* DNA.

scaling An ordering of data in which each measure stands in a specified relationship to other measures in the scale.

schizophrenia A term applied to a number of disturbing behaviours including extreme difficulties in relating to other people, hallucinations, delusions of grandeur or persecution, withdrawal, and erratic, apparently meaningless behaviour.

The term is often erroneously thought to mean 'split personality' in the 'Jekyll and Hyde' sense.

self-perception The individual's view of himself.

semen Male generative fluid containing spermatozoa in suspension.

sensorimotor skills Skills depending on the coordination of muscles and sensory nerves.

sex-linked trait A trait determined by a gene on either of the sex-determining chromosomes.

sex-role stereotyping Fixed concepts of what constitutes acceptable male or female behaviour.

sex typing The tendency of young children to become aware of their sex and behave accordingly.

siblings Brothers or sisters.

social learning theory A theory which suggests that social behaviour is learnt by observing others and imitating behaviour that is rewarded and refraining from that which is punished.

sperm The male reproductive cell.

stereotype An oversimplified and often distorted view of a group of people, e.g. a belief that all members of a particular ethnic group are greedy and dishonest, or proud and industrious.

stimulants Psychoactive drugs that cause arousal.

stress A response to threats and demands to which the individual is subjected by the environment (especially the social environment) often resulting in psychological and physical problems of varying degrees of severity, including anxiety, inability to concentrate, intestinal problems, headaches, depression and high blood pressure. Confusingly, the term is also applied to the external factors causing the response. *See also* anxiety, neurosis.

subconscious Often used as a synonym for 'unconscious', but strictly speaking refers to processes occurring just below conscious awareness.

sublimation A strategy postulated by Freud where individuals are said to cope with unacceptable impulses and anxiety-related energy by diverting them towards acceptable goals.

superego In Freudian psychoanalytical theory, the part of the psyche incorporating the moral standards of the individual and attempting to impose them on the rest of the psyche. In a relatively unindividuated person this would be very close to the perceived moral standards of that person's parents. *See also* ego, id.

suppression A process of self-control whereby the individual is aware of disturbing impulses and tendencies, but actively tries not to dwell on them or to take any action.

syphilis A potentially serious venereal disease that can be sexually transmitted or passed from parent to unborn child; now curable with penicillin.

testosterone The best-known male sex hormone manufactured by the testes; contributes to the growth of male sexual organs and the development of the secondary sex characteristics.

trait Said by personality theorists to be an enduring characteristic or aspect of personality.

tranquillizer A sedative drug used to relieve anxiety, e.g. Valium.

Type A personality Said to be more prone to heart disease: highly competitive tense, goal-oriented, aggressive and impatient.

Type B personality Said to be less prone to heart disease: calm, easygoing, non-aggressive and patient.

tumescence State of being swollen with blood, especially of aroused sexual organs.

ultrasound A method that produces a sound-wave picture of the foetus.

umbilical cord Tube carrying nutrition, via the placenta, to the foetus, and returning waste products for excretion by the mother.

unconditioned stimulus A stimulus (e.g. a puff of air directed at the eye) which automatically elicits an unconditioned response (blinking).

unconscious Said by Freud to be the repository of those mental processes, such as repressed desires or fears, of which the individual is not normally aware. More usually, a process or act which an individual performs without being aware of doing so. *See also* conscious, subconscious.

validity The degree to which a theoretical concept or a test fulfils the function or purpose for which it was developed.

variable In an experiment, one of the conditions controlled and/or measured.

vicarious learning Learning by observing the consequences of the behaviour of others.

withdrawal The physiological condition undergone by a drug-addict denied access to a particular drug.

X chromosome A chromosome that, when paired with another X chromosome, determines that a child will be female. If combined with a Y chromosome, it will be male.

XYY syndrome A rare condition in which a male has an extra Y sex chromosome, resulting in a very tall male, sometimes of below average intelligence. A link with criminality has been suggested.

Y chromosome The chromosome that, if paired with an X chromosome results in a male child.

zygote A fertilized ovum.

Useful Addresses

CHILD HEALTH

American Academy of Pediatrics
PO Box 1034
Evanston, IL 60204

American Association for Childhood Education
  International
3615 Wisconsin Ave NW
Washington, DC 20016

Association for Children with Learning Disabilities
5225 Grace St
Pittsburgh, PA 15236

American Health Foundation
320 East 43rd St
New York, NY 10017

National Association of Children's Hospitals and Related
  Institutions
1308 Delaware Ave
Wilmington, DE 19805

National Foundation for Sudden Infant Death Inc.
1501 Broadway
New York, NY 10036

National Institute of Child Health and Human
  Development
National Institutes of Health
Bethesda, MD 20014

Office of Child Development
Department of Health, Education, and Welfare
PO Box 1182
Washington, DC 20013

Parents Anonymous
250 West 57th St
Room 1910
New York, NY 10019

OLDER ADULT

American Association of Retired Persons
1090 K St NW
Washington, DC 20049

American Health Foundation
320 East 43rd St
New York, NY 10017

American National Red Cross
National Headquarters
Washington, DC 20006

Gray Panthers
PO Box 3177
Washington, DC 20010

Institute of Gerontology
University of Michigan/Wayne State University
5434 Church St
Ann Arbor, MI 48104

Social Security Administration
944 Altmeyer Bldg
6401 Security Blvd
Baltimore, MD 21235

DIET

The Diet Workshop
1975 Hempstead Turnpike
East Meadow, NY 11554

Weight Watchers International Inc.
175 East Shore Road
Great Neck, NY 11023

Take Off Pounds Sensibly (TOPS)
4575 South 5th St
PO Box 4489
Milwaukee, WI 53207

Overeaters Anonymous
3730 Motor Ave
Los Angeles, CA 90034

American Health Foundation
320 East 43rd St
New York, NY 10017

SMOKING

Action on Smoking and Health
PO Box 19556
2000 H St NW
Washington, DC 20006

American Health Foundation
320 East 43rd St
New York, NY 10017

National Cancer Institute
Office of Cancer Communications
Building 31, Room 10A25
Bethesda, MD 20014

American Cancer Society
777 Third Ave
New York, NY 10017

ALCOHOLISM AND DRUG ABUSE

Al-Anon Family Group Headquarters
PO Box 182
Madison Square Station
New York, NY 10010

Alcoholics Anonymous
PO Box 459
Grand Central Station
New York, NY 10017

National Clearinghouse for Drug Abuse Information
PO Box 1701
Washington, DC 20013

National Institute on Alcohol Abuse and Alcoholism Inc.
PO Box 2345
Rockville, MD 20852

MENTAL HEALTH

American Group Psychotherapy Association Inc.
1865 Broadway
New York, NY 10023

American Psychiatric Association
1700 18th St NW
Washington, DC 20009

Blue Cross Association
840 North Lake Shore Drive
Chicago, IL 60611

Division of Mental Retardation
Council for Exceptional Children
1920 Association Drive
Reston, VA 22901

National Institute of Mental Health
Bethesda, MD 20014

VISION

American Foundation for the Blind
15 West 16th St
New York, NY 10011

American Optometric Association
7000 Chippewa St
St Louis, MO 63119

American Printing House for the Blind
1839 Frankfort Ave
Louisville, KY 40206

The Library of Congress
Division for the Blind and Physically Handicapped
1291 Taylor St NW
Washington, DC 20542

National Association for Visually Handicapped
305 East 24th St
New York, NY 10010

National Eye Institute
National Institutes of Health
Bldg 31, Room 6A-27
Bethesda, MD 20014

National Society for Prevention of Blindness
79 Madison Ave
New York, NY 10016

Recording for the Blind Inc.
215 East 58th St
New York, NY 10022

HEARING

American Speech and Hearing Association
9030 Old Georgetown Rd
Washington, DC 20014

The Deafness Research Foundation
366 Madison Ave
New York, NY 10017

National Association of the Deaf
814 Thayer Ave
Silver Spring, MD 20910

National Hearing Aid Society
24621 Grand River
Detroit, MI 48226

Office of Deafness and Communicative Disorders
Rehabilitation Services Administration
Department of Health, Education and Welfare
Washington, DC 20201

Superintendant of Documents
US Government Printing Office
Washington, DC 20402

HEALTHY TRAVEL

Center for Disease Control
US Public Health Service
Atlanta, GA 30333

International Association for Medical Assistance to
  Travelers
350 Fifth Ave
New York, NY 10001

World Medical Association
1841 Broadway
New York, NY 10023

FIRST AID

American National Red Cross
National Headquarters
Washington, DC 20006

Council on Family Health
633 Third Avenue
New York, NY 10017

National Safety Council
425 North Michigan Ave
Chicago, IL 60611

Save Your Child's Life
PO Box 489
Radio City Station
New York, NY 10019

SPECIFIC DISEASES

United Cerebral Palsy Associatons Inc.
66 East 34th St
New York, NY 10016

American Diabetes Association Inc.
1 West 48th St
New York, NY 10020

Epilepsy Foundation of America
1828 L St NW
Washington, DC 20036

Committee to Combat Huntington's Disease
250 West 57th St
Room 2016
New York, NY 10019

Cystic Fibrosis Foundation
3379 Peachtree Rd NE
Atlanta, GA 30326

National Foundation March of Dimes
1275 Mamaroneck Avenue
White Plains, NY 10605

National Hemophilia Foundation
25 West 39th St
New York, NY 10018

American Heart Association
7320 Greenville Ave
Dallas, TX 75231

Citizens for the Treatment of High Blood Pressure Inc.
5530 Wisconsin Ave Suite 1630
Chevy Chase, MD 20015

National Foundaton for Iletis and Colitis
295 Madison Ave
New York, NY 10017

National Institute of Arthritis, Metabolism and Digestive
  Diseases
National Institutes of Health
Building 31, Room 9A08
Bethesda, MD 20014

United Ostomy Association Inc.
1111 Wilshire Blvd
Los Angeles, CA 90017

National Association of Patients on Hemodialysis and
  Transplantation
505 Northern Boulevard
Great Neck, NY 10021

National Kidney Foundation
116 East 27th St
New York, NY 10016

National Multiple Sclerosis Society
257 Park Ave
New York, NY 10010

Muscular Dystrophy Association, Inc.
810 Seventh Ave
New York, NY 10019

Myasthenia Gravis Foundation
230 Park Ave
New York, NY 10017

American Parkinson Disease Association
147 East 50th St
New York, NY 10022

National Psoriasis Foundation
6415 Southwest Canyon Court
Portland, OR 97221

Lupus Erythematosus Foundation Inc.
44 E 23rd St
New York, NY 10010

SEX AND BIRTH CONTROL

Association for Voluntary Sterilization Inc.
708 Third Ave Seventh Floor
New York, NY 10017

American College of Obstetricians and Gynecologists
One East Wacker Drive
Chicago, IL 60601

Planned Parenthood Federation of America, Inc.
810 Seventh Ave
New York, NY 10019

National Woman's Health Coalition
1120 Lexington Ave
New York, NY 10021

National Clergy Consultation Service
55 Washington Square
New York, NY 10012

Association for the Study of Abortion, Inc.
120 West 57th St
New York, NY 10019

PREGNANCY

American College of Nurse-Midwives
1000 Vermont Ave NW
Washington, DC 20005

American College of Obstetricians and Gynecologists
One East Wacker Drive
Chicago, IL 60601

Maternity Center Association
48 East 92nd St
New York, NY 10028

HANDICAPPED

American Coalition of Citizens with Disabilities Inc.
1224 Dupont Circle
Room 308
Washington, DC 20036

National Center for Law and Handicapped Inc.
1235 North Eddy St
South Bend, IN 46617

National Easter Seal Society for Crippled Children and
  Adults
2023 West Ogden Ave
Chicago, IL 60612

National Information Center for the Handicapped
Box 1492
Washington, DC 20013

National Wheelchair Athletic Association
40–24 62nd St
Woodside, NY 11377

Paralyzed Veterans of America
7315 Wisconsin Ave
Suite 300 W
Washington, DC 20014

President's Committee on Employment of the
  Handicapped
Washington, DC 20210

DRUGS AND PHARMACEUTICALS

American Pharmaceutical Association
2215 Constitution Ave NW
Washington, DC 20037

Food and Drug Administration
5600 Fishers Lane
Rockville, MD 20852

Pharmaceutical Manufacturers Association
1155 Fifteenth St NW
Washington, DC 20005

US Government Printing Office
Washington, DC 20402

HEALTH INSURANCE

Blue Cross Association
Box 4389P
Chicago, IL 60680

Health Insurance Institute
277 Park Ave
New York, NY 10017

Physicians' Forum Inc.
510 Madison Ave
New York, NY 10022

DEATH AND DYING

American Cancer Society
777 Third Ave
New York, NY 10017

Euthanasia Educational Council
250 West 57th St
New York, NY 10019

Hospice Inc.
765 Perspect St
New Haven, Conn. 06511

Make Today Count
218 South Sixth St
Burlington, IA 52601

BLOOD AND ORGAN DONATION

American Association of Blood Banks
1821 L St NW
Washington, DC 20036

American National Red Cross
National Headquarters
Washington, DC 20006

National Kidney Foundation
116 East 27th St
New York, NY 10016

National Rare Blood Club
164 Fifth Ave
New York, NY 10010

DOCTORS

American Academy of Family Physicians
1740 West 92nd St
Kansas City, MO 64113

American College of Physicians
4200 Pine St
Philadelphia, PA 19104

American Medical Association
535 Dearborn Ave
Chicago, IL 60610

American Osteopathic Association
212 East Ohio Street
Chicago, IL 60611

Blue Shield
Community Relations
756 Milwaukee St
Milwaukee, WI 53202

DENTISTS

American Dental Association
211 East Chicago Ave
Chicago, IL 60611

American Society of Oral Surgeons
211 East Chicago Ave
Chicago, IL 60611

Health Research Group
2000 P St NW
Washington, DC 20036

HOSPITALS AND NURSING HOMES

American Association of Homes for the Aged
529 Fourteenth St NW
Washington, DC 20004

American Health Care Association
1200 15th St NW
Washington, DC 20005

American Hospital Association
840 North Lake Shore Drive
Chicago, IL 60611

Consumer Commission on the Accreditation of Health
  Services Inc.
381 Park Ave S
New York, NY 10016

Institute of Gerontology
University of Michigan/Wayne State University
543 Church St
Ann Arbor, MI 48104

Further Reading

INFANCY AND CHILDHOOD

Connolly, K. and Bruner, J. (Eds) (1973) *The Growth of Competence*. New York: Academic Press.

Bayley, N. and Schaefer, E. S. (1964) Correlations of maternal and child behaviors with the development of mental abilities: Data from the Berkeley Growth Study. *Monographs of the Society for Research in Child Development* **29** (6). (Whole 97).

Bowlby, J. (1952) *Maternal Care and Mental Health*. Geneva: World Health Organization.

Schaffer, H. R. and Emerson P. E. (1964) The development of social attachments in infancy. *Monographs of the Society for Research in Child Development* **29** (3).

Ross, A. O. (1980) *Psychological Disorders of Children* (2nd edn). New York: McGraw-Hill.

Lewis, M. (Ed.) (1976) *Origins of Intelligence*: Infancy and early childhood. New York: Plenum Press.

Klaus, M. H., Jerauld, R., Kreger, N.C., McAlpine, W., Steffa, M. and Kennel, J. H. (1972) Maternal attachment: Importance of the first post-partum days. *New England Journal of Medicine* **286**, 460–463.

Flavell, J. H. (1977) *Cognitive Development*. Englewood Cliffs, NJ: Prentice-Hall.

Bernstein, J. E. (1977) *Books to Help Children Cope with Separation and Loss*. New York and London: R. R. Bowker.

Endler, N. S., Boutler, L. R. and Ossler, H. (Eds) (1976) *Contemporary Issues in Developmental Psychology* (2nd edn). New York: Holt, Rinehart & Winston.

Evans, R. I. (Ed) (1973) *Jean Piaget: The Man and his Ideas*. New York: E. P. Dutton.

Brown, R. (1973) *A First Language: The Early Stages*. Cambridge, MA: Harvard University Press.

Yando, R., Seitz, V. and Zigler, E. (1979) *Intellectual and Personality Characteristics of Children*: Social class and ethnic group differences. Hillsdale, NJ: Lawrence Erlbaum Associates.

Brown, G. and Desforges, C. (1979) *Piaget's Theory: A Psychological Critique*. London: Routledge & Kegan Paul.

Donaldson, M. (1978) *Children's Minds*. London: Collins.

Lyons, J. (1976) *Chomsky*. London: Collins.

Rutter, M. (1972) *Maternal Deprivation Reassessed*. Harmondsworth: Penguin.

ADOLESCENCE

Alison, J., Blatt, S. J. and Zimet, C. N. (1969) *The Interpretation of Psychological Tests*. New York: Harper & Row.

Anatasi, A. (1976) *Psychological Testing* (4th edn). New York: Macmillan.

Elashoff, D. and Snow R. E. (1971) *Pygmalion Reconsidered*. Worthington, Ohio: Charles A. Jones.

Blane, H. T. and Hewitt, L. E. (1976) Alcohol and youth:

An analysis of the literature, 1960–1975. Report for NIAAA Contract, ADM 281-75-0026.

Eron, L. D., Huessman, L. R., Lefkowitz, M. M. and Walker, L. O. (1972) Does television violence cause aggression? *American Psychologist*, **27**, 253–263.

Frankiel, R. V. (1959) *A Review of Research on Parent Influences on Child Personality*. New York: Family Service Association of America.

Jensen, A. R. (1969) How much can we boost IQ and scholastic achievement? *Harvard Educational Review* **39**, 1–123.

Lane, H. (1976) *The Wild Boy of Aveyron*. Cambridge, MA: Harvard University Press.

Comstock, G. A. and Rubinstein, E. A. (Eds) (1972) *Television and Social Behavior*, Vol. 3: Television and adolescent aggressiveness. Washington, DC: US Government Printing Office, 35–135.

Petersen, R. C. and Stillman, R. C. (Eds) (1978) *Phenylcyclidine (PCP) Abuse: An Appraisal*. National Institute of Drug Abuse Research Monograph, 21, Rockville, MD, 66–118.

Carter, M. (1966) *Into Work*. Harmondsworth: Penguin.

Child Study Association of America (1971) *Your Child and Drugs*. New York: Child Study Press.

Coleman, J. C. (1975) *Relationships in Adolescence*. London: Routledge & Kegan Paul.

Josselyn, I. M. (1971) *Adolescence*. New York: Harper & Row.

Klagsburn, F. (1970) *Youth and Suicide: Too Young to Die*. New York: Pocket Books.

Storr, C. (1975) *Growing Up: A Practical Guide to Adolescence for Parents and Children*. London: Arrow Books.

Yankelovich, D. (1974) *The New Morality: A Profile of American Youth in the 70's*. New York: McGraw-Hill.

YOUNG ADULTHOOD

Arieti, S. (1976) *Creativity: The Magic Synthesis*. New York: Basic Books.

Armor, D. J., Polich, J. M. and Stambul, H. B. (1976) *Alcoholism and Treatment*. Santa Monica, CA: Rand.

Becker, W. (1964) Consequences of different kinds of parental discipline. *In* Hoffman, M. L. and Hoffman L. (Eds) *Review of Child Development Research*, Vol. 1. New York: Russel Sage.

Bennett, I. (1960) *Delinquent and Neurotic Children*. New York: Basic Books.

Brecher, E. M., and Editors of Consumer Reports. (1972) *Licit and Illicit Drugs*. Boston: Little, Brown.

Cleland, C. C. (1978) *Mental Retardation: A Developmental Approach*. Englewood Cliffs, NJ: Prentice-Hall.

Wallerstein, J. S. and Kelly, J. B. (1980) *Surviving the Breakup—How Children and Parents Cope with Divorce*. New York: Basic Books.

Goodwin, D. W. (1976) *Is Alcoholism Hereditary?* New York: Oxford University Press.

Gotteman, I. I. and Shield, J. (1972) *Schizophrenia and Genetics*. New York: Academic Press.

Hetherington, E. M. (1972) The effects of father absence

on personality development in adolescent daughters. *Developmental Psychology* **7**, 313–326.

Kempe, C. H. and Helfer, R. E. (Eds) (1972) *Helping the Battered Child and his Family*. Philadelphia: Lippincott.

Klonoff, H. (1974) Marijuana and driving in real-life situations. *Science* **186**, 317–324.

Lamb, M. (Ed.) (1976) *The Role of the Father in Child Development*. New York: Wiley.

Mishler, E. G. and Waxler, N. E. (1968) *Interaction in Families: An Experimental Study of Family*. New York: Wiley.

Moore, T. W. (1975) Exclusive early mothering and its alternative: The outcome to adolescence. *Scandinavian Journal of Psychology* **16**, 255–272.

Petersen, R. C. (Ed.) (1977) *Marihuana Research Findings*. National Institute of Drug Abuse Research Monographs **14**, Rockville, MD.

Robins, L. N. (1966) *Deviant Children Grown Up*. Baltimore: Williams & Wilkins.

Albee, G. and Rolf, J. (Eds) (1977) *Primary Prevention of Psychopathology* Vol. 1. Burlington, VT: Waters.

Sutherland, N. S. (1976) *Breakdown*. New York: Stein & Day.

Tart, C. T. (Ed.) (1969) *Altered States of Consciousness*. New York: Wiley.

Wallach, M. A. and Wallach, L. (1976) *Teaching all Children to Read*. Chicago: University of Chicago Press.

Zigler, E. and Valentine, J. (Eds) (1979) *Project Head Start: A Legacy on the War on Poverty*. New York: Free Press.

Marris, P. (1964) *The Experience of Higher Education*. London: Routledge & Kegan Paul.

Jelliffe, D. B. and Jelliffe, E. F. P. (1978) *Human Milk in the Modern World*. Oxford: Oxford University Press.

Kitzinger, S. (1971) *Giving Birth: The Parents' Emotions in Childbirth*. London: Gollancz.

La Lèche International (1970) *The Womanly Art of Breastfeeding*. New York: Tandem.

Read, G. D. (1933) *Natural Childbirth*. London: Heinemann.

Hayes, J. and Nutman, P. (1981) *Understanding the Unemployed*. London: Tavistock Publications.

Pahl, J. M. and Pahl, R. E. (1971) *Managers and their Wives*. London: Allen Lane.

Seabrook, J. (1982) *Unemployment*. London: Quartet.

MIDDLE YEARS

Berkun, M. M., Bialek, H. M., Kern, R. P. and Yagi, K. (1962) Experimental studies of psychological stress in man. *Psychological Monographs* **76**, 534. (Whole 15).

Biller, H. N. (1970) Father absence and the personality development of the male child. *Developmental Psychology* **2**, 181–201.

Blatt, B. (1973) *Souls in Extremis*. Boston: Allyn & Bacon.

Brown, G. W., Birley, J. L. and Wing, J. K. (1972) Influence of family life on the course of schizophrenic disorders: A replication. *British Journal of Psychiatry* **121**, 241–258.

Dement, W. C. (1974) *Some Must Watch While Some Must Sleep*. San Francisco: W. H. Freeman.

Greenblatt, M. and Schuckit, M. A. (Eds) (1976) *Alcoholism Problems in Women and Children*. New York: Grune & Stratton.

Janis, I. L. (1973) *Victims of Group Think*. Boston: Houghton Mifflin.

Janis, I. L. and Mann, L. (1977) *Decision Making*. New York: Free Press.

Jarvik, L. F., Eisdorfer, C. and Blum, J. E. (Eds) (1973) *Intellectual Functioning in Adults*. New York: Springer.

Mendelson, J. H. and Mello, N. K. (Eds) (1979) *The Diagnosis and Treatment of Alcoholism*. New York: McGraw-Hill.

Selye, H. (1976) *The Stress of Life* (rev. edn). New York: McGraw-Hill.

Snyder, S. H. (1974) *Madness and the Brain*. New York: McGraw-Hill.

Terman, L. M. and Oden, M. (1959) *The Gifted Group at Midlife*. Stanford, CA: Stanford University Press.

Thomas, A. and Chess, S. (1977) *Temperament and Development*. New York: Brunner/Mazel.

Assersohn, R. (1982) *Express Money Book of Prosperous Retirement*. London: Quartet/Daily Express.

Bailey, C. (1982) *Beginning in the Middle*. London: Quartet.

Brown, G. and Harris, T. (1978) *The Social Origins of Depression*. London: Tavistock.

Fuchs, E. (1978) *The Second Season: Love and Sex for Women in the Middle Years*. New York: Doubleday.

Weissman, M. M. and Paykel, E. S. (1974) *The Depressed Woman*. Chicago: University of Chicago Press.

Masters, W. H. and Johnson, V. E. (1970) *Human Sexual Inadequacy*. Boston: Little, Brown.

OLDER ADULTS

Baldessorini, R. J. (1977) *Chemotherapy in Psychiatry*. Cambridge, MA: Harvard University Press.

Block, J. (1971) *Lives Through Time*. Berkeley, CA: Bancroft.

Bloom, B. S. (1964) *Stability and Change in Human Characteristics*. New York: Wiley.

Park, C. C. and Shapiro, L. (1976) *You Are Not Alone*. Boston: Little, Brown (Paperback: Consumers' Union).

Parkes, C. M. (1972) *Bereavement: Studies of Grief in Adult Life*. New York: International Universities Press.

White, R. W. (1976) *The Enterprise of Living* (2nd edn). New York: Holt, Rinehart & Winston.

Cumming, E. M. and Henry, T. (1961) *Growing Old*. New York: Basic Books.

Butler, R. N. and Lewis, M. I. (1976) *Sex After Sixty*. New York: Harper and Row.

Rubin, I. (1976) *Sexual Life After Sixty*. New York: Harper & Row.

Pizer, H. (1983) *Over Fifty-Five, Health And Alive*. New York: Van Nostrand-Reinhold.

Atchley, R. C. (1972) *The Social Forces in Later Life*. Belmont CA: Wadsworth.

Hershey, D. (1974) *Life Span and Factors Affecting It*.

Springfield, IL: Charles C. Thomas.

Birren, J., Finch, C. E. and Hayflick, L. (Eds) (1975) *Handbook of the Biology of Ageing.* New York: Van Nostrand-Reinhold.

Exton-Smith, A. N. and Evans, J. G. (1977) *Care of the Elderly.* London: Academic Free Press.

Shanas, E. and Sussman, M. B. (Eds) (1977) *Family, Bureaucracy and the Elderly.* Durham, NC: Duke University Press.

Binstock, P. H. and Shanas, E. (Eds) (1977) *Handbook of Aging and the Social Sciences.* New York: Van Nostrand-Reinhold.

Mannay, J. D. J. (1975) *Aging in American Society: An Examination of Concepts and Issues.* Ann Arbor, MI: Institute of Gerontology.

Botwinick, J. (1973) *Aging and Behavior.* New York: Springer.

Spencer, M. G. and Dorr, C. J. (Eds) (1975) *Understanding Aging: A Multidisciplinary Approach.* New York: Appleton-Century-Crofts.

GENERAL

Barlett, F. (1958) *Thinking.* New York: Basic Books.

Bandura, A. (1977) *Social Learning Theory.* Englewood Cliffs, NJ: Prentice-Hall.

Blanck, G. and Blanck, R. (1974) *Ego Psychology: Theory and Practice.* New York: Columbia University Press.

Block, N. J. and Dworking, G. (Eds) (1976) *The IQ Controversy.* New York: Pantheon.

Boring, E. G. (1950) *History of Experimental Psychology.* New York: Appleton-Century-Crofts.

Resnick, L. B. (Ed.) *The Nature of Intelligence.* Hillsdale, NJ: Lawrence Erlbaum.

Eibl-Eibesfeldt, I. (1971) *Love and Hate.* New York: Holt, Rinehart & Winston.

Gardner, H. (1978) *Developmental Psychology.* Boston: Little, Brown.

Talbot, N. B., Kagen, J. and Eisenberg, L. (Eds) *Behavioral Science in Pediatric Medicine.* Philadelphia: W. B. Saunders.

Gove, W. R. (Ed.) (1975) *The Labelling of Deviance.* New York: Sage/Halstead Press.

Hall, C. S. and Lindzey, G. (1978) *Theories of Personality.* (3rd edn). New York: Wiley.

Harper, R. A. (1975) *The New Psychotherapies.* Englewood Cliffs, NJ: Prentice-Hall.

Hilgard, E. R. (1977). *Divided Consciousness.* New York: Wiley Interscience.

Wynne, L. C., Cromwell, R. L. and Mastthysse, S. (Eds) *The Nature of Schizophrenia: New Approaches to Research and Treatment.* New York: Wiley.

Kinsch, W. (1977) *Memory and Cognition* (2nd edn). New York: Wiley.

Kovel, J. (1976) *A Complete Guide to Therapy.* New York: Pantheon.

Loehlin, J. C., Lindzey, G. and Spuhler, J. N. (1975) *Race Differences in Intelligence.* San Francisco: W. H. Freeman.

Loftus, G. R. and Loftus, E. F. (1976) *Human Memory: The Processing of Information.* Hillsdale, NJ: Lawrence Erlbaum.

Maddi, S. R. (1976) *Personality Theories: A Comparative Analysis.* (3rd edn). Homewood, IL: Dorsey Press.

Magaro, P. A., Gripp, R. and McDowell, D. J. (1978) *The Mental Health Industry.* New York: Wiley.

Marks, I. M. (1978) *Living with Fear.* New York: McGraw-Hill.

Maslow, A. H. (1971) *The Farther Reaches of Human Nature.* New York: Viking Press.

Melzack, R. and Wall, P. D. (1965) Pain mechanisms: A new theory. *Science* **150**, 971–979.

Munroe, R. L. and Munroe, R. H. (1975) *Cross Cultural Human Development.* Monterey, CA: Brooks/Cole.

Naranjo, C. and Ornstein, R. (1977) *On the Psychology of Meditation.* Baltimore: Penguin. (New York: Viking, 1971)

Nathan, P. E. and Harris, S. H. (1980) *Psychopathology and Society.* (2nd edn) New York: McGraw-Hill.

Nye, R. D. (1975) *Three Views of Man: Perspectives from Sigmund Freud, B. F. Skinner and Carl Rogers.* Monteray CA: Brooks/Cole.

Ornstein, R. E. (1977) *The Psychology of Consciousness.* New York: Harcourt, Brace, Jovanovich.

Previn, L. A. (1978) *Current Controversies and Issues and Personality.* New York: Wiley.

Resnick, L. B. (Ed.) (1976) *The Nature of Intelligence.* New York: Wiley.

Rogers, C. R. (1961) *On Becoming a Person.* Boston, MA: Houghton Mifflin.

Rosenbaum, C. P. (1970) *The Meaning of Madness.* New York: Science House.

Nicholi, A. M., Jr (Ed.) (1978) *The Harvard Guide to Modern Psychiatry.* Cambridge, MA: The Belknap Press of Harvard University Press.

Schachter, S. (1971) *Emotion, Obesity, and Crime.* New York: Academic Press.

Seligman, M. E. P. and Hager, J. L. (1972) *Biological Boundaries of Learning.* New York: Appleton-Century-Crofts.

Schneidman, E. S. Farberow, N. L. and Litman, R. L. (1970) *Psychology of Suicide.* New York: Science House.

Siegler, M. and Osmond, H. (1974) *Models of Madness, Models of Medicine.* New York: Macmillan.

Skinner, B. F. (1978) *Reflections of Behaviorism and Society.* Englewood Cliffs, NJ: Prentice-Hall.

Smith, C. U. M. (1970) *The Brain.* New York: G. P. Putnam.

Madow, L. and Snow, L. H. (Eds) *The Psychodynamic Implications of the Physiological Studies on Dreams.* Springfield, IL: Charles C. Thomas.

Szasz, T. S. (1961) *The Myth of Mental Illness.* New York: Harper & Row/Hoeber Medical Division.

Tyler, L. (1965) *The Psychology of Human Differences* (3rd edn) New York: Appleton-Century-Crofts.

Vernon, P. E. (Ed.) (1970) *Creativity.* Baltimore, MD: Penguin.

Webb, W. B. (1975) *Sleep, The Gentle Tyrant.* Englewood Cliffs, NJ: Prentice-Hall.

Index

Page numbers in *italics* refer to relevant illustrations or captions; those in **bold** indicate the sites of major discussions

abortion: artificially induced 13, 112, 174; spontaneous 16; *see also* miscarriage
accommodation 58–9
acne *100*, 107, *128*, 135
acrosome 15
ACTH 102
active state 30
acute illness 54
Adam's apple *see* larynx
adaptation 58; by infants 35
adenine *18*
adolescence 25, 77, **97–135**, *98*, *99*, 265; anxieties during 106–7; drug abuse during **118–23**; end of **132–4**, 137; health problems during **135**; marriage during *126*, 145; maturation rates during 107; nutritional needs during 106; and parental relationships **114–17**, 126, 127, 131, 132–3, 190, *192*; peer groups during 114, **124–6**, 127; physical changes during **100–103**, *100–101*, *102*, *103*, **104–106**, *104*, 135; psychological problems during **127–31**, 133; sex during 107, **108–13**, *111*, 126; *see also* maturation, puberty
adolescent growth spurt 25, *100*, *103*, 104–5, 106, *128*
adolescent identity crisis 100
adrenal (suprarenal) glands *102*, 104
adrenalin (epinephrin) 102
adrenocorticotropic hormone 102
adulthood: *see* middle age, old age, young adulthood
ageing 190, 220, 222, 225, 226, **228–37**, *231*; myths about **255**; *see also* maturation, old age
ageing parents 192, 253
aggression: in childhood 63, 64, *91*, 92; in infancy 39
AID (artificial insemination by donor) 13
alcohol, drinking of 258; during adoleseence 118–*119*, *122*, 130; during breast-feeding 27; and depression 206–7; during middle age 200, 217; during old age 238; during pregnancy 18–19; *122*
alienation 116, 133

alimentary canal (gut) 26, 27; *see also* intestines
allergies 135
alveoli (in breasts) *27*
amenorrhea 166
American Planned Parenthood 112
amniocentesis 18, *172*
amnion (amniotic sac) *12*, *17*, *20*, *174*
amniotic fluid *17*, 18, 170, *174*
amphetamines 118, *123*
anaemia 95, 135, *166*
anaesthetics (during labour) 22, 176
anal stage 89
androgens *102*, 104
androgyny 104
angina *201*, 223
anorexia nervosa *128*, 129–30, 135
antenatal care 167, 170, 171, 175
antenatal classes *see* childbirth classes
antenatal clinics 167, *172*
anthropoid apes 28, 35
antibiotics 135, 223
antibodies 26
anti-depressants 195, 211
antidiuretic hormone 102
anti-histamines 135
anus *155*
anxiety 90, 164; during adolescence 106–7, 127, 135; after bereavement 211, 212, 213; and institutionalization 252; during labour 178; in old age 241, 242; during pregnancy 170, **172–3**, 175; about sex 194; and unemployment 216; *see also* depression
apathy: and depression 206; and institutionalization 251, 253; and shock 212
appetite, diminishing 229, 233, 242; *see also* eating problems
areola 106, 166
Aristotle 19, 97
arousal *see* sexual arousal
art (children's): drawing *61*, 74–5; painting *81*
arteries 223, 231, 263; hardening of *see* arteriosclerosis
arteriosclerosis 228, 233; cerebral 246
arthritis 222, 243, 263
artificial insemination by donor 13
Ashanti 210
aspirin *123*, 135
assimilation 58–9
asthma 26, 95, *201*, 226
Atlas, Charles *128*
attention deficit syndrome *see* learning difficulties

attention-seeking *90*
attention span 82
Australian Aborigines 28

babbling (in infancy) 49, 53
bacteria: in alimentary canal 26, 27; on skin 23
balance (in infancy) 49
baldness *201*
Ball, Florie 255
Bank Street College of Education 74–5
barbiturates *123*
barmitzvah *116*
Baruch, Bernard 225
bed-wetting 93, 185; *see also* incontinence
Benzedrine *123*
bereavement *see* widowhood
Bereiter, Carl 74
Bijou, Sidney 47–8
Binet, Alfred 87
biological clocks 21, 104
Birren, James 227
birth 13, *21–3*, *21*, 166, **174–81**, *180–81*; father's role during 177–9; myths surrounding 23; physiological effects of (on baby) 21–2; psychological effects of (on baby) 22; *see also* multiple births, postnatal depression, premature birth, pre-term birth
birth control *see* abortion, contraception
birthmarks 55, *128*
birth rate, illegitimate 178
'birth trauma' 22
bladder *14*, *122*, *155*, *157*, 166, *201*, 232
blastocyst 16
blindness: in childhood 89; in infancy 48; *see also* vision
blood 21; calcium in 102; clotting of 54, 223; 'contamination' by 23; menstrual 23 (*see also* menstruation); sugar in 102, 223, 228, *231*
blood cells 17; *see also* red blood cells, white blood cells
blood circulation 223, 232
blood pressure 102, 155, 156, 170, 228, 231; high *121*, 201, 203, 223, 233 (*see also* hypertension); systolic 105
bloodstream 102, *121*
Bloom, Benjamin 74
blue babies 54–5
body-language 50

body senses 233
bonding *see* mother–infant
  relationship
Booth, Catherine Bramwell *258*
bottle-feeding **26–8**, *28*, *29*;
  psychological effects of 27
bowel *14*
Bowlby, John 72–3, 165
Bradley, Helen 222
brain 104, 232–3, 248; cancer of
  187; inflammation of 95; oxygen
  supply to 231, 246; and sexual
  arousal *154*, *156*, 160; and stress
  201; structure of 76–7; waves 77–8,
  228
brain damage: in adolescence *123*;
  at birth 22; in infancy 48, 55;
  minimal *see* learning difficulties; in
  old age 246
'Brass Tacks' *138*
breast-feeding (suckling) 23, **26–8**,
  26, *27*, *28*, 33, 36, *181*; breast-size
  and 106; frequency of 28;
  psychological effects of 27; *see also*
  demand feeding
breast-milk *see* milk (human)
breasts 171, 194, 229; cancer of 187;
  development of *101*, *103*, 104; size
  of 106, *128*, 170; tissue of 166
breathing difficulties 231
breathing rate *156*
breech birth *20*, 180
bronchitis 54, 223; chronic *121*
Brown, George 202
Buck, Pearl 255
bulimia nervosa 135
bullying (among children) 86
Burns, George 255
Bushmen 28
Butler, Samuel 97

Caesarian section 22, 176, 180
caffeine *123*
calcium (in blood) 102
calorie requirements 186, 197, 232
cancer 187, *211*, *260*; breast 187;
  cervical 187, 203; lung *121*, 187, 256
Caplan, Paula 41–2
carbon monoxide *121*
cardiomyopathy, nutritional *122*
cardiovascular system 231;
  disorders of 195, *260*; of newborn
  child 21–2; and stress *201*; *see also*
  arteries, blood, heart .
Casals, Pablo 255
cataract 233
cell division *16*
cell nucleus *16*

cephalocaudal development *46*
cerebral arteriosclerosis 246
cerebral thrombosis *260*
cerebral–vascular accidents 231
cervix 14, 15, *17*, *155*, *156*, *157*,
  167, *174*; cancer of 187, 203
Chanel, Coco 255
Chaplin, Charlie 222
cheating (among children) 68
Cherry-Garrard, Apsley 189
Chertok, Léon 170
chickenpox 95
child abuse 88, 185
childbirth *see* birth, natural childbirth
childbirth (antenatal) classes 172–3,
  174, 175, 176, *177*
childhood 52, **57–95**, **182–5**, 264;
  health problems in 95; learning
  during 57, 58–9; mental
  development during 74–5;
  development of moral reasoning
  during 67–8; parental influence
  during 64, **68–70**; Piaget's stages of
  58–62; attitudes to school during
  70; entering school **72–5**, **80–81**;
  readiness for school **75–8**; refusal to
  go to school 85–6; social
  development during 63–70, *67*, *69*;
  special problems during **88–94**; *see
  also* education, infancy
child prodigies 71
cholesterol 223, 228, 246
chorion *17*, *20*
chorionic gonadotrophin 172
chromosomal abnormalities 18, *19*,
  55; *see also* Down's syndrome
chromosomes 15, *16*, *20*, 41
chronic bronchitis *121*
chronic depression 129
chronic gastritis *122*
chronic illness 54
churching 23
cilia 14
circadian cycles 30
cirrhosis *122*
cleft palate 54–5
climacterium 202–3; *see also*
  menopause
clitoral hood 156
clitoris *155–6*
club foot 54–5
CNS *see* nervous system (central)
cocaine *123*
codeine *123*
coeliac disease 54–5
cognitive development **58–62**, *59*,
  67, 76, 84
cognitive theory *42*
cohabitation *see* living together

colic 34, 55; evening 30
collagen 231
colostrum 23, 26, *181*
communication: in childhood 57; in
  infancy **35–8**, **50–53**, 55 (*see also*
  speech); in marriage 194
compatibility (in friendships) 193
conception (fertilization) 13, **14–
  16**, *15*, *19*, 108, 112
concrete operational stage **59–62**,
  59
congenital disorders 54–5, *166*; *see
  also* chromosomal abnormalities
conjunctives 95
conservation tasks 60
constipation 95
contraception 108, 111, 112–13,
  165, 264
contraceptive pill *121*, 164, 264
convulsions, infantile 95
cooing (in infancy) 49, 53
coordination: in childhood 82; in
  infancy 56; in old age 232
Copenhagen *163*
cornea 233
coronary artery disease 223, 256
coronary thrombosis *see* myocardial
  infarction
corporal punishment 85
corpus callosum 76
corpus luteum *105*
cortex, adrenal 102
cortex, cerebral 76–7, 246
cortisol 102, 104
counting, learning of *58*
couvade 175
Cowper's gland *155*
cradle-rocking 32–3
crawling *43–44*, *45*, 49
creativity: in adolescence 133; in old
  age 229; in retirement 208; *see also*
  art (children's)
crowning *180*
crying (in infancy) 30–31, *32*, 34,
  36, 49, 50, 55
Cumming, Elaine 217
cystic fibrosis 54
cytosine *18*

dating 146
day-care centres: for the
  elderly *241*; for the young *see*
  education (pre-school)
deafness: in childhood 88, 89; in
  infancy 48; *see also* hearing
death 250, **256–62**, *260*;
  'appropriate' 256–7
De Gaulle, Charles 222

Delauney, Sonia   222
delinquency   63, 68, 73, 127, 129,
   130–31, 133
delta-wave phase   233
demand feeding   28, 31
dementia *see* pre-senile dementia,
   senile dementia
deoxyribonucleic acid *see* DNA
dependence (in infancy)   *35*
depression: in adolescence   129, 130,
   131; after bereavement 211, 212,
   213; in middle age 191, 202, 203,
   204–7, *205*; in old age 231, **240–43**,
   244, 251, 260–61; during pregnancy
   170; and unemployment 216; in
   young adulthood 184, 187, 202; *see
   also* anxiety, postnatal depression
design stage   *74–5*
De Valera, Eamon   255
developmental assessment   48
developmental quotient   46
development tests   46–7
Dexedrine   *123*
diabetes   203, 223, *231*, 242
diarrhoea: in adolescence   127; in
   childhood 95; in infancy 54, 55; in
   middle age 200, 223
Dick Read, Grantly   175, 176
diet   265; in middle age 217; in old
   age 232, 238, 244, 263; in young
   adulthood 186, 187
dieting   *128*, 129–30, 135
diets, special   55, 223; during
   pregnancy 171
digestive system   *121*, 201, 232
diphtheria   95
discipline, parental   **68–70**, 127
disengagement theory   217–18
diuretics   *122*, 135
divorce   117, *126*, 137, *148–9*, 150,
   151, 207, 213; and children 213; in
   middle age 192, 194, 195, 199, 205,
   210–13, *210*, 222
divorce rates   144, 145, *148–9, 213*
DNA   17, *18*
dominant genes   18, *19*
Donaldson, Margaret   82, 84
Down's syndrome
   (mongolism)   *19*, 54–5, *166, 172*
DQ   46
drawing (children's) *see* art
   (children's)
dreaming   *90*, 233; erotic 107, 195;
   see also nocturnal emission, REM
   sleep
drinking *see* alcohol
drugs, abuse of   27, 117, 118–23,
   121, 122–3, 129, 130; and sexual
   problems 164; *see also* alcohol

Duchenne muscular dystrophy   54
ductless glands *see* endocrine glands
dyslexia   79
dysmenorrhea   135

eating problems: in
   adolescence   129–30, 135; in
   middle-age depression *205*; *see also*
   anorexia nervosa, appetite,
   overeating
Ecclesiastes   97
eclampsia   170
eczema   26, *201*
education   58, 63, 218
disabilities **78–82**; elementary-school
   73–4; and employment *134*; and job
   status *139*; further (higher) *133,
   134*, **138–43**, *139*; for gifted
   children 71; pre-school **72–5**, *72*;
   school 62, **72–6**, 79, 133–4; special
   48, 88, *89*; *see also* learning
   disabilities
Education Act (1981)   89
educational handicap *see* learning
   disabilities
EEG (electroencephalogram)   21,
   30, 228
egg (human) *see* ovum
ego   89
egocentricity   45–6, *59, 62*, 82
ejaculation   *14, 100, 102*, 107, 154,
   156, 160–61, 194; female 157; phase
   155, *157, 158*; premature 161–2,
   164; retarded 162, 164
electroencephalogram *see* EEG
embryo *see* foetus
emotional maturity *see* maturation
emphysema   *121*
employment   **138–43**, *138, 139*,
   142–3, *205*, **214–16**, 218, 221
encephalitis   95
endocrine glands   102, 104; *see also*
   adrenal glands, ovaries, pancreas,
   parathyroid glands, pituitary gland,
   testes, thyroid gland
endometrium   *105*, 203
Engelmann, Siegfried   74
environmentalism (and gender
   identity)   39
epididymis   14, *155*
epilepsy   95
epinephrin   102
episiotomy   180
erectile dysfunction
   (impotence)   *122*, 161, 163, 164,
   187, *249*
erection, penile   107, *122*, 154, 159,
   160, 161, 194; phase 155, *156*

Erikson, Erik   93, 265
euthanasia   *250*, 259
evening colic   30
evolution   35
exchange theory   **148–51**
excitement stage (male) *see* erection
   (phase)
exercise: in middle age   **196–7**, *196,
   197*, 217; in old age *238*, **239**, 246;
   during pregnancy **168–9**, 170; in
   young adulthood **186–7**
expressing (of breast-milk)   171
extension (during labour)   *180*
eye   233; *see also* vision
eye-colour, genetic determination
   of   18

Factor VIII   54
Fallopian tubes   14, *15*, 16, *105, 155*
family   182, **190–92**, *191*; extended
   34; nuclear 183
fatherhood   *177–9*, 184; *see also*
   parenthood
feedback loops: in childhood   64–5;
   in infancy 32
feeding in infancy   23, **26–7**, *44*, 55;
   see also bottle-feeding, breast-
   feeding, weaning
fertility   *201*, 204
fertilization *see* conception
fine-muscle control   77, 78
Fiske, Marjorie   191–2, 193, 194,
   203, 206
fixation (by infants)   *38*
fixation (in psychoanalysis)   89
flashcards   83
fleas   95
flora, skin   23
flu *see* influenza
fluoridation   171
foetal alcohol syndrome   19
foetus (embryo)   *12, 39*, 40, *122,
   167*, 170, *172*; abnormalities in 18–
   19; development of **16–19**, *16, 17*,
   166–7, 171; and inoculations   172
follicles   *105*
follicle-stimulating hormone *see* FSH
food fastidiousness   *90*
forceps delivery   22, 176, 180
formal operational stage   *59, 60*, 268
formula-feeding *see* bottle-feeding
fraternal twins   *20*
Freud, Anna   265
Freud, Sigmund   182, 189, 255; on
   child development **89–91**, *90*, 93;
   on emotional maturity 132; on
   gender identity *42*; on sexual
   response 154; on weaning 29

friendships: during adolescence 125–6; in middle age 193–4
frontal lobe (of cortex) 76–7
FSH 102, *105*, *154*
funerals 262
further education *see* education

Galton, Sir Francis 71
games 35, **36–8**, *38*, 45–6, 52
Gandhi, Mahatma 222, 255
Gayton, Richard 178–9
gender identity 39, *40*, 41, *42*; *see also* identity
'generation gap' 116
genes **16–18**, *20*
genital organs 41, *155*; *see also* clitoris, labia, penis, testes, vagina
genital stage 89
genotype 18
German measles 172
gestagens 104
gestation *see* pregnancy
glands, endocrine *see* endocrine glands
glucagon 102
glucose (in blood) 102
glue-sniffing *123*
gluten-free diet 55
glycogen *231*
Goethe, J. W. von 255
gonadotrophins 102, *154*, 172; *see also* FSH, LH
gonads 102, 154
gonorrhea 135
Gordon, Katherine 179
Gordon, Richard 179
grasping (in infancy) *45*, 46, 47, 49
Gray Panthers 222
grief **210–13**; unresolved 211–13
group therapy *216*
growth: during adolescence *101*, *103*, 104–5 (*see also* adolescent growth spurt); during childhood 75; hormone 102; during infancy 25; *see also* maturation
growth spurt *see* adolescent growth
guanine *18*
gut *see* alimentary canal
Gutmann, David 194

habituation 31–2
Hackney Partnership Programme *138*
haemoglobin 21, 228
haemophilia 54, *172*
hallucinogens *123*

handicap: in childhood, mental 88, *89*; in childhood, physical *88*; educational *see* learning disabilities; in infancy, mental 48; in infancy, physical 47–*48*; and sex 195; schools catering for 88, *89*
hard signs 78
hare-lip 23, 54–5
Hatfield, Elaine 150
Hayes, Helen 222
hay fever 226
headaches 200, 223
head lice 95
health: in middle age **196–7**, 217; in old age **226–8**; in young adulthood **186–7**; *see also* exercise, health problems, mental health
health problems: in adolescence **135**; in childhood 95; in infancy **54–5**; in middle age **223**; in old age **263**; *see also* health, exercise, mental health
hearing *227*, 229, 233, 235, 240, 243; *see also* deafness
heart attack *121*, 195, *201*, 223, 243
heart deformities 54–5
heart disease *121*, 174, 187, 202, *211*, 263
heart rate 102, *105*, 155, *156*
Heiman, Julia 159, 160
Hemingway, Ernest 193
Henry, William 217
heredity 25
heroin 118, *123*
herpes II 135
hide-and-seek 46
higher education *see* education
hip dislocation (in infancy) 54–5
hippocampus 77
Hoffman, Martin 68, 70
hole-in-the-heart babies 54–5
homosexuality **112**, *113*
hookworms 95
hormonal abnormalities 41
hormone deficiency 187
hormone replacement therapy 203
hormones 104, 135, *154*, 166, 170, 172, 173, 177; list of major **102**; and the menopause 202
hospitalization 244
hot flushes 202, 203
Hughes, Hector *249*
Hughes, Martin *62*
Hugo, Victor 255
Hunt, J. McV. 74
Huston, Ted 148
hyperactivity *see* learning difficulties
hypernatremia 27
hypertension 201, 223, 233; *see also* blood pressure (high)

hypertonicity 55
hypostatic pneumonia 263
hypothalamus 104, *154*
hypothermia *122*, 263

id 89, 90
identical twins *20*
identifying 70
identity: in adolescence 100–101, 103, 130; in old age 252; sexual 103–4; *see also* gender identity
identity crisis, adolescent 100
illegitimacy 165
illnesses *see* health problems, mental health *and individual illness names*
imitation: during childhood 58, 63, 70; during infancy 37–*38*
impotence *see* erectile dysfunction
incest 88
incontinence *90*, 240; *see also* bed-wetting
indigestion 200, *201*, 223
induced birth 19
induction disciplinary techniques 68, 70, 120
Industrial Revolution 143
Ineichen, Bernard 144
infancy **25–55**, **182–5**; abilities during **35–8**; communication during 35–8; emotional outbursts during 32; feeding during 23, **26–9**, *44* (*see also* bottle-feeding, breast-feeding); handicap in 47–48; health problems in **54–5**; mental development in **43–53**, *52*; motor development in **43–9**, *44–5*; physical development in 25; sex stereotyping during 39, 41–2; speech development in 35, 40–41, 45, 48; **49–53**, *53*; *see also* growth, maturation, sleep patterns, social interactions
infantile convulsions 95
infertility 187
influenza *121*, 223
Initial Teaching Alphabet 84
initiation ceremonies 115, *116*
in-laws 190
insomnia 200; *see also* sleep patterns, sleep problems
institutionalization 89, **251–4**, *254*, 255; 256, 262
insulin 102, 223, *231*
intellectual retardation *see* mental retardation
intelligence 58, *73*, 234, *237*; *see also* IQ
intelligence tests *see* IQ tests

intestines 232; *see also* alimentary canal
involutional melancholia 191
IQ 46–7, 74, 87, 235
IQ tests 46–7, 71, **87**, 235
iron (in baby-feeds) 26, 27
ischemic attacks 246; *see also* brain (oxygen supply to)
isolation *see* loneliness
ITA 84

jargon (baby-talk) 49
job-satisfaction 143
Johnson, Virginia 154; *see also* Masters & Johnson
JTPA Job Corps *138*
Jung, Carl 57, 194, 269
juvenility 77

Kachel, Malley 255
Kagan, Jerome *38*
Kellogg, Rhoda *74*
'kicking' (foetal) *see* womb (activity in)
kicking (in infancy) *44*, 49
kidneys 232; babies' 27; failure of 223, 256; during pregnancy 166
kindergarten *see* education (pre-school)
Kinsey, Alfred 112, 249
Kohlberg, Lawrence 67–8
Korchnoi, Victor 71
Kuhn, Margaret 222

labia: majora *155*; minora *155*, 156
labour *166*, 167, 170, *171*, 173, *180–81*; father's role during 178, 179; pains of **174–7**, 179; stages of *174–5*
labour pains *see* labour (pains of)
lactation 28; *see also* milk (human)
language development *see* speech
lanugo 180
larynx *51*, *102*, 106
laughing (in infancy) 49
Laurence, Ruth Jayne *71*
Lawrence, D. H. *193*
learning 57, 58–9; in old age 229, 235, 255; *see also* education, imitation
learning disabilities (educational handicap) **78–82**, 88–9
Lee, Laurie 82
lens (of eye) 233
leukaemia 95
LH 102, *105*, *154*

Librium 118, *123*
lice 95
Liebermann, Morton 192, 251
life expectancy **258–9**
Lillian, Elsa *249*
limbic system 77
'little strokes' 246
liver 232; cirrhosis of *122*
'liver spots' 55
living together (cohabitation) 144, 149
loneliness: of the elderly *241*, *252*, 254; of young mothers *183*
longevity 258
'look and say' method 83–4
love 111, **146–7**, 148, 222; in middle age **193–5**; in old age **248–9**
love-withdrawal disciplinary techniques 68, 69–70
LSD *123*
lubrication phase 155–*156*, 159, 162, 194
lullabies 33
lung cancer *see* cancer (lung)
lungs *121*, 223, 231
luteinizing hormone *see* LH

Macaulay, Thomas, 1st Baron 71
McGraw, Myrtle 44
Maclean, Duncan 255
maintaining factors (in sexual dysfunction) 164
malnutrition 95, 243, 244
Manpower Services Commission *138*
Mao-tse Tung 255
marijuana *118*, 119, *123*
marital therapy 150–51
marriage *101*, **144–53**, *144*, 148–9, *152–3*, 165, *178*, 199; age at *144*; during adolescence *126*, 145; arranged 146–7, *153*; different customs surrounding 152–3; dissolution of 184, *193* (*see also* divorce); exchange theory of **148–51**; course of in middle age 194; 'mixed' 145, *147*; and retirement 221; social geography of 144; trial *see* living together
Marris, Peter 138–40
Masters, William 154, 267
Masters & Johnson, results of 156, 157, 158, 161, 162, 164
masturbation 107, 108, 109–10, 111, 158, 161, 162, 163, 194, 195
mathematical symbolization 82–3
maturation: during adolescence 99, *100–101*, 107, 126, 135; of brain

40–41, **76–8**; during childhood **75–8**; emotional *132*; during infancy 25, 40–41; of nervous system 21; sexual 99, 104, 106, *109*, *128*; *see also* growth
Mead, Margaret 255
meals-on-wheels 254
measles 95
meditation *171*
medulla (of adrenal gland) 102
meiosis *16*
Meir, Golda 255
memory 264; loss of 229, 236, 245, 246
menarche *see* menstruation
Menninger, Karl 222
menopause 191, 194, 195, 202–3
menorrhagia 135
menstrual blood 23
menstrual cycle *see* menstruation (cycle of)
menstruation 14, 19, 163; commencement of (menarch) *101*, *102*, *103*, 106; cycle of *105*, 106, 166, 167; problems of 106, 107, 135, *201*; *see also* menopause, PMT
mental decline 229, 236–7, 245–6
mental development 234–5; in childhood 74–5; in infancy **43–53**, *52*
mental handicap *see* handicap, mental retardation
mental health 63, 146, 187, 216, **260–62**
mental (intellectual) retardation 19, 54, 88–9
Menuhin, Yehudi 71
mescaline *123*
metabolic rate 102, 232
methadone *123*
Methedrine *123*
middle age **189–223**; and children **190–92**; crisis of **198–9**; depression during 191, 202, 203, **204–7**, *205*; health during **196–7**, 217, *223*; myths of 222; love and intimacy in **193–5**, *193*; stress during **198–204**; and parents 192
mid-life crisis **198–9**
migraine 135
milk 28, 29; cow's 26–7, *28*; human 23, 26–27, *28*, 29, 102, 171, 180, *181*; powdered 27
milk ducts 166
Mill, John Stuart 71
Miltown *123*
mineral supplements 171
minimal brain dysfunction *see* learning difficulties

miscarriage   20, *39*, 40, 112, 173
Mischel, Walter   68
mites   95
mitochondria   15
mitosis   *16*
modelling *see* imitation
Monet, Claude   255
mongolism *see* Down's syndrome
monogamy   152
monozygotic twins *see* multiple
  births
mons pubis   *155*
Montessori, Maria   74–5
morality: in childhood   67–8; the
  new 111–12
moral reasoning, development
  of   67–8
morning sickness   166, 170
morphine   *123*
Morris, Desmond   193
Moses, Anna Mary
  ('Grandma')   255
motherhood   165, 176, 178, 204; *see
  also* parenthood
mother–infant relationship   *22*–3,
  26, 184–5
motor coordination   46, 82
motor development   *43*–9, *44–5*
motor milestones   44
mourning   210; *see also* grief
mouth ulcers   *201*
Mozart, Wolfgang Amadeus   71
multiple births   **20**, *166*
multiple sclerosis   187
mumps   95
muscle cells   16–17
muscular dystrophy   54
myelin   76
myelinization   76
myocardial infarction (coronary
  thrombosis)   223, 243

nail-biting   *90*
narcotics   *123*
nativist stance (and gender
  identity)   39
natural-childbirth techniques   176,
  178
nausea (during pregnancy)   166, 170
Navajo   44
Nembutal   *123*
nerve cells   *16*, 17
nervous system   *260*; central (CNS)
  232–3, 246; of newborn child 21
Neugarten, Bernice   194, 199, 202
neurological disorder   78–9, 82
neurons   232
neurotics   132

nicotine   18, 27, *121*
nipples: female   *27*, *102*, *156*, 166,
  171; male 106
nocturnal emission   107, 162
non-power-assertive discipline   68
noradrenalin (norepinephrin)   102
nursery school *see* education (pre-
  school)

obesity: in adolescence   130; in
  middle age *197*, 201, 203; in young
  adulthood   186, 187
object permanence stage   52
oedema   170
Oedipal period   189
oesophagus   *121*
oestrogen   102, *105*, 106, *154*, 166,
  172, 203
oestrogen-replacement therapy   203
old age   **225–63**; changes during
  228–37; 246; death **256–62**; health
  during **226–8**; health problems
  during **263**; institutionalization in
  251–4, 255; keeping fit during **238–
  9**, *238*, *239*; leisure activities in **208–
  9**, 247; mental changes during 229,
  234–7; myths about **255**; sex during
  243, **248–9**, 255; *see also* senility
old people's homes   *241*
Olivier, Lord   255
O'Neill, Oona   222
operant behaviour   268
oral cavity   *51*
oral stage   89
orgasm   160–61; female 108, 154,
  156–7, 173, 194, 195, 267; male
  107, 155, *156*–7, *159*; multiple 157–
  158
'orgasmic cushions'   157
orgasmic dysfunction   163
orgasmic stage (male) *see* ejaculation
  phase
osteoarthrosis   263
ova *see* ovum
ovarian follicles   *105*
ovaries   *14*, 16, *102*, 104, *105*, *155*;
  cancer of 187; and the menopause
  202
overeating   *90*, *128*, 135
overweight *see* obesity
oviduct   *14*
ovulation   *14*, 102
ovum (egg)   *14*, *15*, 16, *19*, 102,
  105, *167*; *see also* zygote
oxytocin   *27*, 102

pain: during labour   **174–7**, 179;

painkillers, use of during labour   22
palpitations   200, 223
pancreas   *102*, 223
parasites   95, 226
parathormone   102
parathyroid gland   *102*
parenthood   **182–5**, 190
parents, ageing *see* ageing parents
parietal lobe (of cerebral cortex)   76
Parkinson's disease   *201*
Pearlin, Leonard   192
peek-a-boo   36, *38*, 46
peer groups (in adolescence)   114,
  124–6, 127, 131
penis   *14*, 107, *154*, *155*, *156*–7, 164;
  development of *100*, *102*, *103*; *see
  also* erection
perceptual disability *see* learning
  difficulties
'performance anxiety' (over
  sex)   194
perinatal deaths   18, *39*, 40, *166*; *see
  also* abortion, miscarriage
perineum   180
periods *see* menstruation
perspiration   *102*
petting to orgasm   107, 110
phenotype   18, 39
phenylalanine   54
phenylketonuria   54
phenyls   54
phlegm   *121*
phobias   212–13
Piaget, Jean   267, 268; on cognitive
  development **58–62**, *59*, *60*; on
  stages of infancy **45–6**, 52, 67, 82
Picasso, Pablo   255
pictorial stage   *74–5*
pill *see* contraceptive pill
pituitary gland   *27*, *102*, 104, *105*,
  154
placement stage   *74–5*
placenta   16, *17*, *20*, 22, 170, *175*,
  181
play   *69*, 70; *see also* games, social
  interactions
PMT   106, 135
pneumonia   54, 256, 263
polygamy   152
polytechnics   140; *see also* education
  (further)
popularity (in childhood)   63
pornography   158, 160, *163*
'port-wine' stains   55
postnatal depression   22, 179
power-assertive discipline   68–9, 70
PPM   176
precipitating factors (in sexual
  dysfunction)   164

pre-eclampsia 170
pregnancy (gestation) 13, 54, 104, 108, 165, **166–73**, *166, 167, 171, 172,* 176, 182; alcohol abuse during 18–19, *122;* anxiety during **172–3;** biology of **14–19;** emotions during 172; exercise during **168–9,** 170; father's role during 177–9; nausea during 166, 170; premarital 108, 112, 113, 145; problems of 170; sex during 173; signs of 166; smoking during 18, 19, 22, *121;* weight gain during 170–71
premature birth 19, 21
premature ejaculation 161–2, 164
pre-menstrual tension 106, 135
pre-operational stage *59*
prepubertal period (prepubescent stage) *100,* 106
pre-senile dementia 246
pre-term birth 19, 21
primary schools *see* education
problem-solving 234–5
progesterone 102, *105,* 106, 135, 166, 172, 203
progestins 104
Prokofiev, Sergey 71
prolactin *27,* 102
promiscuity, sexual 129
prostaglandin 14
prostate gland *14, 155, 157, 273*
prostatic area *156*
prostatic fluid 157
proximodistal development *46*
psilocybin *123*
psoriasis *201*
psychoactive drugs *see* drugs
psychoanalysis 265; *see also* Freud (Sigmund)
psychoanalytic view of child development **89–91,** *93*
psychological problems: in adolescence **127–31,** 133; in childhood 88
psychoprophylaxis 176
puberty *65,* 98–9, *100–101, 103,* 104, 105, 106
pubic hair *100, 101, 102, 103,* 104
pulling up (in infancy) *44, 45,* 49
punishment *see* discipline, corporal punishment
puzzle-solving *see* problem-solving

quiet alert state 30, 32

Rahe, Richard 201
Ramsey, Ron 211–12

rapid-eye-movement sleep *see* REM sleep
reaching (in infancy) 45, *46, 47,* 49
Read, Grantly Dick 175, 176
readiness tests 75–6
reading, learning of 57, 78, *79,* **83–4;** difficulties with 79, 82
reading tests 75–6
recessive genes 18, *19*
reciprocity (in friendships) 193
red blood cells 18, 54, *121*
redundancy 215
reflex, conditioned *see* conditioned response
refractory period (male) 156, 158
relaxants *123*
remarriage 148–9, 192, 194, 205, *213,* 242
REM sleep 30, *31,* 233
renal gland *157*
repression (in psychoanalysis) 90
reproduction *see* birth, pregnancy, sex
residential propinquity 144
resolution phase (after sexual intercourse): female 156, *157;* male 155, *157, 158*
respiratory system: of newborn child 21–2; and stress *201*
respondent behaviour 268
responsibility in childhood 67
retarded ejaculation 162, 164
retirement 143, 191, 199, 215, **216–21,** *216,* 222, *241;* enforced 240; leisure activities in **208–9,** *247*
reversibility *59,* 60–61, *62*
rheumatic disorders 195, 243, 263
Richardson, Sir Ralph 255
rickets 95
rites of passage 115, *116*
rolling over (in infancy) *44, 46,* 49
Rose, David 77
Rossi, Alice 190, 194
roundworms 95
rubella 172
Rubinstein, Artur 255
Russell, Bertrand 255
Rutter, Michael 88

scabies 95
school *see* childhood, education
scrotum *14, 155, 156*
Seconal *123*
second childhood *230*
second honeymoon 194
second molars *102*
sedatives 118, *123*
self-concept 64–5

Seligman, Martin 206
semen 14, 155, 173, 194
seminal fluid 107, *156*
seminal pool *157*
seminal vesicles 14, *155, 157*
senile dementia 227, 245, 246
senile psychosis 245
senility 231, 244, 245–6, 253, 255, 260, 261
senses 233; development of *36; see also* hearing, touch, vision
sensorimotor stage *46, 59, 60,* 268
sentences, first spoken 49, 50, 51, 53
sex **154–64,** *160;* during adolescence 107, **108–13,** *111,* 126; anatomy of 41; marital 150; in middle age 193; in old age 243, **248–9,** 255; during pregnancy 173; premarital 108, **110–13,** *146; see also* sexual intercourse
sex cells 102; *see also* ovum, sperm
sex crimes *163*
sex education 108, *109*
sex flush 156
sex organs *see* genital organs
sex roles *40,* 42, 103; *see also* stereotyping (sex)
sex stereotyping *see* stereotyping (sex)
sex therapy 108, 164
sexual arousal 106, 108, *154,* 160–61, *162,* 194; female problems of 162–3; *see also* erectile dysfunction, erection, lubrication phase
sexual development *see* maturation
sexual differences, in adolescence *100–101,* **105–7,** 267; in childhood 65; in infancy **39–42,** *39*
sexual dysfunction *see* sexual problems
sexual identity *see* gender identity, identity
sexual inadequacy, feelings of 108; *see also* sexual problems
sexual intercourse *14;* during adolescence 107, 108, **110–13,** *111;* first experiences of 111; *see also* sex
sexuality: during adolescence **108–13,** *110;* in middle age 195
sexually transmitted diseases (STDs) *see* venereal disease
sexual maturity *see* maturation
sexual problems 154, **159–64,** *161,* 187; female **162–4;** male **161–2**
sexual promiscuity 129
sexual relationships in adolescence *100,* 111, 126; *see also* living together, love, marriage, sex

sexual response **154–9**, *156*–7, 161, 194, 248; female 155–6, *158–9*, 195; male 155, *158*, 248; *see also* sexual arousal
sexual stimuli 158–9
shape stage *74–5*
Shaw, George Bernard 255
shock of bereavement 212
sibling rivalry *70*, 117, 185
sickle-cell anaemia 54–5
sight *see* vision
Silberman, Charles 133
similarity (in friendships) 193
Simon, Théophile 58, 87
sinusitis *121*
sitting up (in infancy) *44*, *45*, *46*, 49
skin flora 23
sleep *31*; types of (in infancy) 30; *see also* REM sleep, sleep patterns, sleep problems
sleep patterns (in infancy) 30–31, 55; *see also* insomnia
sleep problems *90*; in adolescence 127, 130; in infancy 33–4, 55; in middle-age depression *205*; in old age 233–4, 242, 263; *see also* insomnia
slums *see* urban ghettoes
smallpox 95, 172
smiling (in infancy) 36, 49
smoking 233, 258; in adolescence 101, 118, **121**, *121*; and breast-feeding 27; in middle age 197, 200, 217, 223; in old age 238; during pregnancy 18, 19, 22, *121*
social interactions: in childhood **63–70**, *67*, *69*; in infancy 37, *38*, 39, 45, 50; in middle age 206
social learning theory *42*
social scripts 66
soft signs 78
solid foods, babies' first *see* weaning
somites 17
Sophocles 255
special education *see* education (special)
speech, development of 35, 40–41, 45, 48, **49–53**, *53*, poor 82, *90*; *see also* sentences, words
sperm **14–16**, *15*, *19*, 102, *154*, *155*, *156*; structure *14*, 15
spina bifida 18, 54–5
spinal block 176
spirits 23
Spitz, Renée 165
Spock, Benjamin 25, 182
sport: in middle age 197; during pregnancy 169, 170; in retirement

209, *247*; in young adulthood *186*; *see also* exercise
standing (in infancy) *45*, 49
STDs *see* venereal disease
stereotyping: age 219, 235; sex 39, 41–2, 66 (*see also* sex roles); social 74
sterility 187
steroids 102
stimulants *123*
Stocks, Mary 255
Stone Age 35
'strawberry' marks 55
stress: in middle age **198–204**, 207, 217, 223; in old age 199, 244, 246; in young adulthood 187; *see also* depression
strokes 201, 223, 231, 233; 'little' 246
Stuart, Richard 150
sucking (in infancy) 32, *33*, 34, 36
suckling *see* breast-feeding
suicide: in adolescence 127, 129, *130–31*, 133; after bereavement 211; after job-loss 214; in old age 242, 259–60
superego 89, 90
suprarenal glands *see* adrenal glands
swaddling *33*
swimming: in infancy 45; in middle age 197, 217; during pregnancy *169*, 170, 171; in retirement 209
syndrome 91
systolic blood pressure 105

talking *see* speech
tampons 163
tantrums *90*
tapeworms 95
tar (from tobacco smoke) *121*
taxonomy (in psychoanalysis) 91, 93
Tawney, R. H. 137
teaching *see* education, learning
technical colleges *see* polytechnics
teething 34, 55
testes *14*, *16*, *154*, *155*, *156*, *157*, 164; cancer of 187; development of *100*, *102*, *103*, 104
testicles *see* testes
testosterone 102, 107, *154*
thought, development of *see* mental development
threadworms 95
thrombus 233
thumb-sucking *33*, *90*
thymine *18*
thyroid gland *102*, 104

thyroitropin 102
thyroxin 102, 104
time-sharing behaviour 94
Titian 255
Tizard, Jack 88
tobacco 118, 119; *see also* smoking
Tobin, Sheldon 251
toilet training 90
Tolstoy, Leo 255
tongue *51*
touch, sensitivity of 229
toxaemia *166*, 170
toys *33*
tranquillizers 118, *123*, 195, 207
Tranxene *123*
'traumatic' experiences 89, **90**; see also 'birth trauma'
trial marriage *see* living together
truancy 85–6
tuberculosis 95
Tuinal *123*
tunica *156*
Turiel, Eliot 66
twins *see* multiple births

ulcers: duodenal *201*, 223; mouth *201*, peptic 226
ultrasound 19
umbilical cord *17*, *21*, *175*
unemployment 220, 247; in middle age *193*, 200, **214–16**, *215*; in youth *133*, *134*, *138*, **141**, 143
unemployment line *215*
universities *134*, **138–40**, 143; *see also* education (further)
urban ghettoes 131, 133
ureter *155*
urethra 14, *155*, *156*, 157
urethral meatus *155*
urinary tract problems 95
urine 232
uterus *14*, 16, *17*, *102*, *105*, *155*, *156*, *157*, 166, *167*, 170, 172, 180

vaccination 95
vagina *14*, *105*, *155*, *156*, *157*, 158–9, 163, 164, *180*; dryness of 194, 202, 203
vaginismus 163–4
Valium 118, *123*
varicose veins 171
vas deferens *14*, *155*, *157*
vasectomy 264
vasocongestion 160, 162
vasodilation *122*
venereal disease (STDs, VD) 108, 111, 112, 135

Verdi, Guiseppe   255
vernix   180
vision   *227*, 228, 229, 233, 235, 240,
   243, 263; *see also* blindness
vitamin deficiency   95
vitamin supplements   171
vitiligo   55
vitreous humour   233
vocabulary (in infancy)   *53*
vocal tract   *51*
vulva   *155*

waking states (in infancy)   30–31
walking (in infancy)   25, 35, *43, 44,
   45*, 48, 49
Walster, Elaine   145
'waters' *see* amniotic fluid
Wayne, John   255
weaning   29, 55
wedding *see* marriage
Weikart, David   74
Weisman, Avery D.   256
wet dreams *see* nocturnal emission
white blood cells   18, 227–8
Whitmore, Kingsley   88
whooping-cough   95
widowhood (bereavement)   194,
   204, 205, **210–13**, *212*, 222
Wight, Isle of   88–9
will, making a 250
wind (in infancy)   36, 55
wisdom teeth   *102*
womb   14, 18, *105*, 156, *174*, 203;
   activity in ('kicking') 166–7
words: first spoken   49, 50–51, 53;
   learning as abstracts 82–3
Wordsworth, William   13
work *see* employment
work ethic   143, 247
worms (parasites)   95
writing, learning of 57, 78, *79*;
   difficulties with 82

yeasts (on skin)   23
Yeats, W. B.   222
yoga   *171*, 197, 217
young adulthood **137–87**; and ageing
   parents 192; establishment phase
   137; health during **186–7**;
   parenthood during **182–5**, prelude
   to **132–4**; transition phase 137; *see
   also* education (further),
   employment, marriage, pregnancy

zygote (fertilized ovum)   *20*

Picture credits

Cover Photograph: The Image Bank

J. Allen Cash 114, 256, 259 **Daily Telegraph Colour Library** 12, 20, 160, 247 bottom right **Mary Evans Picture Library** 23 **The Image Bank** 44, 56, 81 top, 136, 152 bottom, 161, 191 **Camilla Jessel** 89, 234, 248 bottom **London Scientific Fotos** 15 **The Mansell Collection** 34, 75 **Multimedia Picture Library** 19 top, 26, 38, 58, 65, 69, 72, 147, 180, 181 **Petit Format** 16 **The Photo Source** 71 left, 126, 138, 243, 249 **Popperfoto** 71 right **Rex Features** 113, 118, 120, 123, 206, 210, 215, 222, 238, 248 top, 258 **Frank Spooner Pictures** 141 **Tony Stone Associates** 193 **Homer Sykes** 109, 110, 119, 132, 241 bottom, 255 **John Twinning** 183, 252 **Vision International** 14, 21, 22, 29, 32, 35, 37, 40, 43, 47, 48, 52, 53, 67, 77, 85, 88, 91, 96, 116, 124, 139, 142, 165, 168, 169, 177, 197, 224, 237, 247 top and bottom left, 251, 254 **Janine Wiedel** 19 bottom, 70, 80 bottom, 98, 104, 115, 127, 131, 171, 188, 195, 212, 214, 216, 226, 232 **Xenon Photos** Richard Olivier 83, 241 top, Libuse Taylor 74, 79, 149, 227, 229, 230 **ZEFA** 24, 30, 80 top, 81 bottom, 144, 152 top, 153, 172, 185, 192, 208, 209

Acknowledgements

Illustrations and diagrams:

101 from *Carmichael's Manual of Child Psychology,* 3rd edition, P. Mussen (Ed.). Copyright © 1970 by John Wiley & Sons, Inc. Reprinted by permission of John Wiley & Sons, Inc.; **250** reprinted with the permission of Concern for Dying, 250 West 57th Street, New York, New York 10107; **20, 32** from *Elements of Psychology,* 3rd edition, by David Krech, Richard S. Crutchfield and Norman Livson, with the collaboration of William A. Wilson, Jr. Copyright © 1958 by David Krech and Richard S. Crutchfield. Copyright © 1969, 1974 by Alfred A. Knopf, Inc. Reprinted by permission of Alfred A. Knopf, Inc.; **14, 154, 156–7, 158** from *Everyman* by Derek Llewellyn-Jones published by Oxford University Press, 1981; **27** redrawn by permission of Faber & Faber Ltd from *Everywoman* by Derek Llewellyn-Jones, illustrated by Audrey Besterman; **100–1, 117** from *Family Health Guide,* Copyright © 1972, The Reader's Digest Association Limited, London.

Used with permission; **73, 91** from *Introduction to Psychology,* 7th edition, by E. R. Hilgard *et al.,* Harcourt, Brace, Jovanovich Ltd, 1979. (After Bandura, 'Imitation of film mediated aggressive models', from *Journal of Abnormal Psychology,* 66, 8, fig. 1, 1963.); **38** from *Introduction to Psychology* from Clifford T. Morgan *et al.,* McGraw-Hill Book Co., 1979. (Slightly modified from Kagan, 1970.); **60** from *Psycho: Man in Perspective* by Arnold B. Buss. Copyright © 1973 by Arnold B. Buss. Reprinted by permission of John Wiley & Sons, Inc.; **18** from 759 of *Psychology and Life,* 9th edition, by Philip G. Zimbardo, 1975, Scott, Foresman & Co. (From *The New Genetics: The Threads of Life* by G. W. Beadle, Britannica Books of the Year, 1964.); **31, 53** reprinted with permission from Macmillan Publishing Company from *Psychology of the Child and the Adolescent,* 4th edition, by Robert I. Watson and Henry Clay Lindgren. Copyright © 1979 by Robert I. Watson and Henry Clay Lindgren; **162–3** adapted from Robert A. Baron and Donn Byrne, *Social Psychology: Understanding Human Interaction,* 3rd edition. Copyright © 1981 by Allyn & Bacon, Inc. Used with permission; **143, 149, 213** reproduced from *Social Trends 1983* with the permission of the Controller of Her Majesty's Stationery Office.

The publishers also acknowledge their indebtedness to the following books which were consulted for reference:

Adolescent Development: A Life-Span Perspective, Richard M. Lerner and Graham B. Spanier, McGraw-Hill; *Analyzing Children's Art,* Rhoda Kellogg, Mayfield Publishing Co.; *Baby and Child,* Penelope Leach, Michael Joseph; *The Body Machine,* Christiaan Barnard, Hamlyn; *Child's Body,* Diagram; *Developmental Psychology,* Elizabeth B. Hurlock, McGraw-Hill; *Developmental Psychology,* Robert M. Liebert, Prentice-Hall; *Education, Society and Change,* Sandford W. Reitman, Allyn & Bacon; *Family Planning Perspective,* M. Zelnik and J. F. Kantner, 9, 1977; *Focus on Retirement,* Fred Kempe and Bernard Buttle, Kogan Page; *Guide to Family Health,* Macmillan, London and Basingstoke; *Genetic Psychology Monographs,* H. M. Halverson, 1931, 10, 107–286, Journal Press; *The Healthy Body,* Diagram; *Human Development,* Grace J. Craig, Prentice-Hall; *Introduction to Child Development,* Patricia Hicks, Longman; *Journal of Psychosomatic Research,* 1967, 11, 213–18, Pergammon; *Level and Trends of Mortality since*

1950, UN & WHO; *Life Before Death,* Ann Cartwright *et al.,* 1973, Routledge & Kegan Paul PLC; *Life-Span: Individual and Family Development,* Stella R. Goldberg and Francine Deutsch, Wadsworth; *Living Well: The People Maintenance Manual,* Mitchell Beazley; *Man Alive,* G. L. McCulloch, Aldus; *National Data Book and Guide to Sources,* US Department of Commerce: Bureau of the Census; *Physical Activity and Aging,* Roy J. Shepherd, Croom Helm Limited; *Pregnancy and Birth,* Christopher Macy and Frank Falker, Multimedia; *Pregnancy Questions Answered,* Geoffrey Chamberlain, Churchill Livingstone; *Psychology,* John M. Darley, Prentice-Hall; *Psychology: Its Principles and Meanings,* Lyle E. Bourne and Bruce R. Ekstrand, Holt, Rinehart; *Retire and Enjoy it,* Cecil Chisholm, Penguin; *Selfwatching,* Ray Hodgson and Peter Miller, Century; *Sexual Behaviour in the Human Male,* C. Kinsey *et al.,* W. B. Saunders; *Social Trends 1984,* HMSO; *Stress Control,* Vernon Coleman, Pan; *Statistical Abstract of the United States,* US Department of Commerce: Bureau of the Census; *Teach Yourself – Psychology for Today,* Bill Gillham (Ed.), Hodder & Stoughton; *Twins and Supertwins,* Amram Scheinfeld, Chatto & Windus; *Understanding the Unemployed,* John Hayes and Peter Nutman, Tavistock; *What's Happening to the American Family?,* Dar A. Levitan and Richard S. Belous, Johns Hopkins University Press; *Women and Work,* Sheila Lewenhak, Macmillan, London and Basingstoke; *The World Almanac 1984 and Book of Facts,* Newspaper Enterprise.

Multimedia Publications (UK) Ltd have endeavoured to observe the legal requirements with regard to the rights of the suppliers of photographic and illustrative materials.